D0914769

PUTTING PATIENTS FIRST

PUTTING PATIENTS FIRST

Best Practices in Patient-Centered Care

Second Edition

EDITORS

SUSAN B. FRAMPTON

PATRICK A. CHARMEL

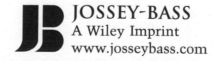

JOSSEY-BASS
A Wiley Imprint
www.josseybass.com

Library of Congress Cataloging-in-Publication Data

Putting patients first: best practices in patient-centered care / editors, Susan B. Frampton, Patrick A. Charmel—2nd ed.
    p.;   cm.
  Includes bibliographical references and index.
  ISBN 978-0-470-37702-4 (cloth)
    1. Medical personnel and patient.   2. Hospital care.   I. Frampton, Susan B.
  II. Charmel, Patrick A.
    [DNLM: 1. Patient-Centered Care—methods.   2. Patient-Centered
    Care—trends.   W 84.5 P993 2009]
    R727.3.P88   2009
    610.69'6—dc22

                                                          2008029694

Printed in the United States of America
SECOND EDITION

HB Printing   10 9 8 7 6 5 4 3 2 1

CONTENTS

PART ONE: ESSENTIAL ELEMENTS OF PATIENT-CENTERED CARE

PART TWO: CURRENT TRENDS IN PATIENT-CENTERED CARE

This book is dedicated to Laura C. Gilpin (1950–2007),
poet, nurse, and friend, and to the love she inspired
in all who knew her and who were touched by
her kindness, caring, and respect.

ACKNOWLEDGMENTS

We would like to express our deepest gratitude to the true pioneers of patient-centered care, including Planetree's founder, Angelica Thieriot, whose eloquent Prologue in this second edition chronicles her personal journey as a patient, which led her to advocate for the rights of all patients. A key colleague in that journey of turning vision into reality was Laura C. Gilpin, to whom this book is lovingly dedicated. Laura's unfailing dedication to patients and to those who care for patients touched everyone she worked with in her early years as a nurse and in her last two decades working with Planetree hospitals around the world. And to the late Harvey Picker (1915–2008), founder of The Picker Institute, an organization, like Planetree, committed to a health care system in which caring, kindness, and respect are believed to be essential elements in the delivery of excellent care.

We continue to be indebted to so many, who, over Planetree's thirty-year history, have helped to nurture, shape, and guide the vision to become the international organization it is today. We are especially grateful to Planetree's founding board of directors, to the initial model sites, and to the organizations, including The Henry J. Kaiser Family Foundation and The San Francisco Foundation, whose support made the establishment of the original Planetree model site possible.

We are especially grateful to affiliate members of Planetree. These hospitals, ambulatory centers, clinics, nursing homes, continuing care centers, integrated health systems, as well as the thousands of nurses, physicians, administrators, managers, librarians, volunteers, and others, through their work each day, are advancing the philosophy and principles of patient-centered, family-centered, and relationship-centered care. We continue to be inspired by the innovation and creativity that this diverse group brings to the patient care experience. Special thanks to our Dutch partners, Planetree Nederland, for their leadership in establishing patient-centered care in the Netherlands, and to Heidi Gil and the staff and leadership team of United Methodist Homes for their commitment to transforming the culture of nursing homes and continuing care centers to a more resident-centered model.

Thanks especially to the patients themselves, who throughout the years have so generously shared their stories and perceptions with us, continually inspiring us to expand the vision of what is possible in health care. We would also like to thank those like-minded individuals and organizations, who through their ongoing work are helping to realize our shared vision.

We truly appreciate the contributions made by so many talented writers in the first edition of *Putting Patients First,* including Bruce Arneill, Susan Edgman-Levitan, Karrie Frasca-Beaulieu, Trevor Hancock, George Handzo, Charlene Honeycutt, Leland Kaiser, Allan Komarek, Kathy Reinke, Carol Ryczek, Phyllis Stoneburner, Dianne Storby, and Jo Clare Wilson. Thank you all for your assistance in making the book a success.

We would also like to acknowledge recent members of the Planetree board of directors for their guidance and support of the organization. Finally, we would like to thank the supportive staff members of Planetree for their work day in, day out, to support our affiliates on their journeys, and in particular to Sara Guastello, without whom this second edition would not have been possible. Her skills, talent, and cheerful diligence were essential to moving this project along and bringing it to successful completion. Thank you, Sara!

Susan B. Frampton and Patrick A. Charmel
The Editors

THE EDITORS

SUSAN B. FRAMPTON, PhD, is president of Planetree, a nonprofit organization. In that capacity, she works with a growing network of hospitals and health centers around the world that have implemented Planetree's unique patient-centered model of care. Prior to her work with Planetree, she spent over twenty years at several hospitals in the New England area. Her work focused on community education, wellness and prevention, planning, and development of integrative medicine service lines. Frampton received her undergraduate training at Rutgers University and both master's and doctoral degrees in medical anthropology from the University of Connecticut. She has numerous publications, including the edited collection *Putting Patients First* (Jossey-Bass, 2003), which won the ACHE Hamilton Book of the Year Award in 2004; chapters in *Patient Advocacy for Health Care Quality* (Jones & Bartlett, 2007); and articles and interviews in *Journal of Alternative and Complementary Medicine, AHA News, Modern Healthcare,* and *Hospitals and Health Networks.* In addition to speaking internationally on culture change, patient-centered design, and health care consumerism, Frampton has presented keynotes on designing patient-centered practices in acute and continuing care and in ambulatory medicine settings for the Medical Group Management Association (MGMA), Healthcare Design Symposium, World Health Organization (WHO) Health Promoting Hospitals group, and Veterans Health Administration.

PATRICK A. CHARMEL, MPH, FACHE, is president and chief executive officer of Griffin Hospital and its parent organization, Griffin Health Services Corporation. He has been associated with Griffin since 1979, when he served as a student intern while attending Quinnipiac University. After graduating from Quinnipiac, Charmel received a master's of public health from Yale University. After serving in a number of administrative positions at Griffin Health Services Corporation, he became president in 1998. He is also the chief executive officer of Planetree, a subsidiary corporation. During his tenure, he has positioned Griffin Hospital as an award-winning, innovative organization, recognized as an industry leader in providing personalized, humanistic, consumer-driven health care in a healing environment. Under his leadership, Griffin has appeared on the *Fortune* magazine list of the 100 Best Companies to Work for in America for nine consecutive years, was named a 2007 Premier/CareScience National Quality Leader, and has received the 2005 and 2007 Health Grades Distinguished Hospital Award for Clinical Excellence. Griffin was also a recipient of the Total Benchmark Solution's Top 100 Quality Award in 2006 and was named one of the Solucient 100 Top Performance Improvement Leader Hospitals in 2007. He is coauthor of *Putting Patients First* (Jossey-Bass, 2003), which received the American College of Healthcare Executives Health Care Book of the Year award in 2004.

In 2005, he was appointed by the U.S. Secretary for Health and Human Services to the twenty-one-member National Advisory Council for Healthcare Research and Quality. He is chairman of the board of directors of the Connecticut Hospital Association and is a member of the board of directors of Qualidigm, a CMS-contracted quality improvement organization. Charmel is vice chair of the board of governors of the Quinnipiac University Alumni Association.

In 2006, Charmel was the recipient of the John D. Thompson Distinguished Visiting Fellow Award at Yale University. He is a recipient of the James E. West Fellow Award from the Boy Scouts of America. He was inducted into the Junior Achievement Free Enterprise Hall of Fame in 2002, and he is a recipient of the Dean Avery Award, given by the *New London Day* newspaper, which recognizes individual commitment to the public's right to know.

THE CONTRIBUTORS

ATHER ALI, ND, MPH, is assistant director of Integrative Medicine at the Yale-Griffin Prevention Research Center, where he supervises research in complementary and alternative medicine (CAM). He is also codirector of the Integrative Medicine Center at Griffin Hospital, where he oversees naturopathic clinical care and residency training. He obtained a bachelor's degree in psychobiology from UCLA, doctor of naturopathic medicine (ND) from Bastyr University, residency in integrative medicine from Griffin Hospital/University of Bridgeport, and a master's in public health, focused on chronic disease epidemiology, from Yale University. He completed a National Institutes of Health (NIH) postdoctoral fellowship, focused on integrative medicine research, and is involved in a number of research projects in CAM and preventive medicine. He is a founding director of integrative medicine at Yale and is Yale University's clinical representative to the Consortium of Academic Health Centers for Integrative Medicine.

CARRIE BRADY, MA, JD, is Planetree's vice president of quality and is responsible for assisting Planetree affiliates in collaborating on patient-centered quality and patient safety strategies and for coordinating the development and implementation of Planetree's patient-centered designation process. Before joining Planetree, Brady spent several years as a vice president of the Connecticut Hospital Association, where her role included coordinating two statewide pilot tests of the Hospital Consumer Assessment of Healthcare Providers and Systems (HCAHPS) patient experience of care survey, developing one of the first patient safety organizations (PSOs) in the nation, and designing a public reporting program for Connecticut hospitals. She has served on several state and national committees, including the National Quality Forum (NQF) Review Committee for Hospital CAHPS, the NQF Serious Reportable Events Maintenance Committee, and the National CAHPS Benchmarking Database Advisory Group. Brady received a JD and a combined MA/BA in sociology from Northwestern University and was a 2005–2006 Patient Safety Leadership Fellow.

RANDALL L. CARTER is Planetree's senior vice president and has provided consultation and programs on patient-centered care, developing healing environments, service, and leadership for health care organizations and physician groups, in addition to audiences in building and design, retail, software, education, broadcasting, and government. Carter serves as a commissioner on the National Health Council's Commission on Putting Patients First and as an expert faculty member for the Patient-Centered Care Institute. Prior to joining Planetree, Carter was a member of the Executive Management Team at Mid-Columbia Medical Center in The Dalles, Oregon. Mid-Columbia was the first systemwide implementation of the Planetree philosophy of care in the United States in 1991. During Carter's tenure at Mid-Columbia, the organization hosted over a thousand organizational site visits and was recognized in numerous publications and health care periodicals, as well as on Bill Moyers' landmark documentary series *Healing and the Mind.*

CAROLYN M. CLANCY, MD, was appointed director of the Agency for Healthcare Research and Quality (AHRQ) on February 5, 2003. Prior to her appointment, Clancy had served as AHRQ's acting director since March 2002 and previously was director of the agency's Center for Outcomes and Effectiveness Research (COER). AHRQ is the lead federal agency for promoting health care quality. Clancy, a general internist and health services researcher, is a graduate of Boston College and the University of Massachusetts Medical School. Following clinical training in internal medicine, she was a Henry J. Kaiser Family Foundation Fellow at the University of Pennsylvania. She was also an assistant professor in the Department of Internal Medicine at the Medical College of Virginia in Richmond before joining AHRQ in 1990. Clancy holds an academic appointment at George Washington University School of Medicine, has published widely in peer-reviewed journals, and has edited or contributed to seven books. She is a member of the Institute of Medicine.

JAMES B. CONWAY, MS, is senior vice president at the Institute for Healthcare Improvement (IHI), after having served as senior fellow from 2005 to 2006. From 1995 to 2005, he was executive vice president and chief operating officer of Dana-Farber Cancer Institute (DFCI). Prior to joining DFCI, he had a twenty-seven-year career at Children's Hospital, Boston, in Radiology Administration, Finance, and as assistant hospital director for Patient Care Services. He holds a master of science degree from Lesley College in Cambridge, Massachusetts. An adjunct faculty member at the Harvard School of Public Health, Conway is the 2001 winner of the first Individual Leadership Award in Patient Safety by the Joint Commission on Accreditation of Healthcare Organizations (JCAHO) and the National Committee for Quality Assurance (NCQA). He is a member of the Institute of Medicine Committee on Identifying and Preventing Medication Errors, a Distinguished Advisor to the National Patient Safety Foundation, and a past member of The Joint Commission Sentinel Event Alert Advisory Group.

JANET M. CORRIGAN, PhD, MBA, is president and CEO of the National Quality Forum, a not-for-profit membership organization established to develop and implement a national strategy for health care quality measurement and reporting. From 1998 to 2005, Corrigan was senior board director at the Institute of Medicine, where she provided leadership for their Quality Chasm Series. Prior to joining IOM, Corrigan was executive director of the President's Advisory Commission on Consumer Protection and Quality in the Health Care Industry. Corrigan received her doctorate in health services research and master of industrial engineering degrees from the University of Michigan and master's degrees in business administration and community health from the University of Rochester. In 2002, she was the recipient of the Institute of Medicine Cecil Award for Distinguished Service, and in 2006, she was appointed a fellow in the American College of Medical Informatics. In 2007, she was awarded the Founders' Award by the American College of Medical Quality, the TRUST Award by the Health Research and Educational Trust, and the Award of Honor by the American Society of Health System Pharmacists.

MARGARET CULLIVAN, MEd, RN, began her career in the academic arena, as a language arts and theater arts instructor at the secondary and college level. A sibling's illness piqued Cullivan's interest in the medical field, resulting in her pursuit of a nursing degree. Combining her medical and educational background, she eventually became director of education at Williamsburg Community Hospital. Presently, Cullivan serves as Planetree coordinator and director of volunteer services/guest service at Sentara Williamsburg Regional Medical Center and is active on local and national boards promoting volunteerism. As liaison for the hospital's nationally recognized auxiliary, she champions their fundraising efforts toward the support of patient-centered care initiatives, such as the chapel, healing garden, and free mammogram and bone density programs.

HEIDI GIL, NHA, CCM, was appointed executive director of Wesley Village in Shelton, Connecticut, in December 2004. She has been with United Methodist Homes since September 2000, previously serving as administrator of Bishop Wicke Health Center. Gil has seventeen years of experience in long-term and sub-acute operations in for-profit and not-for-profit settings, successfully improving financial, clinical, and operational performance. Under Gil's administration, Wesley Village has received several best practices awards, deficiency-free surveys from the State of Connecticut, and a score of 100 percent following the tri-annual JCAHO inspection. Since October 2002, Gil has led the development and implementation of Planetree Continuing Care: Creating Relationship-Centered Caring Environments, making Wesley Village the first leader in adapting the Planetree acute-care model for continuing care. Through the implementation of Planetree, Wesley Village has experienced impressive results in quality measures, employee turnover, net operating income, and overall community satisfaction. As the Plane-tree continuing care director, she is now leading the expansion of the Planetree Continuing Care network and provides consultation services to affiliates nationally and internationally.

CANDACE FORD GRAY, MLIS, has directed the Planetree Health Library in San Jose, California, since its inception in 1987. After earning her MLIS from the University of California Berkeley, she worked in public libraries and managed corporate and hospital libraries. Now executive director of the second-oldest Planetree library affiliate, Gray has given many presentations on health literacy and consumer health information services. She has contributed to revisions of Planetree's *Classification Scheme and Health Resource Center Information and Policy Manual.* She consults with Planetree affiliates and other organizations on developing and operating community health libraries. At the national conference in 2006, Gray received the Planetree Lifetime Achievement Award.

ALEXANDRA HARRISON, PhD, leads the Calgary Health Region's Patient Experience team, which is dedicated to enhancing the experience of care as seen "through the eyes of the patient." The Calgary Health Region is a large, integrated system that provides the full continuum of health care services for more than a million people living in Southern Alberta. Harrison's health care background includes professional practice, management, teaching, and research. She continues to teach as an adjunct faculty member in the Faculty of Medicine at the University of Calgary. Her PhD research demonstrated the critical role that patients and families play in the coordination of health services from the perspective of those who receive care. Prior to joining the Health Region, Harrison had senior roles in medical education at the University of Calgary and the Canadian Medical Association in Ottawa.

STEVEN F. HOROWITZ, MD, served as medical director of the Samuels Planetree Model Unit at Beth Israel Medical Center in New York City, where he was chief of cardiology from 1988 to 2002. He is currently chief of cardiology at the Stamford Hospital in Connecticut and a clinical professor of medicine at New York's Albert Einstein College of Medicine. Horowitz championed the establishment of one of the original Planetree model sites more than fifteen years ago and was instrumental in bringing Planetree to Stamford Hospital. He speaks internationally on his experiences as a physician and cardiologist working to personalize and demystify the hospital experience. Horowitz serves as a national Planetree board member and consultant, and he has worked with the medical staffs of many Planetree affiliates to achieve greater understanding and physician support for patient-centered care. In 2007, Horowitz received Planetree's Lifetime Achievement Award.

F. NICHOLAS JACOBS, MA, is president and CEO of Windber Medical Center and the Windber Research Institute. He holds a master's from Carnegie Mellon University and both master's and bachelor's degrees from Indiana University of Pennsylvania. He has a certificate in health systems management from the Harvard School of Public Health and is also a fellow in the American College of Health Care Executives. He has received several awards, including the Community Rural Health Leader of the Year by the Pennsylvania Rural Health Association. He serves on the boards of the Pennsylvania Mountains Healthcare Alliance and the Hospital Council of Western Pennsylvania. He is the chairman of the Keystone Chapter of the American Red Cross Disaster Relief Services. His writings have been published nationally, and he has been prominently featured in the *Wall Street Journal, Forbes, Fortune, USA Today, Health Leaders,* and *Modern Healthcare.* Jacobs is widely acknowledged as the first health care CEO to create and maintain a blog.

STEVEN L. JEFFERS, PhD, is founder and director of the Institute for Spirituality in Health at Shawnee Mission Medical Center (SMMC), a regional medical center in the suburbs of Kansas City. Jeffers received a BA in religion from Palm Beach Atlantic College, an MDiv from Midwestern Baptist Theological Seminary with a concentration in Greek and New Testament, and a PhD in the Program in the Humanities from Florida State University, where he studied the Greco-Roman classics, the Bible, and world religions. Prior to his current work, Jeffers was a seminary professor with extensive experience in faith congregational ministry. In his role with the institute, he works with physicians, with other health care providers, and with civic, business, and religious leaders of various faith traditions to advocate for the effective, compassionate care of patients and families and the integration of spirituality into the practice of medicine.

H. LEE KANTER, MD, is a practicing cardiologist and electrophysiologist in a twenty-member cardiology practice in Virginia Beach, Virginia. Kanter graduated from the University of Virginia School of Medicine and pursued postgraduate medicine and cardiology training at the University of Michigan and Washington University, respectively. He has been active at Sentara Virginia Beach General Hospital as a physician champion for Planetree and co-chair of the patient-centered care committee. Kanter's current leadership roles include being an active board member of Medical Society of Virginia, president of Virginia Beach Medical Society, and vice president of medical staff, Sentara Virginia Beach General Hospital.

DAVID L. KATZ, MD, MPH, is a board-certified specialist in both internal medicine and preventive medicine/public health and is a fellow of the American College of Physicians and the American College of Preventive Medicine. He is an associate professor (adjunct) at the Yale School of Public Health, director of Yale University's Prevention Research Center, and founder and director of the Integrative Medicine Center at Griffin Hospital in Derby, Connecticut. Katz contributes a monthly nutrition column to *O, the Oprah Magazine;* a weekly health column to the *New York Times* Syndicate; a daily blog to *Prevention Magazine;* and medical consulting to ABC News. He has twice been recognized as a Top Physician in Preventive Medicine by the Consumers' Research Council of America. He has consulted on obesity control and the prevention of chronic disease to the secretary of health, the commissioner of the U.S. Food and Drug Administration, the National Governors Association, and the World Health Organization. He has authored over a hundred scientific articles; numerous chapters, abstracts, essays, and commentaries; and eleven books.

REV. DR. DENNIS KENNY is a psychologist, theologian, and spiritual caregiver. He was the founding director of the prestigious Institute for Health and Healing of the California Pacific Medical Center, which was chosen by *Natural Health* magazine as the leading holistic hospital in the United States. He is the author of *Promise of the Soul* (Wiley), rated the best new self-help book by *Body and Soul* magazine. He has been the spirituality consultant for the Planetree organization. He is currently the director of pastoral care and the director of the Disease Reversal Program at Cleveland Clinic.

GAIL MACKEAN, MPA, PhD, has a long-standing commitment to patient and family-centered care, which has come from her varied and life-long experiences with health, illness, and the health care system, initially as a daughter of a mother living with a chronic, disabling condition and then as a practicing physiotherapist and administrator working in the Canadian health care system; as a parent of two children, one born with complex medical problems requiring ongoing, intense interactions with the health care system; as a parent member of a children's hospital parent advisory committee; and finally as a health services researcher. MacKean currently works as a research and evaluation consultant. She is a member of SEARCH Canada's lead faculty team, has an adjunct appointment with the Department of Community Health Sciences at the University of Calgary, and has close ties to the Calgary Health Region. Her research interests lie primarily in patient and family-centered care and in public participation in health services and policy development.

DWIGHT N. MCNEILL, PhD, MPH, is a vice president of education and research at the National Quality Forum in Washington, D.C., where he is responsible for promoting the attainment of national health care quality improvement priorities through educational forums, publications, and research. Previously, he worked in the federal government on national and state quality reporting and implementing community-wide improvement programs in diabetes, disparities, and asthma. Prior to that, he was involved in the development of Healthcare Effectiveness Data and Information Set (HEDIS), was cofounder and first chairman of the Foundation for Accountability (FACCT), and was director of health care information and planning at Verizon Corporation, where he worked with 140 health plans to measure and improve quality. He received his MPH in psychiatric epidemiology from the Yale University Medical School and his PhD in social policy from Brandeis University.

KIMBERLY NELSON MONTAGUE, MA, AIA, NCARB, is the director of design consultation services for Planetree, where she works with a growing network of hospitals and health centers around the world to help improve their environments in terms of the components for the Planetree Model of Care. Prior to her work with Planetree, she spent over twenty years working as an architect, most recently as a principal with the Albert Kahn Family of Companies. Her portfolio of work includes health care projects ranging from small community-based clinics to large, urban, and teaching hospitals. Her duties ranged from design to development and project management. Montague received a bachelor of science and a master's degree in architecture from the University of Michigan.

WENDY W. PECHE, MA, is a member of the Employee and Organization Development team at Aurora Health Care, Milwaukee, Wisconsin. Peche's role includes the coordination of the system implementation strategy of transforming the culture to patient-centered care. Peche has been passionate about Planetree since 2001, when Aurora's first hospital joined the Planetree membership network. She has been in health care for over thirty years and was at the bedside for the first half of her career. She has a master's degree in administrative leadership and is coauthor of the book *Legendary Team Leadership* (Spring Book Press).

ROBERT F. SHARROW, AIA, ACHA, NCARB, is a health care facility architect in Detroit, Michigan, where he is vice president and director of health care planning at the Albert Kahn Family of Companies, a leading architectural-engineering firm that has designed numerous Planetree facilities. His portfolio of projects includes three completed hospitals and many ambulatory care centers for Aurora Health Care in Wisconsin. He is currently principal for a new replacement hospital project for Elmhurst Memorial Hospital, a Planetree affiliate in Elmhurst, Illinois. Sharrow has a passion for the design of patient-centered care environments and is committed to the development of building designs that embody human-focused care amenities. He has used his profession to develop therapeutic healing spaces that meet the needs of those in the medical profession, patients, and their families.

MICHELE A. SPATZ, MS, earned her master's degree at the University of Illinois Graduate School of Library and Information Science, where she was inducted into Beta Phi Mu, the International Library Science Honor Society. After receiving her degree, Spatz was the first librarian to earn tenure at the University of Illinois College of Medicine in Peoria, working there as reference librarian and then branch library director.

While there, she chaired a regional consumer health information project for central Illinois in the early 1980s. In the fall of 1991, she moved to The Dalles, Oregon, to establish the Planetree Health Resource Center, a community-based consumer health library, for Mid-Columbia Medical Center. She has served as the resource center's director since it opened in June 1992. Spatz is the author of the recently published book *Answering Consumer Health Questions: The Medical Library Association Guide for Reference Librarians* (Neal-Schuman Publishers). She is active locally, regionally, and nationally as a writer, teacher, committee member, and consultant.

ROGER S. ULRICH, PhD, conducts research on the effects of health care architecture, art, and gardens on medical outcomes. He has published widely in both scientific and design journals and is the most cited researcher in the area of evidence-based health care design. His work has influenced internationally the architecture, interior design, and selection of art for major hospitals. Ulrich has worked extensively in the United Kingdom and Scandinavia, especially Sweden, where he has carried out research at the Karolinska Institute of Medicine and other institutions. He has also been visiting research professor in healthcare architecture at the University of Florence, Italy; visiting professor to the Bartlett School of Architecture at the University College London; and Invitation Research Fellow of the Japan Society for the Promotion of Science. Ulrich has also served as senior adviser to the United Kingdom National Health Service for its program to create scores of new hospitals. He is a member of the board of directors of The Center for Health Design, California.

JEAN WATSON, PhD, RN, AHN-BC, FAAN, is Distinguished Professor of Nursing and holds an endowed Chair in Caring Science at the University of Colorado Denver and Anschutz Medical Center Campus. She is founder of the original Center for Human Caring in Colorado and is a fellow of the American Academy of Nursing. She previously served as dean of nursing at the University Health Sciences Center and is a past president of the National League for Nursing. Watson has earned undergraduate and graduate degrees in nursing and psychiatric–mental health nursing and holds her PhD in educational psychology and counseling. She is a widely published author and recipient of several awards and honors, including an international Kellogg Fellowship in Australia and a Fulbright Research Award in Sweden. She holds six honorary doctoral degrees, including three international honorary doctorates from Sweden, United Kingdom, and Quebec, Canada. Her most recent book is *Caring Science as Sacred Science* (F. A. Davis, 2005).

CATHERINE WHALEN is the director of Community Initiatives at Mid-Columbia Medical Center in The Dalles, Oregon. In this capacity, she is the primary community liaison for the medical center, representing organizational resources for local initiatives and guiding strategic priorities for community involvement. She has played a key role in facilitating the awareness and adoption of the *healthy communities concept* at the organizational, city, and county levels. Whalen has been a speaker on the subject of healthy communities and the five-component definition of health at the Oregon Association of Hospital and Health Systems, the Arkansas Rural Health Forum, and Allina Medical Systems. She copresented with Trevor Hancock at the annual Planetree Conference in Rhinebeck, New York. She is currently a member of the Association for Community Health Improvement, an examiner for the Washington State Quality Award, and a past examiner for the Malcolm Baldrige National Quality Award.

PHILIP J. WILNER, MD, MBA, is vice president and medical director for Behavioral Health at Weill Cornell Medical Center of New York-Presbyterian Hospital. He is executive vice chair of the Department of Psychiatry and associate professor at Weill Medical College of Cornell University. Wilner received his bachelor's degree, summa cum laude, from Columbia College and his MD from the College of Physicians and Surgeons, both of Columbia University. He completed his psychiatry internship, residency, chief residency, and research fellowship training at the New York Hospital Cornell Medical Center and his MBA in health care administration at the Zicklin Business School of Baruch College. Since the early 1990s, Wilner has assumed positions of increasing responsibility in clinical management and leadership for the renowned Payne Whitney Manhattan and Westchester Divisions of the Weill Cornell Medical Center of New York-Presbyterian Hospital. Wilner was the recipient of a Reader's Digest Fellowship in 1988 and conducted studies in the biological bases of psychiatric illness. He is a fellow of the American Psychiatric Association and member of the American College of Healthcare Executives and the American College of Physician Executives.

PROLOGUE

WHAT PATIENTS CAN TEACH US ABOUT IMPROVING THE QUALITY OF HEALTH CARE

The genesis for the idea of Planetree came out of a hospital experience I had in the late 1970s. I became seriously ill with an unidentified virus and spent two weeks in a leading hospital in the San Francisco Bay Area. I survived with a fervent intention to change the way hospitals treat patients.

The following year was spent trying to parse out which elements of my hospital experience had been the most negative and figure out how they could be improved. I also set out to speak with anyone who had experience in changing institutions, especially in health care: dreamers, innovators, and paradigm changers.

From those conversations came the members of the original board of Planetree and a specific philosophy of care, an apparently obvious—but in fact forgotten—point of view: hospitals exist to make people better, to help them heal. All the other motives—profit, employment, training, efficiency, and so forth—are ancillary to the main purpose and will only be well served if the principal objective, healing, is kept in focus.

Alienation, fear, hopelessness, loneliness, and dehumanization were the emotions that overwhelmed me during my hospital stay and led me to feel that I would never get out alive.

The first impression came at reception, where seemingly uncaring clerical personnel put my husband and me through endless questionnaires and forms as I fought against nausea and the fear that I would pass out. I was then led to a room that faced an air well, furnished only with a mechanical contraption that served as a bed and a metal chair. I felt that I had arrived at a Gulag.

During the two weeks that I was there, I never saw the same nurse twice. Other than my doctor, who came early in the morning to shake his head and talk about me as if I weren't there (once saying to my husband, "I'm afraid we're losing her"), anonymous people came and went, giving me pills, drawing blood, and answering my fearful questions with "I don't know, you'll have to ask your doctor."

My mother-in-law sent me an orchid, which became the center of my attention. It was the only refuge from the bleak and sterile ugliness that surrounded me. I stared at it as if to save my life.

My fever and general discomfort kept me awake most of the night, but often, overcome by exhaustion, I would fall asleep at dawn only to be awakened an hour later and served a totally unhealthy, inappropriate, and inedible breakfast.

What would I have needed? What would have been truly healing? These thoughts occupied my mind over the next fifteen years as many wiser, more experienced minds than mine joined the effort to continue to evolve the philosophy of care that is Planetree.

During the period of gestation that followed my hospitalization, I spent many hours in the library researching the history of hospitals. The paths we took to arrive at the current state of affairs became clear. From the hospices of the Middle Ages to the horrifyingly septic institutions of the nineteenth century, through largely well-intentioned and useful changes, we had arrived at the modern, efficient, dehumanized institutions that prevailed in the 1970s. As in many other aspects of life, however, the most inspirational hospitals were the original ones, the ancient Greek Aesculapian hospitals.

In sharp contrast to the barren environments of modern hospitals, ancient hospitals were set in sacred groves, on spectacular sites. Their stated purpose was to awaken the vital healing energies with beauty, art, music, theater, and poetry. Through herbal potions and ritual, they connected their patients to their inner wisdom, and after one night of dreaming in the Abaton (as records meticulously carved in stone say), many patients were either healed or understood how to heal themselves and were discharged. For those who needed more care, a regimen of exposure to the arts, appropriate physical therapies, and herbal potions had a notable rate of success. One of the crucial elements, I imagine, was hope and the positive support of the Aesculapian priests, whose vocation it was to heal.

As I reflected on my experience, some of the issues that came up as needing urgent attention were

- The need for an aesthetic environment, especially one that has elements of nature
- The importance of quality human contact, continuity of care, and family involvement
- The crucial need for empowerment, human dignity, and control

All of these are aspects of the physical, human, and psychological environment.

Out of the six hundred or so people I met with in that early period were people who became the founding board. Among them was Dr. John Gamble, then chief of medicine at Pacific Presbyterian Hospital. He had been involved in an earlier attempt to humanize health care, called the Patients Involved and Responsible (PIR) node. His wisdom, leadership, and political expertise were essential to the success of Planetree.

Roslyn Lindheim was a professor of architecture at the University of California at Berkeley. She had a lifelong interest in healing environments and had designed a number of innovative hospital units. As part of her research for Planetree, she checked herself into a hospital for two days, an experience she found terrifying and demoralizing even though she was in perfect health.

Stewart Brand, futurist and publisher of the *Whole Earth Catalogue,* brought his boundless intelligence to bear every time the flow of ideas got snagged on some less-relevant point and put us back on track. His lifetime of thinking outside the box created a matrix for the group's creativity. He also brought us our founding director, the brilliant and effective Ryan Phelan, without whom none of our ideas would have become realities.

Jill Goffstein had founded a very successful alternative school, and Suzanne Arms had single-handedly started the alternative birth movement with her book *Immaculate Deception.* Their boldness was based on experience in making change, and it proved to be invaluable.

Dr. Don Creevy, in his obstetrical practice, modeled the ideal Planetree doctor: one who takes time to thoroughly inform his patients, who grants women their right to have the birth experience they want, who makes it safe for them to do so, and who generally expresses the caring and attention that healing requires.

Victoria Fay brought her impeccable taste and sense of color and design to the first Planetree interiors.

Phelps Dewey knew about business and the financial aspects of institutions—an element of crucial importance to our success.

Dr. Fred Hudson brought us more medical expertise and many powerful contacts in the community.

Dr. Aileen Aicardi, beloved pediatrician, provided her professional viewpoint and wisdom.

Joan Barbour shared her knowledge as a health educator and came up with the name, *Planetree,* in honor of the tree on the island of Cos under which Hippocrates taught the first medical students.

Mary Crowley, Gretchen de Witt, and Betsy Everdell were of immeasurable help in providing us the community support and fundraising capabilities without which the project would not have succeeded.

Lee and Adrian Gruhn and Cyril Magnin were our very first donor board members, our very own angels.

The experience in humanistic care and health education provided by Drs. Jordan R. Wilbur and David Sobel were indispensable for our envisioning of Planetree.

Together, we attempted to address the question of how to create healing environments, a discussion that I am happy to report continues to this day in the many splendid Planetree sites and in the spirit of this book.

Angelica Thieriot

INTRODUCTION

PATIENT-CENTERED CARE MOVES INTO THE MAINSTREAM

In the approximately six years since the first edition of *Putting Patients First* was written, patient-centered care has moved from an emerging trend in the health care delivery systems of countries including the United States, Canada, and the Netherlands to a defining characteristic of quality patient care in an ever-expanding number of countries around the world. This move into the mainstream after decades on the fringe is largely the result of the convergence of several evolving social and economic realities:

1. The aging of baby boomers and the associated rise in consumer expectations around the health care experience

2. Unprecedented access to health information fueled by the Internet

3. The demand for greater transparency in reporting of outcomes and new governmental incentives to report these results for widespread dissemination to the public

4. Increased demand for timely and convenient access to costly medical technologies and pharmaceuticals that continue to drive health care costs—including both out-of-pocket costs for patients and employer contributions—increasingly skyward

As we struggle to balance these pressures within what many patients and providers describe as an understaffed, overwhelmed system, providing caring, kind, and respectful service has become even more of a challenge. What began eons ago as a personal calling to provide care to the ill, distressed, and injured has become a trillion-dollar business in the United States alone, with third-party payers in many cases now determining the nature of the patient-caregiver relationship and the extent of their contact with each other. The healing partnership between patient and physician has been reduced to seven-minute office encounters in many settings, and the majority of nurses in hospitals spend more time on documentation than in actually providing care at the bedside (Advisory Board Company, 2003).

Despite these challenges, a growing number of hospitals, clinics, continuing care facilities, and physician practices have found ways to create exemplary patient and resident-centered cultures. They have transformed the experience of care to include what so many other industries have mastered: choice, convenience, personalization, quality, and service. These aspects of a consumer-centric approach mirror the six core elements that the Institute of Medicine declared to be necessary to the delivery of quality patient care—that it be safe, timely, efficient, effective, equitable, and patient-centered (Institute of Medicine, 2001).

Truly patient-centered organizations have figured out how to address the very human needs of patients who come to us when they are most vulnerable, looking for support, comfort, and hope. These organizations see the big picture and attend to the smallest, and yet often the most meaningful, details of the patient experience. They find ways to decrease emergency room wait times and to provide comfortable, attractive furniture in areas where waiting occurs. They offer twenty-four-hour visitation throughout their facilities and support the active involvement of the patient's family, providing adequate space for them as well as meaningful roles and responsibilities as valued members of the care team. They openly share information with patients and their designated caregivers, encouraging them to review their medical charts and contribute their own progress notes, respecting the fact that we can never know another person as well as we know ourselves. These organizations are converting to electronic medical records and are developing interactive systems that connect information between departments so that patients no longer have to respond to the same requests for personal information over and over again. They have taken down the physical barriers in facilities between patients, families, and staff, while attending to individual privacy, realizing that the needs of patients come first and that addressing those needs in a timely fashion is not a disturbance of our work. It IS our work. These organizations have found creative and successful ways to have staff spend more time interacting with patients and less time in isolated documentation activities and endless and inefficient walking back and forth between patient rooms and the locations of needed supplies. These improvements to the patient care experience have resulted in a slight increase in overall ratings in patient satisfaction in American hospitals between 2002 and 2006 (Press Ganey, 2007).

There is some good news on the patient front, but less progress has been made over the past six years with the most valuable of health care resources—our employees. Good people with caring hearts enter the health professions to serve patients. Disenchanted with an industry that often seems to put the bottom line before human needs, nurses in particular are burning out, and fewer young people are choosing health care professions. Combined with an increase in the demand for health care, these forces are fueling a labor shortage that threatens to undermine health care for years to come (Advisory Board Company, 2003). Joel Seligman, the CEO of New York's Northern Westchester Hospital, summed up the situation well: "I can only hope that the world is beginning to realize that the stress level for health care workers is out of control, and that we need to bring more balance back into the system; no wonder we need tea carts and meditation rooms for staff in hospitals today!"

Even though the majority of health care organizations have not kept pace with the consumer revolution, more and more are beginning to "get it," and as a result, the vision of patient-centered care pioneers like Harvey Picker of The Picker Institute and Planetree's founder, Angelica Thieriot, is slowly being realized. We are beginning to see hospitals respond to consumer demands, improving care delivery systems to provide the most sophisticated technical care in a more personalized, humanized, and demystified manner. Nonetheless, the majority of patients hospitalized today, whether in the United States, Canada, Europe, Latin America, or Asia, still find themselves in provider-focused systems. The CEO of a large metropolitan hospital in the United States suggested that most health centers still deliver more "surgeon-focused care" and "nursing-focused care" than patient-centered care. This comment reflects that many aspects of the hospital experience which thirty years ago left Angelica Thieriot feeling detached, ill-informed, and insignificant during her own healing process persist today.

THE PLANETREE MODEL

As Thieriot herself describes in the Prologue of this second edition, it was a series of traumatic personal health care experiences that served as the impetus for the development of the Planetree model. Founded in 1978 as a nonprofit organization, Planetree vowed to reclaim for patients the holistic, patient-centered focus that medicine had lost. Everything in the hospital setting was to be evaluated from the perspective of the patient. Every element of the organization's culture was to be assessed, based on whether it enhanced or detracted from personalizing, demystifying, and humanizing the patient experience. A premium was placed on making information available to health care consumers, enabling them to be informed partners in their care.

Planetree's first step was to establish a consumer health resource center, which opened in 1981 in San Francisco. The resource center initially offered users a library of over two thousand health books and medical texts, a clipping file of current medical research, a catalogue of support groups and agencies, and a bookstore. Such a wealth of health information resources was an unheard-of luxury at a time when patients were still routinely barred from entering a hospital or medical school library.

The Planetree Health Resource Center became a national model, subsequently helping other organizations establish successful libraries throughout the country. The center developed a widely used consumer cataloging system known as the Planetree Classification Scheme, which continues to be used by health resource centers around the world.

History of the Planetree Model

Access to health and medical information was only one aspect of Planetree's vision for personalizing health care. In June 1985, with funding from The Henry J. Kaiser Family Foundation and The San Francisco Foundation, a major milestone was reached with the opening of the Planetree model hospital unit. The first of five Planetree model hospital sites, the thirteen-bed, medical-surgical unit at Pacific Presbyterian Medical Center in San Francisco, California, was like no other hospital unit in existence at that time. This unit was the culmination of years of grassroots effort to create a truly new model of care in the hospital setting. Its creation launched one of the most far-reaching experiments in the realm of consumer-responsive, patient-centered care ever attempted in this country.

Using findings from numerous focus groups with patients, families, and staff members, the innovative medical-surgical unit was designed to offer the latest medical technology in an environment that was comforting and supportive. The thirteen-bed unit was a pioneering effort to change the way patients experienced hospitals—from impersonal and intimidating institutions to nurturing, healing, and educational environments.

Planetree patients had the opportunity to develop direct communication with their doctors, in which they were encouraged to ask questions, request information, and participate in their care. This open communication benefited both patients and their physicians, in that the prescribed treatment plan continually reflected the patients' own goals.

An atmosphere conducive to healing was created by Planetree's original architect, Roslyn Lindheim. Lindheim, a professor at the University of California at Berkeley, had studied hospitals and therapeutic environments throughout the world and had incorporated the most significant aspects into the model unit. The result was a remarkable transformation of a typical hospital environment into a physical space that promoted healing, learning, and patient participation.

Standard partitions between patients and staff members were removed, leaving open and airy work spaces. Soothing colors were chosen, and each room was decorated differently to be as individual as the patient who occupied it. A patient lounge was created to be a comfortable place where patients, families, and friends could relax, share a meal, or watch a movie. The lounge also served as a satellite resource center, providing medical and health information on the unit.

The Planetree unit included a kitchenette, where patients and family members were encouraged to prepare meals, using hospital food or food they had brought from home. Hungry patients were never told that they would have to wait until hospital staff members delivered the next meal.

Acknowledging that hospitals are often perceived as frightening, unfamiliar places, staff members encouraged the patient's family and friends to spend time there as a comfort to the patient, helping the patient avoid loneliness and isolation. Visiting hours on the Planetree unit were unrestricted, and children were permitted to visit. Family members and friends who wanted to stay overnight were accommodated either in the patient's room or on a sofa bed in the patient lounge nearby.

One specific person was designated by the patient as his or her care partner. The care partner was often the person who would continue to care for the patient after he or she was discharged from the hospital. The care partner worked closely with the nurses in a supportive, supervised environment to learn whatever skills might be needed—to perform tasks as simple as helping a patient bathe or dress or as complex as adjusting a portable ventilator.

The model unit provided a wide variety of educational opportunities for patients and their loved ones, including written materials, audiotapes and videotapes, and personal instruction by the staff.

Patients were given information packets specific to their diagnosis and needs. These packets, provided by the Planetree Health Resource Center, included basic medical information, listings of support groups, and other resources that might be helpful after the patient had gone home. In addition, information about complementary therapies, such as massage or stress management, was provided.

The Planetree philosophy stressed that one of the most valuable learning resources available was the patient's own medical chart. Patients were encouraged to read their charts daily, ask questions and discuss findings, and participate in the decisions affecting their care. Patients were also encouraged to keep written records of their experiences and observations in patient progress notes, which became a permanent part of their medical chart if they so desired.

It was the goal of the Planetree unit to help patients not only get well faster but also stay well longer, possibly avoiding future hospitalizations. With this in mind, Planetree created a self-medication program, enabling appropriate patients to administer their own medications while they were hospitalized. Patients were given fact sheets listing uses and possible side effects, and a pharmacist was available to answer questions. The patient gradually assumed more responsibility, taking the medication at the appropriate time and charting that it was taken. This learning process often avoided the problems that occurred when a patient went home with several medications and was unsure what, when, or how much should be taken.

While reducing the stress of hospitalization, the Planetree unit also educated patients about ways to reduce the stress in their daily lives. Volunteers who were specialists in relaxation, visualization, and massage offered their services at no charge, helping to make the hospital stay more relaxing and rewarding.

While drawing on the latest technology in Western medicine, the model unit also attempted to nurture the healing resources within each patient. Although medicine traditionally draws on the body's resources to heal, Planetree believes that by incorporating the mind and spirit into this process, healing can take place faster and more completely. In an effort to meet the needs of the whole person (body, mind, and spirit), the Planetree unit incorporated the arts into its healing environment.

Research on the Model Unit

The original Planetree unit was structured as a three-year demonstration project, serving as a model for hospitals and health care providers throughout the country. As part of the pilot project, the University of Washington agreed to evaluate the impact of the Planetree unit on the patient experience. The evaluation was also designed to study the level of satisfaction among nurses and doctors on the Planetree unit, its effect on the quality of patient care, and its cost-effectiveness. Significant findings included increases in patient satisfaction with the environment of the unit, the technical quality of the care provided, and the education provided. Study results summarized the project as a "successful example of patient-centered hospital care" (Martin and others, 1998, p. 133).

The success of this unique experiment generated a great deal of interest. Four additional model sites were subsequently implemented between 1987 and 1990 to refine the model in diverse settings.

By the early 1990s, hundreds of tour groups from hospitals across the country and around the world had visited the model sites and worked with the Planetree organization to enhance patient care at their institutions. Managed care was rapidly expanding, hospital budgets were shrinking, the number of beds was declining, and competition for patients was growing. Executive teams were looking for innovative strategies to improve patient satisfaction and differentiate their hospitals in an increasingly competitive health care marketplace. One such team from a community hospital in Connecticut believed that the Planetree model was the right strategy for them. Pioneering a new relationship with Planetree, Griffin Hospital in Derby, Connecticut, became the first Planetree affiliate in 1992. Given this more flexible approach to Planetree implementation, additional hospitals and health systems followed suit, forming what has become a community of patient- and resident-centered hospitals, health systems, and long-term and continuing care facilities. The membership network is a rapidly growing coalition across the United States, Canada, Europe, and beyond, advancing innovative solutions to the changing needs of health care consumers.

Health Care Consumerism

The story of Planetree mirrors the journey of patient-centered care through the evolution of health care delivery during the last three decades. In its earliest days, the model was viewed as a radical, idealistic philosophy that challenged the status quo of a high-tech, provider-focused system. As more and more organizations adopted and refined the model, over twenty years beginning in the mid-1980s, it began to be seen as an innovative differentiation strategy for organizations wanting to demonstrate their superior level of commitment to the holistic needs of patients. More recently, the model is evolving into a systematic approach for defining, implementing, and measuring patient-centered practice in a wide variety of settings. Patient-centered care has become a well-accepted approach to improving health care quality from the increasingly respected perspective of the patient/consumer. No longer passive recipients of care, today's educated consumers are a powerful force for change. They are driving a transformation in health care no less profound than that brought about by the technological breakthroughs of the twentieth century.

The rapid rise in health care consumerism can be linked to several trends. The first has been the steady increase in health care costs. As these costs have risen, so too has the amount consumers are expected to pay out of their own pockets. Employers have shifted more and more of the burden of health care coverage onto employees. In response, individuals have increased both their knowledge and their scrutiny of how their health care dollar is being spent, and they are demanding new levels of value and service (KPMG, 1998; Press Ganey Associates, 1999; Ganey and Drain, 1998).

At the same time, we have undergone an explosion in the amount of information available in all areas—in particular, on health-related topics. The ease of access to this information, especially that provided by the Internet, has created an exceptionally well-informed population (Larkin, 1999; McLaughlin, 2001; Eng and others, 1998; Ernst & Young LLP, 1998). In addition to general health information, the availability of hospital and health care quality data has increased dramatically. The Centers for Medicare and Medicaid Services now collect and publicly report outcomes on a growing number of performance measures, and the HCAHPS survey similarly provides easily accessible data on patient satisfaction with hospitals and health centers across the United States and in parts of Canada and Europe. Consumer access to this information is beginning to influence utilization. Dr. Toby Cosgrove, CEO of The Cleveland Clinic, one of the most highly regarded health care systems in the United States, recently acknowledged the importance of taking patient satisfaction as seriously as excellent clinical care when he appointed a chief experience officer to oversee a new division focused on improving the patient experience. The emerging power of health care consumerism to shape delivery systems is likewise being felt in countries such as the Netherlands, largely held to have one of the finest health care systems in the world. Several of their largest academic medical centers, including The Hague Hospital, are considering widespread implementation of patient-centered practices and use of a satisfaction survey similar to HCAHPS.

What do consumers want from the health care system today? That is something that has not changed since the first edition of this book. The majority still feel confident that they will receive high-quality technical care when they enter most hospitals or health centers. That means that the characteristics that define a superior patient experience from the consumer perspective have little to do with clinical care. Instead, what consumers seek out is respect, kindness, privacy, information, autonomy, choices, care coordination, and inclusion.

Unfortunately, too many patients, residents, and clients do not find these on a regular basis. Although conditions are improving in many areas, as a whole, hospitals and health centers have a long way to go in meeting patients' needs. Nothing less than a complete transformation of health care organizational culture is required. At the heart of this transformation is the need to listen to what both patients and caregivers feel are barriers to health and healing and to find ways of removing these barriers (American College of Healthcare Executives, 1999; Bezold, 1999; Coile and Russell, 2002).

ESSENTIAL ELEMENTS OF PATIENT-CENTERED CARE

Pioneers of patient-centered care like The Picker Institute and Planetree embarked on journeys to identify and remove these barriers to healing through a variety of strategies, including focus group work, analysis of Picker survey data, and the establishment of demonstration projects or Planetree model sites. These early initiatives ascertained certain essential elements of patient-centered care, which have been adapted and refined over time as additional health care organizations found new ways to better meet patient needs (Frampton, 2000, 2001; Freedman, 2001).

Part One of this book, comprising Chapters One through Nine, discusses nine essential elements of patient-centered care, by drawing from the experiences and insights of the organizations that have implemented them over the past two decades. These core elements of patient-centered care have stood the test of time, but their expression has flourished in a thousand different ways. As employees at hospitals, clinics, and continuing care sites across the country and beyond have had the opportunity and responsibility to bring patient-centered care to life in their organizations, a limitless well of creativity has been tapped. Some of their best ideas are presented in the case studies included throughout this book.

In Chapter One, Jean Watson and I explore human interactions and how they can be shaped to create an organizational culture that is truly healing and patient-centered. This involves not only the provision of nurturing, compassionate, personalized care to patients and families but also—and just as important—it involves how staff care for themselves and one another. It also involves how organizations foster cultures that support and nurture their staff. Two case studies are included. The first is focused on Stamford Hospital's employee retreats, which helped to reawaken staff's passion for their chosen professions and set in motion a cultural transformation within the hospital. The second features Alegent Health's innovative ethnographic approach for thoroughly understanding the needs of its patient population in a highly personalized manner.

Candace Ford Gray and Michele A. Spatz present the Planetree model's approach to patient, family, and community education in Chapter Two. Strategies—including development of health resource centers, customized patient information packets, bedside collaborative care conferences, patient pathways, and open medical chart policies—are described, and special attention is paid to the growing role of electronic access to information for patients and providers. Case studies highlight outcomes related to Hackensack University Medical Center's practice of hourly rounding and detail an array of programs that strive to empower patients to be active, informed participants in their own health care, including Cleveland Clinic's MyChart Program, Sentara Virginia Beach General Hospital's Personal Health Books for patients, and Griffin Hospital's popular Mini-Med School program.

In Chapter Three, Alexandra Harrison, Gail MacKean, and Margaret Cullivan examine the role that social support networks play in health and healing. Increasingly short lengths of stay are serving to underscore the vital caregiver role that families can play, both before and after hospitalization. Practices that support involvement of family and encourage the utilization of hospitalization as an opportunity to educate those who will be the patient's caregiver at home are presented, along with strategies for incorporating the patient and family perspective into organizational planning. Also addressed are ways to creatively engage volunteers to provide comfort, companionship, support, and diversions for patients and their loved ones. Case studies describe the efforts of Good Samaritan Hospital and Spectrum Health to involve families as members of the care team.

In Chapter Four, David L. Katz and F. Nicholas Jacobs discuss the role of food and nutrition in hospitals as both an integral factor in health and a powerful symbol of comfort. The mechanics of a number of creative food service programs are described in case studies. The first focuses on Swedish Covenant Hospital's approach to addressing the food preferences of diverse populations and the second on Kadlec Medical Center's twenty-four-hour A La Carte Meal Service.

Exploring the vital role of spirituality in the healing process is the subject of Chapter Five. Steven L. Jeffers and Dennis Kenny highlight studies that have documented the clinical relevance of religion and spirituality, and special attention is paid to ways that caregivers can attend to the spiritual needs that often arise at the end of life. Case studies demonstrate how two sites have worked to address the diverse spiritual needs of their patient populations, including Centre de réadaptation Estrie's incorporation of spiritual practices into the rehabilitation process and Page Hospital's construction of a traditional Native American hogan.

In Chapter Six, David L. Katz and Ather Ali present an overview of the rise in utilization of a variety of integrative approaches in conventional care and the relationship with health care consumerism; dissatisfaction with high-tech, low-touch medical care; and the growing recognition of the mind-body-spirit connection to health. Sharp Coronado Hospital's use of healing touch, clinical aromatherapy, and massage treatments as part of patient care is presented in a case study.

In Chapter Seven, Roger S. Ulrich explains why when it comes to health care art, the decisive criterion is not if it is beautiful or thought provoking, but whether it improves patient outcomes. He then provides evidence-based guidelines for the selection of health care art. Examples of healing arts programs in place at patient-centered organizations reflect that the arts encompass more than the visual arts. In the chapter's case study, a *music-thanatologist* describes the powerful role that music can play in end-of-life care.

Kimberly Nelson Montague and Robert F. Sharrow, two architects who specialize in patient-centered healing design, demonstrate the fundamental role that the physical environment can play in the healing process.

Chapter Eight provides an overview of evidence-based, patient-centered design elements that have been shown to reduce stress and anxiety, increase patient satisfaction, and promote patient privacy and safety. A case study describing newly constructed Midwest Medical Center underscores how such a patient-centered approach to design supports the health and healing of patients. A second case study about Martha's Vineyard Hospital suggests how "greening" can result in a healing setting that is also healthy for our global environment.

In Chapter Nine, Randall L. Carter and Catherine Whalen examine how the healthy communities movement and a patient-centered approach to care can work hand in hand to promote patient empowerment, health, and wellness. Two case studies provide examples of organizations reaching out beyond hospital walls to ensure that the community's broad range of health care needs is met. Sentara Williamsburg Regional Medical Center's Block Buddies Program uses trained volunteers as neighborhood health resource contacts to combat a number of the barriers that hinder health care access. Created in response to drastic Medicaid cuts that threatened to seriously jeopardize patients' ability to get their prescription medications, in just a year and a half, Saint Thomas Hospital's Dispensary of Hope program has dispensed more than 1.25 million dollars' worth of donated sample pharmaceuticals to patients in need.

CURRENT TRENDS IN PATIENT-CENTERED CARE

Part Two of this book, Chapters Ten through Fifteen, builds on the content of the first half of the book by considering patient-centered care in the context of the myriad of other forces influencing the health care industry today, including how it relates to quality and patient safety, public reporting and pay for performance, physician satisfaction, and of course the bottom line. These issues are explored in the context of transforming the culture of health care as we know it.

In Chapter Ten, Patrick A. Charmel presents the business case for patient-centered care. Drawing from case examples of hospitals whose implementation of patient-centered care has resulted in positive outcomes related to patient satisfaction, employee satisfaction, length of stay, readmission rates, and malpractice claims, he makes the case for "doing well by doing good."

In Chapter Eleven, Steven F. Horowitz and H. Lee Kanter share their insights on the physician's role in fostering patient-centered practices and the importance of engaging medical staff in implementation efforts.

Chapter Twelve demonstrates that patient-centered care is hardly limited to acute care hospitals. Authors Heidi Gil, Wendy W. Peche, and Philip J. Wilner describe adaptations to the model that have made patient- or resident-centered care a reality across the health care continuum. Two case studies about long-term care organizations in the Netherlands underscore that although the model of patient-centered care may require adaptations to reflect different cultures, the desire for respectful, compassionate, dignified care is universal.

With its emphasis on patients as partners and empowering patients with information, patient-centered care is inextricably linked to patient safety. In Chapter Thirteen, Carrie Brady and James B. Conway explore opportunities for engaging patients as partners in their care and safety. Best practices presented in case studies include Calgary Health Region's Patient/Family Safety Council and Aurora Sinai Medical Center's Patient Safety Staff Retreats.

Chapter Fourteen examines the influence of public policy on advancing patient-centered care. Carolyn M. Clancy of the Agency for Healthcare Research and Quality and Janet M. Corrigan and Dwight N. McNeill of the National Quality Forum share their insights on the role of government, payers, and the general public in empowering patients as partners and advancing patient-centered care as a national health care priority.

Finally, in Chapter Fifteen, Carrie Brady and I summarize the challenges and opportunities for further development of patient-centered care in healing health care environments. Looking at today's best practices in combination with emerging trends in health care, we suggest where we should focus our attention in order to overcome existing barriers to wider adoption of patient-centered practices.

Most fittingly, this second edition of *Putting Patients First* ends with the words of a patient. Like Angelica Thieriot, Linda Kenney has turned her own traumatic health care experience into a personal crusade to improve health care. She explains why patient-centered care resonates with her, as a patient. Her perspective serves to reinforce just why patient-centered care matters and is a call to action to health care providers, patients, and families alike.

Derby, Connecticut   Susan B. Frampton
August 2008

REFERENCES

Advisory Board Company. *Nursing Executive Center National RN Survey.* Washington, D.C.: Advisory Board Company, 2003.

American College of Healthcare Executives. "Patient- and Family-Centered Care: Good Values, Good Business." *Conference Brochure.* Miami Beach: American College of Healthcare Executives, Mar. 22–23, 1999.

Bezold, C. "Health Care Faces a Dose of Change." *Futurist,* Apr. 1999, *33*(4), 30–34.

Coile, R., Jr., and Russell, C. *FUTURESCAN 2002, A Forecast of Healthcare Trends 2002–2006.* Chicago: Health Administration Press, American College of Healthcare Executives, 2002.

Eng, T. R., and others. "Access to Health Information and Support: A Public Highway or a Private Road?" *Journal of the American Medical Association,* 1998, *280*(15), 1371–1375.

Ernst & Young LLP. "Built to Last Means Built to Change." *Medicare+Choice and the New Health Care Consumerism.* June 1998.

Frampton, S. "Planetree Patient-Centered Care and the Healing Arts." *Complementary Health Practice Review,* 2000, *7*(1), 17–19.

Frampton, S. "Vantage Point: The Planetree Model." In N. Faass (ed.), *Integrating Complementary Medicine into Health Systems.* Gaithersburg, Md.: Aspen, 2001.

Freedman, D. H. "Redesigning the Hospital Environment." In N. Faass (ed.), *Integrating Complementary Medicine into Health Systems.* Gaithersburg, Md.: Aspen, 2001.

Ganey, R., and Drain, M. "Patient Satisfaction: What You See Is What You Get." *Trustee,* Nov./Dec. 1998, *51*(10), 6–10.

Institute of Medicine. *Crossing the Quality Chasm: A New Health System for the Twenty-First Century.* Committee on Quality of Health Care in America. Washington, D.C.: National Academy Press, 2001.

KPMG. "Consumerism in Health Care: New Voices." *Consumerism in Health Care Research Study Findings.* Jan. 1998, pp. 6–24.

Larkin, H. "Programs to Boost Patient Satisfaction Pay Off in Many Ways, CEO's Say." *AHA News,* June 21, 1999, p. 1.

Martin, D., and others. "Randomized Trial of a Patient-Centered Hospital Unit." *Patient Education and Counseling,* 1998, *34*(2), 125–133.

McLaughlin, N. "Great Expectations: Providers Better Pay Attention to Educated Patients." *Modern Healthcare,* Feb. 2001, p. 24.

Press Ganey Associates. "One Million Patients Have Spoken: Who Will Listen?" *Satisfaction Monitor,* 1999.

Press Ganey Associates. "Patient Perspectives on American Health Care." *Hospital Pulse Report,* 2007.

PUTTING PATIENTS FIRST

PART

1

ESSENTIAL ELEMENTS OF PATIENT-CENTERED CARE

CHAPTER

1

HUMAN INTERACTIONS AND RELATIONSHIP-CENTERED CARING

JEAN WATSON AND SUSAN B. FRAMPTON

This chapter does the following:

- Explores the role of human caring in creating optimal human interactions in health care environments
- Describes the Relationship-Centered Care/Caring model and how this supports a patient-centered approach to healing partnerships

Note: This chapter draws heavily on two previous works: J. Watson, *Nursing: The Philosophy and Science of Caring* (2nd ed.), Boulder: University Press of Colorado, 2008; and L. Gilpin, "The Importance of Human Interactions," in *Putting Patients First* (1st ed.), San Francisco: Jossey Bass, 2003.

■ Describes tools and techniques employed at Planetree affiliates that foster optimal healing relationships

INTRODUCTION

When Angelica Thieriot, the founder of Planetree, was confronted with an acute illness that required hospitalization, she felt it was more frightening to be hospitalized than to face a life-threatening health crisis. "First do no harm" is the golden rule of health care. Yet many patients leave hospitals, as Thieriot did, feeling abused, traumatized, and dehumanized. In an attempt to alleviate physical suffering, many health care environments seem to create—or at least exacerbate—emotional suffering. Planetree's goal has always been to change the way patients experience hospitals and other health care settings. This experience is fundamentally rooted in the interactions and relationships between patients, families, and health caregivers.

Clinical care and health care practices are grounded in human communication, human interactions, and relationships. At the same time, approaches to system solutions are often disconnected from relationships and caring. "The current dilemmas in health care are often located within a framework that emphasizes the outer forces of economics, staffing shortages, and technological-medical issues, or system/institutional needs" (Watson, 2004b, p. 249). This disconnection between the current focus in addressing health care issues (read that as *sick care*) conflicts with and greatly differs from the deeply human-to-human caring relationships and human-to-human connections that give meaning and purpose to nurses, patients, all other health practitioners, and systems alike.

In spite of, or because of, the dissonance between and among the diverse external forces affecting health care and the human caring relational dimensions, it becomes mandatory to recognize and acknowledge that any authentic solution to health problems has to arise from a deeply human discourse—a discourse that philosophically and theoretically underpins and guides health and healing for professional-disciplinary practices and system changes. The Planetree model of care provides a framework for shifting the discourse toward more humane and caring practices for practitioners and systems.

Whereas the health care system excels at measuring and improving the "what" and the "why" of medical care, patients themselves are more concerned with the "how" and "by whom." In a technological era that values the objectivity of science, little regard has been given to the subjective experience of patients. Subjectivity is often relegated to the realm of *patient satisfaction* and referred to as *soft science*. Although patient satisfaction is viewed as vital to the hospital's financial health, it is rarely perceived as having an effect on the health outcomes of those who receive care. New medications, procedures, and other advances in medical care are often studied extensively, whereas the manner in which these advances are delivered is intentionally factored out. As Leland Kaiser points out, "If it doesn't matter how the care is delivered, why do pharmaceutical companies conduct double-blind studies?" (personal interview, April 11, 2001).

What underlies many of the issues raised in focus groups and satisfaction surveys with patients and caregivers alike is an area that medical science finds difficult to define, much less to quantify. It involves the vague and elusive but vital area of human interactions. How do we communicate caring? How do we ensure that patients feel respected? How do we encourage patients to ask questions? How do we honor patients' dignity when dignity may be defined differently by each patient?

When a nurse or other caregiver enters a patient's room to give a medication, deliver a meal, or complete any task, what really takes place? Medical science would have us believe that completing the task alone is enough. Quality is seen as a measure of how skillfully and efficiently each task is performed. But from the patient's perspective, every task is more than the delivery of medical services. It is an opportunity for a caring human interaction and forms the basis for a healing partnership between patient and caregiver.

These relationships are central to attending to the humane, ethical considerations that affect subjective human experiences, perceptions, and meanings related to hospitalization or treatment regimes (Shattell, 2002). Whether the relationships are caring or not has consequences for both patients and practitioners, especially nurses (Halldorsdottir, 1991; Swanson, 1999).

These relationships and their impact on the care experience are captured in the shift from externally generated problem solutions to inner-oriented, ontological, human-caring relational changes, at several levels (Tresolini and Pew-Fetzer Task Force, 1994):

- Practitioner-to-patient relationship

- Practitioner-to-practitioner relationship

- Practitioner-to-community relationship

- Practitioner-to-self relationship

Each of these levels is informed and affected by one's understanding and exploration of human caring as the ethical and philosophical foundation for professional practice, as well as an action component. Caring relationships at all levels affect health and healing outcomes and become the basis for understanding the critical nature of patient communications, for developing human (caring-ontological) competencies, and for cultivating relationship-centered caring at all levels of one's life and work.

RELATIONSHIP-CENTERED CARE/CARING

Planetree has always believed that the way care is delivered is as important as the care itself, and the Relationship-Centered Care (RCC) model focuses its full attention on this issue. RCC emerged from the original Pew-Fetzer Task Force, an interdisciplinary project that sought to advance all health professional education beyond the conventional biomedical, technical orientation and toward an expanded model for healing. This focus acknowledged that *relationships* are critical to the care provided by all health practitioners, regardless of discipline or subspecialty and holds a central place in education and practice (Tresolini and Pew-Fetzer Task Force, 1994, p. 11). Further, this term conveys the importance of human-to-human interaction, of human-to-human caring and connections, as the foundation of any therapeutic or healing activity. Relationship-centered care/caring likewise locates health care within a context of multiple and diverse relationships, which put into action "a paradigm of health that integrates caring, healing, and community" (Tresolini and Pew-Fetzer Task Force, 1994, p. 19).

This philosophy brings forth deeply human connections and opens up the subjective/intersubjective world and the relational connections between and among all aspects of one's life and one's interactions. This model therefore does not and cannot stand outside in some detached, abstract construction of practitioner-patient-community relationships. Rather, this model invites the full self of practitioner to engage in the full self of the patient, whereby the subjective world of both are brought closer together (Tresolini and Pew-Fetzer Task Force, 1994, p. 22) through a human-to-human intersubjective caring connection (Watson, 1999).

Concepts and Consequences of Caring/Noncaring

The caring literature in nursing science studies has identified concepts and outcomes related to constructs such as empathy, compassion, communication, hope, trust, respect, faith, love, patient-centeredness, and relationship-centeredness (Quinn and others, 2003). The work of Swanson (1999) in particular has relevance to the significance of caring and its effects, for better or worse, depending on the presence of caring in practice models. For example, her 1999 work synthesized 130 database articles, chapters, and books on caring, published between 1980 and 1996. These studies included both empirical and theoretical-interpretive studies. Swanson summarized and categorized her findings into five levels:

- Capacity for caring (characteristics of caring persons)

- Concerns and commitments (beliefs and values that underlie nursing)

- Conditions (what affects, enhances, or inhibits the presence and practice of caring)

- Caring actions (what caring means to nurses and clients and what it looks like)

- Caring consequences (outcomes of caring—for both patients and nurses)

The overall summary of Swanson's findings related to consequences of caring for both patient and nurse has implications for all health professionals, as captured in Figures 1.1 and 1.2.

- Emotional-spiritual well-being (dignity, self-control, personhood)
- Physical well-being (enhanced healing, saved lives, safety, energy, lower costs, greater comfort, less loss)
- Trust relationship, less alienation, greater family involvement

- Humiliation, frightened, out of control, despair, helplessness, alienation, vulnerability, lingering bad memories
- Decreased healing

FIGURE 1.1. *Consequences of Caring/Noncaring: Patients.*

Source: Swanson, 1999, p. 54.

- Emotional-spiritual (sense of accomplishment, satisfaction, purpose, gratitude, preserved integrity, fulfillment, wholeness, self-esteem, living one's own philosophy, respect for life and death, reflective, love of nursing)

- Increased knowledge

- Hardened, oblivious, robot-like
- Depressed, frightened, worn down

FIGURE 1.2. *Consequences of Caring/Noncaring: Nurses.*

Source: Swanson, 1999, p. 54.

As illustrated in these figures, one's stance toward and practice of caring at the individual and system level can for better or for worse either facilitate healing or create distress for both parties. Thus, caring and one's relationship can be constructive or destructive, healing or nonhealing.

Halldorsdottir's research is considered a timeless study of this caring/noncaring relationship continuum (Halldorsdottir, 1991). Through her research, she identified five levels, or types, of *caring relationships.* These ranged from Type 1, which she named *biocidic* (toxic, life-destroying, leading to anger, despair, and decreased well-being), to Type 5, *biogenic* (life-giving and life-sustaining). The biogenic is of course the ideal kind of caring, which allows for an authentic human-to-human connection that is gratifying for both patient and nurse. As Halldorsdottir put it:

This Biogenic mode involves loving benevolence, responsiveness, generosity, mercy and compassion. A truly life-giving presence offers the other interconnectedness and fosters spiritual freedom. It involves being open to persons and giving life to the very heart of man as person, creating a relationship of openness and receptivity yet always keeping a creative distance of respect and compassion. The truly life-giving or biogenic presence restores well being and human dignity. It is a transforming personal presence that deeply changes one. For the recipient there is experienced an inrush of compassion, often like a current [1991, p. 44].

- Type 1, *biocidic,* or life destroying (toxic, leading to anger, despair, decreased well-being)
- Type 2, *biostatic,* or life restraining (cold or treated as a nuisance)
- Type 3, *biopassive,* or life neutral (apathetic or detached)
- Type 4, *bioactive,* or life sustaining (classic nurse-patient relationship, as kind, concerned, and benevolent)
- Type 5, *biogenic,* or life giving (transpersonal caring)

FIGURE 1.3. *Caring Relationships: Uncaring to Caring.*

Source: Halldorsdottir, 1991, pp. 37–49.

Figure 1.3 identifies the five types and the continuum of caring/ noncaring.

The biogenic caring relationship is considered congruent with *transpersonal caring* and Watson's *caring moment* (Watson, 1985, 1999; Quinn and others, 2003), in that the relationship is affecting both patient and nurse in a way that paradoxically transcends the moment, while both being fully present in the moment.

As Quinn and others (2003, p. A69) remind us from another point of view, these models of caring and their effect and consequences can be supported by the "enormous literature in psychoneuroimmunology, social support, love, and systems and chaos theories. . . . For example, social support has been shown to affect health status, as has love. The . . . (caring) relationship might be viewed as a type of critical social support and a particular kind of love, offered in moments of intense disequilibrium and vulnerability" toward healing. As supported by both Swanson and Halldorsdottir's work, caring has consequences, which can either be life-giving or life-draining, healthy as well as destructive for both.

A conscious, informed, intentional approach to better our understanding of caring and relationship is necessary for true professional practices if we are to assume ethical as well as empirical-practical responsibility for sustaining caring at the individual, system, and societal levels.

It is through relationships and caring that health professionals and nurses in particular are to sustain caring and healing practices through the formal cultivation of such relational caring competencies, moving closer to biogenic–transpersonal caring. At the same time, it has to be acknowledged that "the biggest 'psychosocial' problem facing us may be the need for our own personal transformation—to understand and promote change within ourselves" (Tresolini and Pew-Fetzer Task Force, 1994, p. 24).

Practitioner-to-Self Relationship

The practitioner-to-self relationship is grounded in self-awareness, self-reflection, and specific lifelong practices, which cultivate a caring consciousness, loving-kindness, and equanimity toward self. Cultivating a loving, caring relationship with self generates such feelings toward others. This is referred to as *caritas* (Watson, 2008), drawing upon the Latin association, which makes a connection between caring and love, reminding us that caring is something precious and fragile and has to be cultivated. One of Watson's original core *carative factors* (1979, p. 9) for a caring model was "cultivation of sensitivity to one's self and others," which in turn helps "develop a helping-trusting human caring relationship" and instills faith, hope, and trust.

In this framework of starting with self and one's relationship with self, we acknowledge, "To be human is to feel. . . . but all too often people allow themselves to think their thoughts, but not to feel their feelings" (Watson, 1979, p. 16). Further, we rarely build in a self-responsibility to pay attention to our feelings to the extent that we are able to cultivate skill in witnessing and reflecting on our own behavior, reactions, moods, and emotions. We rarely are taught about honoring our emotions, witnessing them, becoming familiar with them. Through this process of attending to and reflecting on our emotions, we are allowing them to pass through us, to be released or channeled, rather than holding and freezing the emotions. It is in lack of self-awareness and through fighting our emotions, holding onto them, justifying them, and so on, that our feelings torture or control us with internal psychic fights. Conversely, when we cultivate an emotional awareness and even an *emotional intelligence* of self-acceptance, self-love, and patience, we are learning how to generate an inner peace and calm for self, thereby becoming a healing presence for self and others.

It is through this beginning point of attending to our self-awareness that we cultivate our spiritual growth and our ability to witness our dynamic changing feelings. We also learn that our feelings often control us. We learn to see how often we freeze and set our emotions, creating more discomfort for our self and others. In contrast, when we honor our relationship with our self in kind, caring, loving ways, we learn that our feelings give us insight into our shared human condition. We learn in this model that we all have emotions and feelings, but *we are not our emotions and feelings* (Watson, 1999).

The development of self-growth and sensitivity to self evolves from emotional work and emotional insights. This effort requires the nurturing of judgment, taste, values, and sensitivity in human relationships in general. The development of feelings of caring and compassion can expand and deepen through the study of the humanities: arts, aesthetics, drama, film, and literature, as well as through diverse life experiences with persons with different values, cultures, belief systems, and geographical and national settings, which can cultivate compassion and understanding that take us beyond our limited perceptions and set opinions about judging others. The recognition and development of such understanding generates knowledge and wisdom, which leads to self-growth; self-acceptance; and the practices of patience, loving-kindness, equanimity, and forgiveness toward self first, then toward others.

In this model, we are awakened to the process of learning from self and one another how to be more human—how to identify our inner self with others, finding the dilemmas of others in ourselves. "What we learn from it is self-knowledge. The self we learn about or discover is every self. It is universal—the human self. We learn to recognize ourselves in others" (Watson, 1979, p. 59).

People are often afraid to look within because they fear that if they are honest, they will see only imperfections, which can be threatening. It seems easier to push back feelings, to deny them, to refuse to deal with them or to become consumed by them. All of these are harsh approaches toward self. Those who are not sensitive to their own feelings find it difficult to be sensitive to the feelings of others. Those who repress their own feelings may be unable to allow others to express or explore their feelings. However, caring and compassionate approaches to one's own feelings, allowing for imperfections, accepting self with both strengths and weaknesses, all become part of honoring one's own humanity (Watson, 1979).

We learn through this process how to avoid making negative judgments and critical reviews toward self and others—realizing that the feelings of others are not unlike our own feelings. We also learn that the feelings of others do not have to threaten us, making us want to cut off someone else's feelings. Through cultivating a loving-kindness toward self, we become more caring, loving, and kind toward others; as we become less judging of our own emotions, we become more open, more receptive, more allowing, more honoring and thus more therapeutic and more healing for self and other. Such emotional learning is foundational to relationship-centered caring practices and is the ground from which healing and health emerge.

Practitioner–to-Patient Relationship

The practitioner-to-patient relationship is directly affected by and generated from one's relationship with self. The foundation for a caring-healing relationship with other requires deepening one's own humanity, with cultivation of specific skills, knowledge, and values. These specific aspects of relationship and communication flow directly from self and one's own ability to BE PRESENT to self and other. Thus self-awareness and being authentically present become the most basic starting point for relationship-centered caring.

Being Present: A Caring Moment

Being present requires specific knowledge and skills related to the human dimensions of *being-in-right-relation* with self. It requires cultivation of mindfulness and a consciousness of caring and healing—in the moment. Being present requires being authentically oneself, not a role model or a professional facade with distant, clinical preconceived judgments and impressions. It requires staying in the other's frame of reference with active, attentive listening, without judgment. It requires hearing the message and voice of other—hearing the tone behind the words, listening to and seeing the body language. Relationship-centered caring (RCC) from practitioner to patient requires listening with the third ear, listening to the inner voice of one's own intuition. This skill requires recognizing the patient's life story and its meaning to the person, realizing that listening to a patient's story may be the greatest healing gift we can offer.

This authentic *presencing of being* creates a *caring moment,* where the practitioner is open to receive other, connecting with the spirit of other, beyond just the body physical-ego other. RCC within a caring moment finds the practitioner centered, conscious, mindful, intentional, and available to what is presenting itself in the communication/relationship—in the moment. This process is what creates a *caring moment,* which in turn can become a healing moment. A caring–healing moment affects both practitioner and patient, in the moment, but extends beyond the moment, for better or for worse, depending on the practitioner's presence and basic starting point. This depth of understanding both *caring* and *relationship* is the basis for biogenic caring and transpersonal healing moments and possibilities.

The practitioner relationship-centered caring model acknowledges that caring and relationship cannot be based solely on an individualistic model of caring but makes explicit that caring begins with self and radiates out from self to other, to family, to community, to planet Earth, even to the cosmos, affecting the entire infinity field of humanity (Levinas, 1969; Watson, 2005). This notion of caring as *caritas* extends beyond an individual conveying a deeper level than conventional thinking. This concept of caritas makes the relationship between caring and love and extends to nature and the larger universe (Watson, 2005, 2007).

Caritas to Communitas

In extending caring to a model of caritas, or *clinical caritas* (Watson, 2004a), the underlying values are made explicit. This notion of caritas/ deep caring is consistent with Nightingale's sense of *calling* for those in nursing and health care generally as a commitment to a professional and personal covenantal ethic of compassionate human service that is guided by an "altruistic-humanistic value system" (Watson, 1979). It is acknowledged in this extended framework that caring is a phenomenon that is to be cherished. It is fragile, delicate, and precious, requiring attention and cultivation to sustain. "When caring and love come together to serve humankind, we discover and affirm that caring-healing work is more than just a job, but a life-giving and life-receiving (biogenic) career for a lifetime of growth and learning" (Watson, 2007).

As this model becomes more explicit, we are more able to integrate the past with the present and the future. Such maturity and evolution requires (consistent with the Pew-Fetzer Task Force report): transforming self and those we serve, including our institutions and the professions themselves. As we more publicly and professionally assert a model of caring relationship, grounded in notions of caritas and biogenic/ transpersonal dimensions of caring for self and other, we locate our self and health care within a new emerging cosmology of caring and loving as part of healing relationships. Through this shift, we call forth a sense of reverence and sacredness with respect to self, other, and all living things, thus invoking and transposing caritas to extend to *communitas* in thinking and actions, as a new and deep form of caring relationship (Watson, 2005). When caritas, love, and caring manifest at the community level, the notion of a moral community emerges. Such a community of caring consciousness for self and others exemplifies the concept of communitas.

Communitas

This interconnection between caritas and communitas makes explicit that we belong to a shared humanity and are connected with one another. In this way, we share our collective humanity across time and space and are bound together in this infinite universal field, which holds the totality of life itself.

The attention to cultivation of practitioner to community relationship is based further on an ethic and ethos of shared humanity, which reminds us that we learn to be more human by seeing our self in the other, and vice versa, realizing that one level of humanity reflects back on the other. This ethic and ethos is located within an emerging cosmology referred to as a *unitary consciousness* (Watson, 1999), noting that everything in the universe is connected, not separate and disconnected. Thus, we learn to be more open, more available, more present to the wonders of life itself, bonding us through the very breath of life, honoring the fact that we share the very air we breathe. Caritas and communitas define an emerging global ethic of caring-healing through relationships, belonging, and connectedness, which helps us restore the sacred in the midst of everyday existence.

Developing and sustaining deeper understanding of community—within both a concrete, local, and immediate sense and a universal communitas sense—forms the foundation for effective human caring. It is in recognizing, honoring, and incorporating a caring-communitarian ethic and ethos into our practice models that we help sustain individual and community. Further, it is through giving expanded attention to community relations that we bring forth our belongingness, our connectedness, and our shared human conditions. It is through this awareness and awakening that we cultivate more compassion, wisdom, and skills for caring relations, individually and collectively. It is through this awakening that we become agents and instruments for a moral community of caring. Thus, in this model we are moving toward a greater appreciation for the role of community and social support in health and healing.

ROLE OF SOCIAL SUPPORT IN HEALTH AND HEALING

Positive interactions between patients and staff members are fundamental, but do they demonstrably contribute to health and healing? Is there evidence that caring and kindness are better medicine? Few studies have been done in a hospital setting to examine the health benefits of interactions with staff members, but there are many other examples suggesting that social connections have a positive effect on health outcomes.

In a seventeen-year follow-up on the 6,848 adults who participated in an Alameda County study, it was found that women who were socially isolated had a significantly elevated risk of dying of cancer of all sites, and men with few social connections also showed significantly poorer cancer survival rates (Reynolds and Kaplan, 1990). David Spiegel, in his book *Living Beyond Limits* (1993), cites many studies linking cancer survival to social support. Spiegel proposes several possibilities for the positive effects, including the notion that social support may affect the quality of a patient's basic activities, such as eating and sleeping, and may help patients interact more effectively with their physicians. He also suggests that social support may serve as a buffer against stress, possibly decreasing the production of stress hormones such as cortisol and prolactin. Stress is known to have a deleterious effect on the immune system. Heart disease, the leading cause of death in the United States, has also been closely correlated with a low level of social support. At Duke University, a study of nearly fourteen hundred men and women diagnosed with coronary artery disease found that 50 percent of those who were socially isolated died within five years, compared with 17 percent of those living with a spouse (Williams and others, 1992). Many other studies report findings that loneliness, isolation, and lack of social support contribute to illness and premature death (Blazer, 1982; Berkman, Leo-Summers, and Horwitz, 1992; Wiklund and others, 1988). Dean Ornish, in his book *Love and Survival* (1988), cites many studies supporting the link between social connectedness and health outcomes.

Social support also seems to alleviate the physiological effects of stress. Kamarck, Manuck, and Jennings (1990) found that when women were asked to complete a mental math problem alone, their systolic blood pressure and heart rate were significantly higher than if they were allowed to have a friend with them. In a similar study, participants were asked to give a speech, either alone, in the presence of a supportive person, or in the presence of a nonsupportive person. Those with a supportive person present during the speech experienced the least change in blood pressure, whereas those in the presence of a nonsupportive person exhibited the greatest rise in blood pressure—even more than those who gave the speech alone (Lepore, Mata Allen, and Evans, 1993).

Several studies define social connectedness as being married, having a confidant, meeting with others in ongoing support groups, or participating in other activities that could foster and maintain long-term relationships. (The importance of these relationships will be covered in depth in Chapter Three, which discusses the role of family and friends.) One could make the case that a brief interaction with a nurse, laboratory technician, or other health care provider might not be enduring or significant enough to have any effect on the patient. But the Lepore study suggests that positive support during stressful events can minimize stress, whereas a nonsupportive person can exacerbate the stress. The stress of giving a speech might be comparable to what patients experience when undergoing a frightening medical procedure.

It is not uncommon in focus groups to hear descriptions from patients of how one caring person, even one brief interaction with a caring person—someone who listened to or supported the patient at a difficult time—changed the patient's experience. Not infrequently, patients state that the person who listened or seemed most caring was a hospital housekeeper. This is one reason why Planetree considers everyone who works in a hospital or in any related health care field to be a caregiver. From a patient's perspective, the title or job description of someone caring is of less importance than the fact that the caregiver is providing emotional support.

Until we have additional evidence regarding the potential health benefits of human interactions, we can build a strong argument for the importance of caring interactions and their impact on measures of patient satisfaction. Many questions asked on a typical patient satisfaction survey solicit the patient's perceptions about the manner in which care was delivered. How helpful was the staff in various departments? How willing were nurses and physicians to answer questions? How well were family members kept informed? Rarely are questions asked about the medical care itself. Was the surgical procedure performed correctly? Did you receive the correct medications? Were falls prevented? The quality of the medical care itself is usually tracked through incident reports, performance improvement measures, and reviews of adverse patient outcomes. Patient satisfaction, though not considered "hard science," is currently the best measure of the effects of human interactions on the patient's overall hospital experience.

The first study of patient satisfaction at a Planetree site was conducted by the University of Washington at the initial Planetree model unit. In this randomized, controlled trial of 618 patients hospitalized between 1986 and 1990, patient outcomes on the Planetree unit were compared with those on other medical-surgical units. Planetree patients were found to be significantly more satisfied with their hospital stay, their nursing care, the social support they received, the environment on the unit, and the education they were given (Martin and others, 1998).

More recent comparisons of patient satisfaction at Planetree-affiliated hospitals with national benchmark data are explored fully in Chapter Ten, and they indicate clearly the relationship between the quality of caring and satisfaction scores.

There is a misconception that supportive interactions require more staff or more time and are therefore more costly. Although labor costs are a substantial part of any hospital budget, the interactions themselves add nothing to the budget. Kindness is free. Listening to patients or answering their questions costs nothing. It could be argued that negative interactions—alienating patients, being unresponsive to their needs, or limiting their sense of control—can be very costly in lost patient revenues and perhaps litigation. Angry, frustrated, or frightened patients may be combative, withdrawn, and less cooperative, requiring far more time than it would have taken to interact with them initially in a positive way.

Ethnography Program

Like many health care organizations, Alegent Health has historically relied heavily on surveys and focus groups to explore the perceptions of patients about the care they received. Although the data gathered has provided useful snapshots of the patient experience, it has fallen short of Alegent's goal of thoroughly understanding the needs of its patient population. In 2006, the system began supplementing its traditional feedback mechanisms with ethnographic research, which meant fully participating in the patient experience with patients—going to their home, traveling with them to a procedure, and staying with them for the duration of their visit. This approach forced Alegent to abandon preconceived notions, to set aside prior knowledge of internal processes in place, and to closely observe what their patients actually do, how they behave, and how they interact with others. Armed with this knowledge, Alegent's leadership recognized they would be poised to better understand their patients and to respond quickly and appropriately to best meet their needs.

Alegent introduced this new approach to improve its oncology service line and was supported in the effort by an outside anthropological

FOR EXAMPLE

consulting group. With all legal clearances in place, eight oncology patients were observed "in the field." An at-home interview was followed by two weeks of ongoing observation during treatments, office visits, diagnostic tests, and the like. The experiences of the patients were chronicled via continuous audio and video recordings of their interactions, as well as picture journaling to further document the project team's observations. This fieldwork also extended to the patients' caregivers, including interviews with staff, medical professionals, and ancillary personnel that the patients encountered throughout their hospital/treatment center visits.

Quantified, this data collection process produced more than 1,500 data points, each reflecting either an implied or an expressed patient need. A two-day ideation process followed, for which a diverse group of cancer survivors, staff, community leaders, and members of the project team were convened to examine the data collected and brainstorm solutions. The result was that those 1,500 data points were synthesized into 350 tangible ideas for improvement. The observations were particularly useful for guiding the design of the system's first Image Recovery Center. They confirmed that when cancer patients look better, they start to feel better, and when they start to feel better, their sense of control comes back, and with it comes a renewed sense of self-confidence. Today, Alegent's Image Recovery Center reflects these findings, promoting healing on the outside through such services as free head shaves for patients who have begun to lose their hair, skin care products, wigs, massages, manicures and pedicures, and relaxation areas. The information gathered has also guided the revision of several internal processes to help streamline the experience for patients and their families.

CONTRIBUTED BY MYRA RICCERI, ALEGENT HEALTH

PUTTING CONCEPTS INTO ACTION

Achieving high patient satisfaction is likely the goal of every hospital. Mission statements from hospitals large and small, urban and rural, for-profit and nonprofit, usually include words such as *caring, compassionate, respect,* and *dignity*—all of which reflect the quality of human interactions. But putting these concepts into practice can be a difficult task. Providing patients with what they want—being valued and respected, having a sense of control, and being provided with opportunities to participate—cannot be achieved solely by implementing programs or policies. Care partner programs, unrestricted visiting hours, and open-chart policies are of little use if they are implemented in an environment that has not addressed the quality of fundamental human interactions.

Personalized Care

The Planetree model has focused extensively on working with hospital staff members by conducting retreats for all hospital employees, to encourage supportive interactions with each patient. This chapter's case study on Stamford Hospital's retreat process underscores the effectiveness of placing staff in the role of the patient in order to sensitize them to the vulnerability and loss of control so often experienced by patients. In addition, some hospitals have tried to identify and define specific behaviors or interactions that are perceived to be beneficial, but many Planetree sites focus on the concept of providing each patient with personalized care. *Personalized care*—that each patient is a unique individual with different preferences and needs—is a vital concept to be reinforced with caregivers. What is appropriate for one patient may be inappropriate for another. One patient may wake up at 5 AM, ready for a bath and breakfast, whereas another patient may routinely stay awake until 3 AM and wish to sleep until noon. Positive interactions require personalizing the care.

Although most of us would endorse the concept of personalization, practical implementation of the concept in the health care setting can be difficult. Standardization rather than personalization has been the rule for decades. Even if there are no written policies, many unwritten perceptions form the dominant organizational culture at many institutions. Patients are weighed at 5 AM. Bed baths are given in the morning. Blood products are usually administered at night. There is typically no medical reason for the timing of these standard hospital procedures. Patients who wish to sleep late can be weighed at the same time each evening so that the information is available when the physicians make rounds in the morning. Bed baths can be given in the evening. Blood products can be administered during the day so that the patient's sleep is not disturbed by frequent checks of vital signs. Common sense is often overridden by corporate culture. "That's not the way we do things here" and "That would inconvenience the medical staff" are frequent refrains when efforts are made to implement change. Organizational transformation helps staff members question every hospital routine, even those held most sacred, so that personalization becomes standard.

Staff Retreats

When Stamford Hospital in Stamford, Connecticut, made the decision in 2004 to implement the Planetree model of care, its motivation to join was three-fold: to reinforce its commitment to patient-centered care, to increase patient satisfaction, and to support a core strategic initiative—transforming the organizational culture.

The first charge given the new Planetree coordinator was to lead staff retreats. An organizational decision was made to embrace patient-centered care by starting at the top. By participating in the retreat process, the leadership team learned a lot about themselves and the patient care experience and reaffirmed their commitment to sharing that passion and knowledge with Stamford Hospital's twenty-four hundred employees. The question posed was how to accomplish this without losing any of the positive momentum that had been generated. An aggressive plan to get all employees to a retreat within eighteen months was put in motion. Even though many perceived this as an overly ambitious and improbable goal, others knew that time was of the essence and that such a high-impact, concerted effort would be the best way to build and sustain the momentum. Patient and employee satisfaction scores told the story of the need to embrace the Planetree philosophy: patient satisfaction was in the bottom quartile, and employee satisfaction was not much better. Consisting of sixteen managers and staff members, the team of retreat facilitators was ready for the challenge.

Early on, a beautiful venue in the next town was selected to hold retreats. A hundred-year-old convent overlooking Long Island Sound proved to be a spiritual oasis for employees. Just being in the space made everyone feel special, relaxed, and at peace.

Everyone was welcomed—skeptics and believers alike; and at times, it was not easy. However, senior management was supportive and kicked off each retreat. Experiential exercises and brainstorming sessions where staff members shared ideas, role-playing, and a three-course lunch were components of the eight-hour day.

Months passed and it got easier. Employees were calling to sign up for a retreat and to join Planetree committees, and some who had attended a retreat asked if they could facilitate. Knowing their opinion counted, that they could affect the culture change, and that senior leadership supported these changes was liberating!

In the midst of this, Stamford Hospital introduced some major image changes, launching a new logo, mission, vision, and values. And for the first time, employees took part in the planning. People talked about living these organizational values and "being Planetree."

Three years later, the results were palpable. Both patient satisfaction and employee satisfaction rose to the top quartile. Encouraged by these results, Stamford Hospital's Planetree journey continues widespread engagement by a hospital community with a shared commitment to improving the patient experience and creating a better work environment for themselves and their peers.

CONTRIBUTED BY DEBORAH FEDELI, STAMFORD HOSPITAL

Patient Advocacy

Another important aspect of personalized care is patient advocacy: What do we do with the information obtained regarding what the patient wants? Who will support patients in obtaining what they perceive they need? Who will be the patient's advocate?

Nurses frequently fill the role of patient advocate but often at a significant price. "Going to bat" for a patient sometimes means challenging the health care system or breaking established rules. In many hospitals, this puts the nurse in an awkward situation. Being a "good" caregiver from the patient's perspective may mean being a troublesome employee from management's perspective. In an organization that supports personalization and patient advocacy, nurses and other caregivers no longer have to bend or break rules to support the needs of patients.

Appreciation and Recognition of Staff

Many books have been written about the need to develop reward-and-recognition programs to acknowledge good work by staff members. Many hospitals have implemented employee-of-the-month programs and annual awards or bonuses. Although all of these have their merit, they may fail to address the underlying culture that in many typical hospitals is focused more on punitive measures than on staff acknowledgment and recognition. In focus groups with the staff, a common refrain is that although reprimands from managers and coworkers are frequent events, appreciation is shown only once a month at official ceremonies. Of particular concern is the growing feeling that hospital employees express about the use of patient satisfaction scores in a punitive manner. Nursing and other staff lament the use of such data to "knock us over the heads" when scores fluctuate downward even a single percentage point.

Organizational transformation, though not a quick fix, can profoundly change a hierarchical, punitive culture into one with an "attitude of gratitude." Reward-and-recognition programs are vital as formal, organizational expressions of appreciation, but they are most effective when integrated into a culture in which the appreciation and acknowledgment of others is expressed freely and frequently and is not a mandated, quantified goal for managers. For example, even though written expressions of gratitude from managers to staff members are laudable, they quickly lose credibility and value when staff members discover that they are measured requirements that their supervisors must attain in order to obtain their annual bonus.

The terms most often used—*reward, recognition,* and *award*—have subtle implications that they originated in a hierarchical environment. Rewards come from the top down. Managers recognize worthy staff members. As hospitals become less hierarchical, such terms as *gratitude, appreciation,* and *acknowledgment* will become more common. Small gestures of appreciation, such as simply saying thank you more often, can become part of a new less-hierarchical culture.

Whereas it is vital that managers and administrators acknowledge employees who best embody the organizational values, it is equally important that coworkers acknowledge one another and that all staff members feel comfortable expressing gratitude to anyone. Departments can thank other departments via notes, gifts, or celebrations. Staff members can express their appreciation not only to coworkers but also to managers, administrators, and physicians. To be effective, this culture change needs to be role-modeled first by every administrator, manager, and supervisor so that it becomes second nature to all employees.

Celebrations of organizational successes, even of small accomplishments, provide wonderful opportunities to recognize the essential role that staff members play in helping the organization succeed. Whenever the hospital or individual departments achieve goals, reach desired benchmarks, or receive media attention, opportunities can be created to honor staff members for their accomplishments. They are not merely doing their jobs; they are doing their jobs exceptionally well.

Massage for the staff is another way that hospitals can express appreciation for the efforts of their caregivers. At several Planetree affiliates, a massage therapist brings a massage chair to a staff lounge so that caregivers can relax and feel nurtured during a break. Some hospitals provide gift certificates to staff members for massages as thank-you gifts to recognize their contribution to the hospital.

These simple human interactions can provide an environment of gratitude in which staff members are frequently reminded that they are valued and that their work is appreciated.

Communication and Participation

Two-way communication (being informed and being heard) is another interaction that contributes to staff satisfaction. When staff members are informed, they are better able to participate in creating a work environment in which they can thrive. A structure needs to be established, however, that solicits their input and encourages their ideas and solutions.

Lack of information leads to rumors and speculation. At focus groups, some employees have complained that their only source of information about the hospital comes from the local newspaper. In the old hierarchical model, staff members were kept uninformed because of the misconception that they didn't need to know, wouldn't be able to understand the information, or might be needlessly upset, particularly if the hospital was experiencing financial difficulties. In reality, staff members are usually quick to perceive problems and are fearful and frustrated when uninformed. Withholding information or—as is more often the case—not making the effort to provide it creates anxiety, mistrust, and an "us-versus-them" environment.

Employee newsletters, e-mail, written communications, and frequent town-hall-style meetings are useful tools for keeping hospital staff informed. Expecting information to pass unimpeded through several levels and still reach the staff is wishful (and hierarchical) thinking. It is not uncommon for administrators to provide information to managers who are in turn expected to pass the information along to the staff. Some managers are effective at relaying the information but many are not. Direct communication is the most reliable. It is also helpful for managers to understand the importance of conveying information.

To be most effective, communication needs to be two-way: staff members want to be kept informed, but they also need an opportunity to be heard. Having a voice in how care is delivered and having opportunities to participate creates an environment in which staff members can be the exceptional caregivers they want to be. It is a misconception that the benefit of staff input is simply to win their support and buy-in. The opinions, ideas, suggestions, and creative solutions of caregivers are tremendous assets in creating a healing environment for patients and an optimum working environment for the staff.

Good leadership is vital in creating an environment that supports staff participation. The hospital's leadership also plays a key role in supporting the transformation of the organization. One of the central roles of leadership is to support and articulate the highest vision of the organization. Focusing on financial success is essential, but if that is the ultimate vision of the organization, it may be difficult to enlist staff members to achieve that goal. Most caregivers did not choose their jobs or professions with the goal of helping an institution's bottom line. Nor do patients choose to come to a hospital for the purpose of enhancing its financial viability. Organizational transformation is only possible when everyone who is part of that organization has a clear vision of the ultimate goal. For the vision to become a reality, staff members must feel valued themselves so that they can communicate a sense of caring to patients.

Understanding of all these dimensions and vicissitudes of relationship and caring is the basis for creating a more integrated model of caring-healing, of *caritas* to *communitas*. The relationship that practitioners form with self, with patient, with community, and with other practitioners is critical and requires balanced attention to transform education and practice as well as practitioners themselves, be they students or skilled clinicians. (Tresolini and Pew-Fetzer Task Force, 1994, p. 37). The Planetree model and its emphasis on putting patients first serves as a moral and spiritual template for transforming the human interactions in health care, which ultimately serves as the core for sustaining caring, all relationships, and humanity itself.

REFERENCES

Berkman, L., Leo-Summers, L., and Horwitz, R. "Emotional Support and Survival After Myocardial Infarction: A Prospective, Population-Based Study of the Elderly." *Annals of Internal Medicine,* 1992, *117*(12), 1003–1009.

Blazer, D. "Social Support and Mortality in an Elderly Community Population." *American Journal of Epidemiology,* 1982, *115*(5), 684–694.

Gilpin, L. "The Importance of Human Interactions." In S. B. Frampton, L. Gilpin, and P. A. Charmel (eds.), *Putting Patients First: Designing and Practicing Patient-Centered Care.* San Francisco: Jossey-Bass, 2003.

Halldorsdottir, S. "Five Basic Modes of Being with Another." In D. A. Gaut and M. Leininger (eds.), *Caring: The Compassionate Healer.* New York: National League for Nursing, 1991.

Kamarck, T., Manuck, S., and Jennings, J. "Social Support Reduces Cardiovascular Reactivity to Psychological Challenge: A Laboratory Model." *Psychosomatic Medicine,* 1990, *52,* 42–58.

Lepore, S., Mata Allen, K., and Evans, G. "Social Support Lowers Cardiovascular Reactivity in an Acute Stressor." *Psychosomatic Medicine,* 1993, *55,* 518–524.

Levinas, E. *Totality and Infinity.* (A. Lingis, trans.) Pittsburgh, Pa.: Duquesne University Press, 1969.

Martin, D., and others. "Randomized Trial of a Patient-Centered Hospital Unit." *Patient Education and Counseling,* 1998, *34*(2), 125–133.

Ornish, D. *Love and Survival.* New York: Harper Perennial, 1998.

Quinn, J., and others. "Research Guidelines for Assessing the Impact of the Healing Relationship in Clinical Nursing." *Alternative Therapies Journal,* 2003, *9*(3), A65–A79.

Reynolds, P., and Kaplan, G. "Social Connections and Risk for Cancer: Prospective Evidence from the Alameda County Study." *Behavioral Medicine,* 1990, *16*(3), 101–110.

Shattell, M. "Eventually It'll Be Over: The Dialectic Between Confinement and Freedom in the Phenomenal World of the Hospitalized Patient." In S. Thomas and H. Pollio (eds.), *Listening to Patients: A Phenomenological Approach to Nursing Research and Practice.* New York: Springer, pp. 214–236, 2002.

Spiegel, D. *Living Beyond Limits.* New York: Fawcett, 1993.

Swanson, K. "What Is Known About Caring in Nursing Science: A Literary Meta-analysis." In A. S. Hinshaw, S. Feetham, and J. Shaver (eds.), *Handbook of Clinical Nursing Research.* Thousand Oaks, Calif.: Sage, 1999, 31–60.

Tresolini, C. P., and Pew-Fetzer Task Force. *Health Professions Education and Relationship-Centered Care.* San Francisco: Pew Health Professions Commission, 1994.

Watson, J. *Nursing: The Philosophy and Science of Caring.* Boston: Little, Brown, 1979.

Watson, J. *Nursing: Human Science and Human Care—A Theory of Nursing.* Boston: Jones & Bartlett, 1985.

Watson, J. *Postmodern Nursing and Beyond.* New York: Elsevier, 1999.

Watson, J. Theory of Human Caring Web site. 2004a. [http://hschealth.uchsc.edu/son/faculty/caring.htm].

Watson, J. "Commentary: Relational Core of Nursing Practice." *Journal of Advanced Nursing,* 2004b, *47*(3), 241–250.

Watson, J. *Caring Science as Sacred Science.* Philadelphia: F. A. Davis, 2005.

Watson, J. Theory of Human Caring Web site. 2007. [http://hschealth.uchsc.edu/son/faculty/caring.htm].

Watson, J. *Nursing: The Philosophy and Science of Caring.* (2nd ed.) Boulder: University Press of Colorado, 2008.

Wiklund, I., and others. "Prognostic Importance of Somatic and Psychosocial Variables After a First Myocardial Infarction." *American Journal of Epidemiology,* 1988, *128*(4), 786–795.

Williams, R., and others. "Prognostic Importance of Social and Economic Resources Among Medically Treated Patients with Angiographically Documented Coronary Artery Disease." *Journal of the American Medical Association,* 1992, *267*(4), 520–524.

CHAPTER

2

ACCESS TO INFORMATION: INFORMING AND EMPOWERING DIVERSE POPULATIONS

CANDACE FORD GRAY AND MICHELE A. SPATZ

This chapter does the following:

- Emphasizes ways in which the Planetree model for education empowers patients to be active participants in their care with information that meets their individual information needs and requests

- Describes why patient education and information are essential to patient safety

- Identifies a number of specialized resources and services in place at patient-centered hospitals that foster an atmosphere conducive to learning and collaboration
- Discusses the essential elements and benefits of an open medical chart policy
- Identifies strategies for assisting patients and their loved ones in navigating information available online
- Discusses ways in which a health resource center can support not only patients' health information needs but also those of the community-at-large

In the late 1970s, the concept of patient-centered care was not yet born. When Planetree founder Angelica Thieriot, along with her family members, experienced three separate hospitalizations, she was completely frustrated by the lack of information about the medical conditions affecting her and her loved ones. It is hard to believe today, but at the time she was hospitalized, hospital libraries were closed to the public, nurses were instructed not to tell patients their vital signs, other medical information was routinely withheld, and of course, the Internet was many years away.

Under Angelica's guidance, access to health and medical information became a founding tenet of Planetree. Information is provided both at the bedside and in the community where patients live. This chapter focuses on Planetree's unique approaches to offering information to patients and health care consumers.

ACCESS TO INFORMATION AT THE BEDSIDE

When people become patients, they generally discover that they need new information in order to live with, manage, or recover from their illness or condition. Some patients may take their health for granted until an unexpected health crisis refocuses their attention. Other patients are well-informed, arriving with computer searches or laptops in hand, ready to discuss the latest treatment options with their physicians. And still others are uninformed and hard to engage in a dialogue about self-care. Family members, vital to providing care for patients at home, may feel unprepared to take on the unexpected role of caregiver. Addressing each patient's cultural and linguistic background presents additional educational challenges. The diverse characteristics of patients and their families often present challenges to health care professionals attempting to provide information and obtain informed consent (Giloth, 1993). Nevertheless, the Institute of Medicine (IOM) lists "access to information" as a primary principle in creating health care for the twenty-first century (Institute of Medicine, 2001).

A Patient-Centered, Patient-Driven Model

Since the opening of its first model unit in 1985, Planetree's goal for health care organizations has been going beyond simply providing quality medical care to creating an environment in which patients and their families are offered the tools, skills, and knowledge they need to be active partners in their care. Illness is seen both as an educational opportunity and an opportunity for personal transformation. Patients are brought together with numerous health professionals, including nurses, physicians, pharmacists, dietitians, librarians, physical therapists, social workers, and chaplains, who are willing to share their knowledge in an environment conducive to learning. The Planetree model for education is both patient-centered and patient-driven, encouraging patients to ask questions and participate in the decision-making process, with the goal of enabling them to direct their own care. The Planetree approach expands the traditional protocol from providing standardized educational resources about a patient's condition to offering information based on the personal interests and requests of the patient. For instance, patients may have questions about lifestyle changes, coping skills, or the illnesses of other family members.

Despite an information-rich society and mandates by The Joint Commission to provide patients with health and medical information, patient focus groups and surveys reveal that many hospital education programs are failing to meet patients' needs and expectations (Gerteis, Edgman-Levitan, Daley, and Delbanco, 1993). Although providing education is a goal of health care facilities, the diversity of patients' educational needs coupled with the severity of their illnesses, tight budgets, and low staffing often causes educational efforts to be minimal or done "on-the-fly." Patient teaching is typically left until the day of discharge when a patient and his or her family may be too distracted to concentrate, overwhelmed by the volume of information and instructions.

Planetree recognizes that knowledgeable patients are more likely to follow the advice of their physicians and that self-care and caregiver skills that have been practiced repeatedly in the hospital setting are more likely to be correctly performed at home. Moreover, because they are in partnership with their health care team, patients are less likely to file lawsuits. Studies show that lack of information and communication in the health care setting prompts some angry patients to sue (Lichtstein, Materson, and Spicer, 1999; Colon, 2002). Similarly, informed patients tend to be more compliant, follow self-care instructions better, and understand when to seek additional counsel about their health concerns (Barrier, 2003).

There is a perception that patient and family education is expensive. Yet the cost of *not* educating patients is staggering. National attention is now focused on the problem of health literacy, defined by *Healthy People 2010* as "the degree to which individuals have the capacity to obtain, process, and understand basic health information and services needed to make appropriate health decisions." The Institute of Medicine, in its landmark report, *A Prescription to End Confusion,* states that "studies have shown that people with low health literacy understand health information less well, get less preventive care—such as screenings for cancer—and use expensive health services such as emergency department care more frequently" (Institute of Medicine, 2004). The economic burden of not meeting the needs of patients with health literacy challenges costs the United States an estimated $106 billion to $236 billion annually, according to a University of Connecticut report (Vernon, 2007).

The Joint Commission white paper *"What Did the Doctor Say? Improving Health Literacy to Protect Patient Safety"* (2007a) asserts that there is a "fundamental right and need for patients to receive information—both orally and written—about their care in a way in which they can understand this information." The white paper goes on to assert, "The safety of patients cannot be assured without mitigating the negative effects of low health literacy."

Engaging patients in their learning needs is part of the recommended strategy to meet national patient safety goals and to reduce the nation's health care costs. The Joint Commission (2007a) advocates such elements as these:

- Adopting disease management practices, including individualized education and multidisciplinary team outreach to patients, which are known to reduce the incidence of error and positively affect health outcomes

- Providing self-management education customized to the learning and language needs of individual patients

"If an individual understands and can act upon medical instructions, unnecessary emergency department visits and hospitalizations can be reduced, which in turn lowers overall healthcare costs," notes Diane Pinakiewicz in *Low Health Literacy: Implications for National Health Policy* (Vernon, 2007). In today's world, it is too costly *not* to educate patients.

Elements of a Patient and Family Education Program

Although health care organizations vary in their implementation of the Planetree model, many have incorporated the following elements into their patient and family education programs.

Educational Relationships. One of the most important aspects of an educational environment is the relationship among the patient, the family, and the professional health care team. Two-way communication is essential with nurses and other staff who are educating and informing as well as asking and listening. Staff members play a vital role in creating an atmosphere conducive to learning throughout the patient's stay. Patients and families often need encouragement from staff to ask questions and seek information. Fear of appearing ignorant or of offending physicians or staff members keeps some patients silent. Creating a positive relationship between staff and patients removes barriers of fear and uncertainty, thus setting the stage for patient learning and collaboration in their care—and meeting the clear communication criteria of *National Patient Safety Goals* (The Joint Commission, 2007b). Goal 13 specifically states that care providers should "encourage patients' active involvement in their own care as a patient safety strategy," and 13A asserts that providers should also "define and communicate the means for patients and their families to report concerns about safety and encourage them to do so" (The Joint Commission, 2007b).

Sometimes, the best teachers are other patients and families, who can share similar experiences about coping with illness. By having a kitchen on the unit, which draws people together, or an arts program, which offers concerts and other events, Planetree hospitals enable patients and families to support one another and exchange information about coping and caregiving.

Open Medical Chart Policy. One of the most valuable educational resources and an integral tool in reaching national patient safety goals is the patient's own medical record. Encouraging patients to read their own chart helps create an environment of trust and openness, often initiating a dialogue between patients and caregivers (Grange, Renvoize, and Pinder, 1998).

At many Planetree hospitals, patients are actively encouraged to read their medical record. The first time patients read their record, nurses review the information with them to answer questions and explain abbreviations. A frequently heard comment from patients after reading the chart is, "My doctor already told me this." The medical record provides reassurance that information is not being withheld and assists with clear communication and keeping caregiver-patient communication channels open.

Many patients who read their medical record read it only once. Others choose to read it daily, reviewing orders and test results. One patient with severe liver damage was able to track improvements in his liver function tests while he was hospitalized and not consuming alcohol. Seeing the evidence that his liver was recovering offered him hope that changing his lifestyle could improve his prognosis. This was the impetus for his requesting information about joining Alcoholics Anonymous.

In addition to reading their chart, some patients choose to document their perspective in the Patient's Progress Notes, which, at their request, becomes a permanent part of the medical record. To protect confidentiality, only the patient has access to his or her own medical record. If the patient would like a family member to have access to the chart, he or she can sign a form, releasing medical information to the designated person.

An open medical record is also a valuable asset in risk management. Patients have prevented numerous errors by noticing that important information, such as allergies, was missing from the record or by pointing out discrepancies in medication orders.

There is also evidence to suggest that an open medical record policy can positively influence overall patient satisfaction. A review of information collected along with HCAHPS data from January 2006 to March 2007 indicated that patients at Griffin Hospital who were told that they could read their medical record were more likely to be "very satisfied" with their overall hospital experience: 87.8 percent of those told of their ability to read their medical records were "very satisfied," compared with 77.1 percent who were not told. Additional data encompassing HCAHPS scores from three other Planetree affiliate hospitals (plus Griffin Hospital) further indicate that patients who are told they can read their medical chart are both more likely to recommend the hospital to others (Figure 2.1) and more likely to give the highest hospital ranking (9 or 10) (Figure 2.2) (Frampton, Horowitz, and Stumpo, forthcoming).

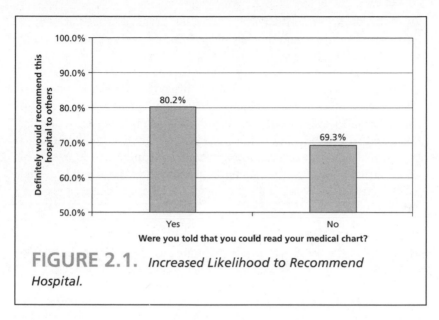

FIGURE 2.1. *Increased Likelihood to Recommend Hospital.*

Note: n = 3504.

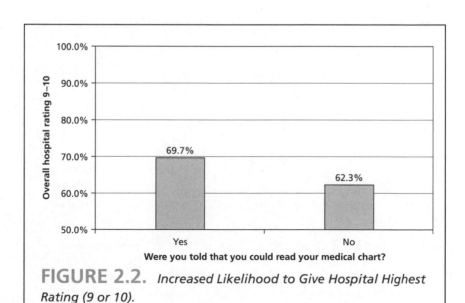

FIGURE 2.2. *Increased Likelihood to Give Hospital Highest Rating (9 or 10).*

Note: n = 3504.

Care Coordination Conference. Care coordination conferences further encourage good communication. This brief meeting, usually scheduled shortly after admission and often lasting no longer than ten minutes, includes the physician, the nurse, the patient, and ideally a member or members of the patient's family. The purpose of the conference is to clarify the goals and expectations of the treatment plan. The expected day of discharge and discharge planning may also be discussed so that educational needs can be anticipated and resources provided. The care coordination conference ensures that all members of the health care team, including the patient and family, are involved in the decisions determining the patient's care and have congruent expectations.

Hourly Rounds. Patient education happens in a variety of ways at the bedside. Hourly rounds lay the foundation for compassionate care and important information exchanges by strengthening the nurse-patient relationship through anticipatory attention to patients' needs. Originating in England, where they are called *patient comfort rounds* (Castledine and others, 2005), hourly rounds follow a recommended protocol. Nurses complete scheduled tasks, such as changing a dressing or giving medications, and "check the three Ps: potty, position and pain" ("Hourly Rounds Keep Call Lights Quiet," 2006). During these tasks, information regarding the patient's condition and education regarding self-care may be shared. Before leaving, the nurse asks the patient if he or she needs anything and reassures the patient of hourly return visits. A multi-hospital study showed that the consistent interaction and strong relationship built by hourly nursing rounds increased patient satisfaction and also significantly reduced patient falls and call light use. Nurses participating in the study reported greater work satisfaction, stating that they had more time to care for patients because call lights came less frequently. They also reported a quieter work environment (Meade and others, 2006). As discussed in the following case study, Hackensack University Medical Center has had an hourly rounding program in place since 2006.

Bedside Report. Bedside report moves the important conversation that nurses have at shift change from a peer-to-peer interaction to an interaction that includes the person at the center of discussion: the patient. The careful communication exchanged during a report is an essential component of good patient care and also a priority benchmark of national patient safety goals. By including the patient in these crucial conversations,

Hourly Rounding

Hackensack University Medical Center (HUMC) in Hackensack, New Jersey, has been working since early 2006 to implement hourly rounding hospital-wide as a means of enhancing the nurse-patient relationship and emphasizing that any nurse-patient interaction is an opportunity for caring and the exchange of information. In the two years since, it has seen promising results linking the practice to improved outcomes.

The outcomes demonstrated on one HUMC specialty unit provide compelling data that reinforce the difference between a nurse "checking" on a patient and a nurse specifically and routinely addressing the patient's pain, potty, and positioning needs (Studer Group, 2008). The results from this unit suggest that the practice makes an impact not only on patient satisfaction but also on a number of clinical metrics. Since the implementation of hourly rounding on the unit, results on patient satisfaction have significantly improved, including the following:

- Results for "likelihood of recommending the hospital" increased to the 92nd percentile nationally by the second quarter of 2007 (when compared with the unit's specialty), up from the 52nd percentile in the first quarter of 2006.
- Scores on the question of "how well patients' pain was controlled" increased to the 90th percentile nationally in the second quarter of 2007, up from the 39th percentile in the first quarter of 2006.
- Scores on the question of "promptness to call bell" increased to the 93rd percentile in the second quarter of 2007, up from the 47th percentile in the second quarter of 2006.
- In addition, the number of incidences of pressure ulcers on the unit was reduced to zero as of the third quarter of 2006.
- Patient falls in the first three quarters of 2007 were down by almost 10 percent.
- When checking the patient perception of care through Discharge Call Manager, 96 percent of patients on the unit indicated they had been seen every two hours or less.

The organization's HCAHPS survey data for the unit further emphasize the value of hourly rounding with scores (capturing patients reporting

FOR EXAMPLE

"always") in several key areas considerably higher for the unit as compared with the entire hospital, including the following:

• Responsiveness of hospital staff: 26 percent higher
• Composite score for communication with nurses: 11 percent higher
• Composite score for pain: 8 percent higher
• Overall rating: 12 percent higher

Note: Data is based on an internal drill down of results from 2007 patients and is not case-mix-adjusted publicly reported information.

These metrics continue to be measured, and their results shared and celebrated to reinforce the importance of hourly rounding, not as one more "to do" item for nurses, but as a truly patient-centered practice that is key to providing quality patient care.

CONTRIBUTED BY DENA MCDONALD AND NINA SETIA,
HACKENSACK UNIVERSITY MEDICAL CENTER

bedside report helps ease patient anxiety by addressing important points of care, concern, and progress. These bedside sessions inform, educate, and ideally empower the patients about their diagnosis or condition (Caruso, 2007).

Sharp Coronado Hospital and Healthcare Center in Coronado, California, implemented nursing report at the patient's bedside in 2005. Their quick and to-the-point report facilitates the smooth transition of nursing staff, letting patients know who their next caregiver is and providing reassurance that incoming staff understand each patient's plan of care. Successes include fewer dry IV bags and infiltrated IV sites and fewer falls. On a more dramatic note, during one change of shift at the bedside, the departing nurse noticed a change in the patient's color and alertness. Upon investigation, they discovered she was in tachycardia. Had there not been nursing report at the bedside, this patient may not have received timely treatment. It is an incident such as this one that clearly illustrates the patient safety value of nursing bedside report.

Patient Pathways. Planetree embraces patient pathways as another tool of patient empowerment and education. A patient pathway provides a roadmap for the care team and the patient to reach a desired destination— the patient's successful discharge and the ability to appropriately manage his or her condition. Patient pathways have been defined as "a patient education tool patterned after a clinical pathway that is used to educate patients about their expected hospital stay and answer frequently asked questions" (Parker, 1999). A patient pathway provides a snapshot of a typical hospital stay and course of treatment for a specific diagnosis, anticipating and allaying the concerns of patients.

Satellite Libraries. Many Planetree hospitals facilitate learning with a unit or satellite library. These smaller libraries, in easily accessible areas, provide a range of educational resources, often focusing on the specific needs of the unit, such as information on cancer or cardiology. Depending on space, they often include books and pamphlets, multimedia, and a computer for online searching. A copier and printer enable patients and families to take information home with them. The resources are diverse and may include inspirational, humorous, and first-person accounts, as patients and family members sometimes benefit more from supportive materials rather than from disease-specific information.

Information Packets. For hospitals with Planetree Health Resource Centers, personalized information packets are offered to patients on any health or medical topic. Health information specialists make patient information rounds or visits to newly admitted patients. During a typical visit, the health information specialist talks with a patient and inquires about any information needs relating to the patient's diagnosis or condition. Through focused interaction, the health information specialist determines the patient's level of understanding and cognitive ability.

After completing patient rounds, the health information specialist returns to the Resource Center and assembles a personalized packet of information, consisting of patient-friendly, trusted materials selected for their ability to answer concerns. Elements of an information packet often include an overview of the diagnosis or condition, treatment information, complementary therapies if requested, nutrition, coping and lifestyle materials (for instance, stress reduction techniques or how to talk with your children), local support groups, and relevant classes. No two patient packets are alike—each packet is tailor-made for an individual with unique skills, needs, and interests. If not delivered to the patient's bedside, they are mailed to the patient's home within forty-eight hours of request.

Outpatient Information Packets. In most health care settings, clinic patients' information needs are often addressed through standard educational materials such as pamphlets and brochures. Planetree Health Resource Centers personalize this service by providing a brief information packet to clinic patients. Prescription-like pads are used by physicians and other clinic care providers to request patient-specific information. Then the completed slip is faxed to the Health Resource Center for fulfillment. At Mid-Columbia Medical Center in The Dalles, Oregon, a pop-up box feature was programmed onto the Next-Gen® electronic medical record, prompting the clinician to request information on the patient's diagnosis or medical condition. Clinicians may request information on a low-cholesterol diet for a patient with hypercholesterolemia, for example, as well as local exercise programs, using the electronic request form. NextGen® then automatically faxes the information request form to the Health Resource Center for fulfillment, and the customized information is mailed to the patient's home.

FOR EXAMPLE

The Personal Health Book

Sentara Virginia Beach General Hospital (SVBGH), which has been implementing the Planetree model for six years, recognizes that providing patient-centered care means considering patient needs, preferences, and expectations and working to ensure that the delivery of care is contingent upon these needs. Realizing that patients today are much more educated, more inquisitive, and more likely to ask why and how, SVBGH introduced the *Personal Health Book* to empower patients through education, reinforce the need for them to take responsibility for their health, and improve communication between caregivers by providing the latest and most accurate medical information.

The *Personal Health Book* is issued exclusively to inpatients who have chronic medical conditions that will result in ongoing treatment. Divided up into sections, including My Diagnosis and Personal Medical History, My Treatment Plan, My Medical Information, My Nutritional Information and Needs, My Exercise Plan and Physical Limitations, My Community Resources, and My Spiritual Resources, the books are given to patients at least twenty-four hours after they are admitted. Families and patients are strongly encouraged to participate in populating the book, which encourages them to ask key questions they need to be aware of, such as, "What is my Digoxin level today?" Patients are instructed to take their book with them to every medical visit, which offers the health care provider an opportunity to get accurate and pertinent information specific to the patient's health status and current treatment plan. It also allows the members of the health care team to have a visual understanding of test results, medications, consult reports, and the like, which are specific to the patient's care, just as it did in the case of one SVBGH patient, a California resident vacationing in the area.

Two days into her vacation, Jane had a cardiac arrest and was brought to SVBGH. She was immediately taken to the Cardiac Catheterization lab, where the interventional cardiologist was able to successfully place a stent in her blocked artery. She was admitted to the Cardiac Coronary Care Unit, and over the next few days she recovered without any complications. Jane had diabetes, and this was managed concurrently with her cardiac condition. She received her *Personal Health Book,* which included all of this pertinent information. Jane and her daughter were both astounded at the detailed yet organized information they received. When the nurse reviewed with her the medication section, Jane cited how easy it was to be able to remember all of the medications she had to take, as they were recorded clearly in her book along with their possible side effects. Two weeks after discharge, SVBGH received a call from Jane, during which she reported how impressed her local doctors were with the dictated history and copies of all the tests that the patient had compiled in her *Personal Health Book,* with her California physician stating, "I didn't need to call the physician because all of my questions were answered in the patient's *Personal Health Book.*"

CONTRIBUTED BY THE PATIENT-CENTERED CARE COMMITTEE OF
SENTARA VIRGINIA BEACH GENERAL HOSPITAL

E-Information. Hospitals are increasingly allowing patients and family members to bring laptops into the hospital during their stay. Many Planetree hospitals, such as Sentara Virginia Beach General Hospital, offer free wireless Internet access to patients and visitors. Pediatric units are adding social networking capabilities so young patients can interact with peers during their hospitalization. Patients and family members are often interested in looking online for additional health information. However, most individuals need assistance in learning how to sort the junk from the gems that would be relevant to their particular medical situation. Guidance in evaluating online health information is a service for which Health Resource Center librarians are ideally suited. However, hospitals and clinics can suggest that patients who are interested in looking for health information begin their search from trusted links provided on the hospital or clinic Web site.

FOR EXAMPLE

Cleveland Clinic's MyChart Program

Lori Izeman felt poorly. Her doctor thought it might be mononucleosis. At twenty-one, she was living away from home for the first time. So she was happy when her parents sent her a surprise—a giant chocolate kiss. Settling down to enjoy the treat, she picked up a magazine and glanced at a health article titled, "Ten Symptoms of Diabetes." In that moment, *Lori's life changed forever . . .*

"Of the ten symptoms listed, I realized I had eight," she says. Ripping the story out of the magazine, she hurried to her doctor, who confirmed that Lori had Type I diabetes, a chronic disease with no known cause and no known cure.

Suddenly, the carefree young woman was immersed in a world of insulin injections, blood glucose monitoring, and a concern for health reaching far beyond that of other people her age. She also learned that even though diabetes is serious, there was no reason why she shouldn't lead a long and happy life. The key was careful health management.

That's where My**Chart** comes in. An online service offered by Cleveland Clinic, My**Chart** gives patients personalized and secure access to their medical records. With My**Chart**, patients can make doctor appointments, view personal health records, get test results, and request prescription renewals.

Today, Lori is the busy mother of four. She uses My**Chart** to manage all her tests, medications, and appointments. Like many people with diabetes, she has multiple medical problems, takes more than one medication, sees more than one specialist, and schedules numerous appointments.

"My**Chart** makes it all very convenient," says Lori. "It gives me timely health checkup reminders—much like the maintenance schedule you get with a new car. I know what I need to do, and when, to maintain my health.

"Thanks to My**Chart**, I can readily access all my medical records released to me by my Cleveland Clinic doctors," she adds. "For someone with Type I diabetes, that's really important—especially since the information is portable. When I was first diagnosed, I was afraid to travel. Now I feel comforted knowing I can show any doctor in any country my health information on My**Chart**."

Lori is also enthusiastic about Cleveland Clinic's Health Information Center, which provides comprehensive write-ups on symptoms and the latest treatments for virtually any disease or condition. One day, she developed an unusual symptom. "I was freaking out because I learned it indicated I had a disease that could attack the joints," she says.

For better information, she accessed Cleveland Clinic's Health Information Center through My**Chart**. "It turned out to be not nearly as scary as I'd thought," she says. "There is so much confusing health information on the Internet, and it's difficult to know what to believe. But you can look up any medical condition in the world on My**Chart** and get information straight from Cleveland Clinic's reliable health information database. It's written in a simple, understandable way."

Contributed by Steve Szilagyi, Cleveland Clinic

ACCESS TO INFORMATION IN THE COMMUNITY

Unlike the situation thirty years ago when Planetree was founded, health care consumers now face a deluge of health information. The sheer volume available (and even pushed at the general public) is overwhelming. Direct-to-consumer (DTC) advertising of prescription drugs (allowed by the FDA since 1997 but still prohibited in Europe) is routine, yet "pharmaceutical websites, and by extension DTC advertising, . . . show little inclination to clearly and completely communicate side effects of drug usage" (Davis, 2007, p. 38). Media headlines focus undue attention on less-significant medical studies, and talk-show marketing of health-related books is endless. The single greatest change in health information availability, however, has come with the Internet.

The Value of Community Health Libraries in the Information Age

Unfortunately, assuming that consumers can educate themselves about their health concerns by using Internet resources overlooks two critical issues: the accessibility and the quality of health information online.

Many lay persons are unable to access health information online. "Information Searches That Solve Problems," a 2007 Pew Internet and American Life Project (PI&ALP) report, found that more than a third of Americans have low access to the Internet: they either do not use the Internet at all or they only have dial-up connections. Unsurprisingly, "the low-access population is older, poorer, and less well-educated than the general population," characteristics of many people who have the potential to benefit most from appropriate health education (Estabrook, Witt, and Rainie, 2007). Even savvy consumers with high-speed access to the Internet are often frustrated by the amount of time it takes to find a site that appropriately addresses their specific concerns.

The quality of online health information is also problematic. According to another PI&ALP report, "Online Health Search 2006," 80 percent of American Internet users have searched for health information. However, most used a general search engine, rather than a recommended health Web site, and only 15 percent always checked the information's source and date (Fox, 2006). Review of the medical literature offers multiple studies that conclude that much of the health information on the Internet is incomplete, inaccurate, misleading, or at a literacy level well above the average health care consumer's reading level.

Planetree Health Resource Centers address these challenges in a number of ways: providing health information in a variety of formats and educational levels; having high-speed Internet stations freely available to patrons; training consumers, one-on-one or in groups, how to research health topics online and then evaluate the results; initiating a discussion about trusted resources when patrons come in with previously obtained printouts; and featuring articles on Web site evaluation in newsletters, near resource center computers, and on their own Web sites.

In addition to providing health information services for patients and community members, library staff also help their hospital affiliate uphold another Planetree tenet: *healthy communities.* By serving on hospital and community boards and committees, Health Resource Center staff offer organizing skills, literature searches, and a valuable nonclinical perspective, which support patient safety initiatives and community health projects. Also, the majority of Planetree-affiliated hospitals are nonprofit and must meet a periodic tax exempt benchmark by proving their true *community benefit.* Funding a health resource center that is free and open to the public helps meet that community benefit standard. For-profit hospital affiliates may also declare appropriate health library education activities as part of their annual Medicare cost reimbursement report.

Nuts and Bolts of Planetree Libraries

Successful Planetree libraries are free, open to the public, and promoted to the entire community as well as to the hospital's patients and families. The scope of health and medical information available is both broad and deep. Coverage of all health promotion topics and medical conditions, with materials that range from easy-to-read to professional and technical literature, is the ideal. Planetree libraries include information on complementary therapies and strive to provide evidence-based resources. *Health* is broadly defined to include physical, emotional, social, and spiritual well-being, so Planetree collections address such diverse topics as parenting teenagers, using "green" cleaning products, and grieving the death of a pet.

Even though the library is designed to be easy to use (often using the unique Planetree Classification Scheme), a medical librarian is always available to help patrons navigate a sizeable print, media, and database collection that is reflective of local languages and health care traditions. Health Resource Center staff field questions that may be straightforward and simple ("My son has mononucleosis. What precautions and self-care tips should we know about?") or challenging ("What are the risks and benefits of a lumbar 5 foraminotomy—lateral, not canal?") After a reference interview, staff helps a patron select materials appropriate to his or her skills and needs. When collections are sufficiently extensive, borrowing is encouraged.

Why Planetree Resource Centers Are Special

The hallmark of Planetree consumer health libraries is the individualized attention that each patron receives. Planetree Health Resource Center staff understand the importance of providing health information tailored to each individual's concerns. Individuals who seek help at Planetree Health Resource Centers vary widely in their literacy levels, educational background, learning styles, English fluency, prior knowledge about their topic, and their level of stress. Furthermore, people often come with unexpressed needs, or even concerns they may not have recognized. For example, someone researching a spouse's Parkinson's disease may only request materials describing the treatment and progression of Parkinson's. The sensitive library professional could subsequently suggest, "Now, what about something for you today?" and then offer resources for coping with caregiver stress.

Planetree Health Resource Centers are designed to provide a warm, welcoming atmosphere—a safe place where people stressed by a health care concern can focus on their learning needs in a calm and supportive environment. It is a place where all visitors can read and seek understanding at their own pace and gain perspective on their personal situation. Staff and volunteers provide information in a caring and nonjudgmental manner. "You were so kind to my mother and me" is a typical patron comment. Visitors may spontaneously offer one another suggestions and encouragement in the resource center.

Exploring the Various Models

The Planetree model for health libraries and resource centers can be adapted to fit the needs of the sponsoring hospital. Two successful models are (1) a combined library for both consumers and professionals in a hospital setting and (2) a stand-alone, community-based library. In some cases, forging partnerships with the community's public library makes the most sense. Planetree affiliate West Park Hospital in Cody, Wyoming, is raising funds and committing resources for a specialized health and medical collection in the county's newly expanded public library.

Whatever the model, Planetree recommends that resource centers and libraries employ a master's prepared librarian to direct the services and manage the collection of resources. In graduate school, librarians are trained in collection development policies and activities, which contribute to a resource center that is vibrant and inclusive and meets the needs of diverse users. Once resources are obtained, another vital, but often overlooked, professional skill is required: the ability to organize—catalogue—a collection in a way that maximizes its usefulness.

Perhaps the most important skill a professional librarian brings is expert communication skills in conducting the *reference interview*—helping visitors sort out and articulate the information needed to cope with, manage, or make decisions regarding their own health or the health of a loved one. Just as in a public library, a professional librarian in the medical setting has the skill set needed to respond to complex reference questions using current, authoritative sources. Librarians also educate visitors, empowering them to locate reliable information and thus helping them increase their self-sufficiency.

Medical librarians are vital in the recruitment, training, and retention of appropriate library volunteers, who can assist professional staff and the public. It is important to note that the concepts of information, advice, and advocacy are related. Librarians provide health and medical information and encourage patrons to advocate for their own health care, but they do not give advice. Those subtle yet critical differences are sometimes lost on well-intentioned volunteers.

Promotion and Outreach

People who know the services of a health library value them immensely. Yet, because the need for health and medical information often arises unexpectedly, and the use of a health library may be only episodic, promoting health resource center services requires an ongoing, multifaceted campaign. "Why didn't I know about you before?" is commonly heard when an individual in need discovers the library.

As is typical of marketing successes, most clients hear about health resource center services through word of mouth. "My mother (neighbor, friend, colleague) told me how much help you can get here." Encourage satisfied clients as they leave to help spread the word; they'll be pleased to be an ambassador. Building relationships with public librarian colleagues is vital because people from all cultural, educational, and language backgrounds regard their neighborhood library as a primary source of information. Make sure public librarians have a referral device at hand to give to their patrons with unmet health information needs.

Relationships with pharmacists, nurses, and other health care colleagues will foster champions, who will regularly refer their patients. Every community has many health and service groups that need to know of services for their clients. Planetree librarians regularly make presentations at meetings of community organizations, linking library services to community vitality. The Planetree Health Library in San Jose, California, hosts meetings of book clubs, support groups, and women's service groups, which introduce the collection and services to brand-new people who might otherwise be unaware of the library.

The people who most need assistance in understanding medical conditions are often the hardest to reach. Delivery of effective health information services to persons whose first language is not English, to older adults isolated by lack of mobility, or to those who struggle with basic literacy requires special strategies. Health resource centers partner with groups whose primary mission is serving vulnerable populations (mobile health vans, Meals on Wheels, public health departments, literacy programs, and health ministries) with a customized health-information-by-mail service.

Many people are unfamiliar or uncomfortable with medicine. The hospital and health care system are foreign to them. Resource centers help people make sense of and negotiate a world that can be confusing, cold, and quick. People can take a deep breath in a Planetree library, and those who have visited one are grateful for the help they received, according to on-site surveys. In a community survey that Mid-Columbia Medical Center performed to identify its most valued community programs, the Planetree Health Resource Center ranked first.

FOR EXAMPLE

Mini-Med School

Today's health consumer is bombarded with reports about the latest medical breakthroughs, promises about how technology will transform patient treatments, and direct-to-consumer promotions for medications and other medical products. With so much information available, it is no wonder that patients have difficulty navigating the road to patient empowerment. In response to this phenomenon, Griffin Hospital offered its first Mini-Med School program in fall 2006.

The essence of the Mini-Med School Program is to bring physicians and the community together in a way that fosters education and understanding. The free program consists of a series of ten consecutive Thursday evening sessions (offered in both the spring and the fall), designed for a general audience ranging from adolescents interested in pursuing health care careers to senior citizens seeking information on how to live longer, healthier lives. Each two and a half hour session is divided into two presentations, with a break for refreshments in between. Physician presentations all follow a common PowerPoint template, and copies of the presentations, which participants can keep in the three-ring binder provided at the first session, are distributed each week for note taking.

In addition to getting a basic understanding of human anatomy and the pathology of various diseases, participants also learn about strategies for disease prevention. Physician presenters stress a number of common themes, such as the harmful effects of smoking, the importance of regular health screenings, and the impact of lifestyle choices on overall health. An excellent means of engaging the hospital's physicians, the Mini-Med School provides each presenter an opportunity to share his or her area of expertise and interact with participants during the Q&A session that concludes each presentation.

The culmination of the program is a "graduation," at which participants who attended 70 percent or more of the sessions receive diplomas and T-shirts, as well as other fun prizes, to recognize their commitment to the program. Underwriting support is provided by several pharmaceutical companies and medical device manufacturers, which helps defray the cost of these items, as well as copying, refreshments, and other ancillary costs. Physicians volunteer their time to the program.

Both the individual sessions and the overall program have received consistently positive reviews from the more than 250 "Mini-Med Students" who have participated to date. The ongoing community interest and demand is evidenced by the fact that the inaugural session had more than 150 people on the waiting list due to meeting space limitations, and each subsequent session has been filled to capacity.

The health empowerment benefits for Mini-Med School participants are clear, but the hospital and its physicians also benefit from the goodwill the program engenders in the community, as well as opportunities for exposure to a large number of potential new patients. To date, about a third of participants have never been to the hospital, and nearly half have traveled from outside the hospital's primary service area to attend. With word of mouth such a powerful factor in health care decision making, the Mini-Med School has become an important part of both the hospital's health empowerment and its marketing imperatives.

CONTRIBUTED BY TODD LIU AND KEN ROBERTS, GRIFFIN HOSPITAL

CONCLUSION

Access to information is a core Planetree principle—one deeply rooted in its history. From open charts and bedside shift changes to health resource centers, patient-centered hospitals continually strive to recognize and meet the information needs of diverse patients in a variety of meaningful ways. The wider world of health care now understands what Angelica Thieriot knew all along—that information is not just a nicety. Vital for patient safety, it relieves patient anxiety and fosters care partnerships between patients and health care professionals. The core component of empowering patients and health care consumers through information and education remains at the heart of Planetree patient-centered care.

REFERENCES

Barrier, P. A. "Two Words to Improve Physician-Patient Communication: What Else?" *Mayo Clinic Proceedings,* 2003, *78*(2), 211–214.

Caruso, E. M. "The Evolution of Nurse-to-Nurse Bedside Report on a Medical-Surgical Cardiology Unit." *Medical Surgical Nursing,* 2007, *16*(1), 17–22.

Castledine, G., and others. "Clinical Nursing Rounds, Part 3: Patient Comfort Rounds." *British Journal of Nursing,* 2005, *14*(17), 928–930.

Colon, V. F. "Ten Ways to Reduce Medical Malpractice Exposure." *The Physician Executive,* 2002, *28*(2), 16–18.

Davis, J. "Pharmaceutical Websites and the Communication of Risk Information." *Journal of Health Communication,* Jan.–Feb. 2007, *12*(1), 29–39.

Estabrook, L., Witt, E., and Rainie, L. "Information Searches That Solve Problems: How People Use the Internet, Libraries, and Government Agencies When They Need Help." Washington, D.C.: Pew Internet and American Life Project, 2007. Accessed Jan. 15, 2008, from [www.pewinternet.org/pdfs/Pew_UI_LibrariesReport.pdf].

Fox, S. "Online Health Search 2006." Washington, D.C.: Pew Internet and American Life Project, 2006. Accessed Dec. 17, 2007, from [www.pewinternet.org/PPF/r/190/report_display.asp].

Frampton, S., Horowitz, S., and Stumpo, B. "Open Medical Records." *American Journal of Nursing,* forthcoming.

Gerteis, M., Edgman-Levitan, S., Daley, J., and Delbanco, T. (eds.). *Through the Patient's Eyes: Understanding and Promoting Patient-Centered Care.* San Francisco: Jossey-Bass, 1993.

Giloth, B. (ed.). *Managing Hospital-Based Patient Education.* Chicago: American Hospital Association, 1993.

Grange, A., Renvoize, E., and Pinder, J. "Patients' Rights to Access Their Healthcare Records." *Nursing Standard,* 1998, *13*(6), 41–42.

Healthy People 2010. Section 11: Health Communication. Washington, D.C.: Office of Disease Prevention and Health Promotion, U.S. Department of Health and Human Services.

Accessed Dec. 17, 2007, from [www.healthypeople.gov/document/html/volume1/11HealthCom.htm].

"Hourly Rounds Keep Call Lights Quiet." *Nursing,* 2006, *36*(2), 33.

Institute of Medicine, Committee on Quality of Health Care in America. *Crossing the Quality Chasm: A New Health System for the Twenty-First Century.* Washington, D.C.: National Academies Press, 2001.

Institute of Medicine. *Health Literacy: A Prescription to End Confusion.* IOM Report Brief. Washington D.C: Institute of Medicine, Apr. 2004. Accessed Dec. 17, 2007, from [http://www.iom.edu/?id=21119].

(The) Joint Commission. *What Did the Doctor Say? Improving Health Literacy to Protect Patient Safety.* Chicago: The Joint Commission, Feb. 2007a. Accessed Dec. 17, 2007, [www.jointcommission.org/Public Policy/health_literacy.htm].

(The) Joint Commission. *National Patient Safety Goals.* Chicago: The Joint Commission. 2007b. Accessed Dec. 17, 2007, from [www.jointcommission.org/PatientSafety/National-PatientSafetyGoals/08_dsc_npsgs.htm].

Lichtstein, D., Materson, B., and Spicer, D. "Reducing the Risk of Malpractice Claims." *Hospital Practice,* 1999, *34*(7), 69–72, 75–76, 79.

Meade, C. M., and others. "Effects of Nursing Rounds on Patients' Call Light Use, Satisfaction, and Safety." *American Journal of Nursing,* 2006, *106*(9), 58–70.

Parker, C. "Patient Pathways as a Tool for Empowering Patients." *Nursing Case Management,* 1999, *4*(2), 77–79.

Studer Group. "Hourly Rounding: Lessons Learned." *Hardwired Results,* 2008, (9), 9.

Vernon, J. A., and others. *Low Health Literacy: Implications for National Health Policy.* North Adams, Mass.: Partnership for Clear Health Communication, National Patient Safety Foundation. Accessed Dec. 17, 2007, from [www.npsf.org/askme3/pdfs/Case_Report_10_07.pdf].

CHAPTER

3

HEALING PARTNERSHIPS: THE IMPORTANCE OF INVOLVING PATIENTS, FAMILIES, AND VOLUNTEERS

ALEXANDRA HARRISON, GAIL MACKEAN, AND MARGARET CULLIVAN

Note: We are pleased to acknowledge the contribution of Joanne Ganton of the Calgary Health Region and Beverley Johnson, CEO of the Institute for Family-Centered Care, for their review of the chapter and helpful suggestions.

This chapter does the following:

■ Identifies core elements for developing partnerships between patients, families, and health care providers

■ Highlights specific patient-centered practices that engage families as active participants in patient care, including care partner programs, family presence protocols, self-management programs, and patient-directed visitation

■ Discusses strategies for integrating the patient-client and family voice into organizational planning, decision making, and quality improvement

■ Identifies opportunities for volunteer involvement in advancing a patient-centered approach to care

INTRODUCTION—THE IMPORTANCE OF PARTNERSHIPS

Health care involves people caring for others in a privileged relationship with those who are served. Most individuals are part of a social network that is vital to maintaining their physical and mental health. It is the family, as defined by the patient, who provides most of the care needed when the patient is in the community. With the increase in chronic diseases, hospitalization is becoming only one aspect of an ongoing experience of care. Including the expertise of the patient and the patient's family in the acute care environment is becoming increasingly important—for both the patient and the care providers. This chapter describes and discusses opportunities for healing partnerships between health care providers, volunteers, patients, and their families. These partnerships take place at multiple levels, ranging from providing individual patient care to setting the strategic priorities for the health care organization. Such partnerships are critical to the development of high-quality, safe patient care; a better health care experience for patients and their loved ones; and a more rewarding work experience for health professionals, hospital workers, and volunteers. This chapter highlights some promising practices that serve as a reference point for looking toward a bright vision for the future.

Partners in Care

There are many definitions and descriptions of patient- and family-centered care. Central to most definitions is the development of true collaborative relationships or partnerships between patients, families, and health care providers. Core principles (MacKean, Thurston, and Scott, 2005) include the following:

■ Placing patients and their family at the center of every care decision

■ Providing care that is focused on the person as an individual, in the context of family and community, rather than on the disease

■ Considering patients and their families as the experts on their own needs and values

■ Enabling patients and their families to be active participants in the decision making around their own (or their family member's) care

■ Developing a truly collaborative relationship between health professionals and patients and their families that is based on mutual respect

Partnership is about working together to achieve something that would be impossible to do on your own, and it is characterized by the following:

■ Identification of a common goal to work toward and a joint evaluation of progress

■ Mutual respect about what each partner brings to the partnership

■ Open and honest communication and two-way sharing of information

■ Shared planning and decision making

■ Ongoing negotiation about the role that each partner can and wants to play over time (Jeppson and Thomas, 1997; MacKean, Thurston, and Scott, 2005; Thompson, 2007)

Considering these characteristics of a true partnership, it is clear that optimal levels of involvement for patients should not be determined by professionals, and the emphasis must be on rights rather than on obligations (MacKean, Thurston, and Scott, 2005; Thompson, 2007). Determining the optimal level of patient involvement means open and honest communication and ongoing negotiation, as this statement from a health care professional illustrates:

I learned about asking patients what was important to them rather than telling them what was important to me. And I learned that when

people and families come to us, we cannot separate their physical bodies from their emotional and social worlds. More than anything else, I learned that all of us who work in health care should recall the platinum rule "Do unto others as they want you to do" [Crocker and Johnson, 2006, p. 145].

Patient and family involvement is a complex, multifaceted, and dynamic concept, which evolves in the context of a true partnership. The extent to which a particular patient or a patient's family member wishes to be involved and the role they play depend on the specific circumstances and often change over time (Thompson, 2007). Viewing healing partnerships as central to quality patient care and positive health care experiences represents a shift in thinking. Health care providers are no longer on a pedestal, viewed as the keepers of all knowledge. Rather, multiple types of expertise are acknowledged and valued. This is particularly evident as patients live longer with a chronic condition and their expertise and their confidence in managing their condition grows. This approach is asking a great deal from health care providers, however, in that they need to learn how to coach as well as how to "do" (Harrison and Verhoef, 2002). The advantage is that healing becomes a shared journey, with mutual support, which can be infinitely more rewarding for everyone.

The Importance of Family as Partners

According to Dr. Richard Antonelli, University of Connecticut School of Medicine, "Respecting families as partners is fundamentally important. It starts with your heart. I can honestly say that families have been some of my most influential teachers in the twenty five years I have been in medicine. . . . Families must be thought of as full partners in advising on matters of quality, compassion, and cultural effectiveness" (Crocker and Johnson, 2006, p. 159).

Considerable evidence collected over the past twenty years has increased our understanding of what patients want and value from the health care system. Involvement of families and friends is something that patients have repeatedly identified as important. In the book *Through the Patient's Eyes* (Gerteis, Edgman-Levitan, Daley, and Delbanco, 1993), the authors remind us that patients often depend on their family to advocate for them, want their family with them to provide comfort and emotional support, and need and want their family to be involved in their care and decision making related to their care.

Research indicates that patients prefer having family members involved in their care more often than actually occurs in practice (Botelho, Lue, and Fiscella, 1996; Gerteis, Edgman-Levitan, Daley, and Delbanco, 1993; Rotman-Pikielny and others, 2007), and that families want the same things as patients do: information, respect, and emotional support (Vom Eigen and others, 1999; MacKean, Thurston, and Scott, 2005). The family often has considerable expertise about the patient. It is important that they understand what is going on and that they be purposely involved, as they are often providing care and support for the patient at home.

Increasingly, it is being recognized as good practice to have patients choose who they want involved during their hospital stay, including who should have access to their medical records. Respecting the *patient's* definition of family should be incorporated into any written policies or guidelines on family presence and participation. In his book *No Need to Trouble the Heart,* Patrick Conlon tells his story of caring for the man he loves through an acute life-threatening illness, requiring a prolonged hospital stay. In this passage, Conlon describes his efforts to level out some of the power imbalance inherent in our health care culture and the kind of expertise that families bring:

> *Truth is, I refused to be anyone's subordinate through this crisis, an early decision. The ride was hard enough. Nor did I want to pretend to know any more than I did about his clinical condition. They knew the illness, yes, but I knew Jim. I could reach back through thirty years for all the personal stuff, the foibles, behaviours and patterns, and might help complete him for them [Conlon, 2006, p. 85].*

The Benefits of Partnerships

Since the 1950s and 1960s, research has shown the negative effects of restrictive visiting policies on hospitalized children and their families (Ahmann, Abraham, and Johnson, 2003). There is a growing body of evidence that suggests people in hospitals, not only children, benefit from having their families with them and involved in their care. Some positive outcomes, identified to date in the published literature, are summarized in Table 3.1.

TABLE 3.1. **Benefits of Involving Patients and Families.**

	Benefits identified in the literature
Patients and families	• More knowledgeable and competent patients and families (American Academy of Pediatrics Policy Statement, 2003)
	• Better health care experience or improved patient/family satisfaction (Rotman-Pikielny and others, 2007; American Academy of Pediatrics Policy Statement, 2003)
	• Less anxiety or stress (American Academy of Pediatrics Policy Statement, 2003)
	• Improved patient outcomes, both physiological and functional (Wetzels and others, 2007)
	• Improved growth of very low birth weight infants (Johnston and others, 2006)
	• Less pain medication necessary for children (American Academy of Pediatrics Policy Statement, 2003)
	• Improved emotional health for patients and families (Sloper,1999; King, Law, King, and Rosenbaum, 1998; Dunst and Trivette, 1996; Ahmann, 1998)
	• Improved family outcomes
	• Decreased stress (Bru and others, 1993; Tuller and others, 1997)
	• Improved mental health (American Academy of Pediatrics Policy Statement, 2003)

Health care providers

- Improved satisfaction with quality of work life for health care providers (American Academy of Pediatrics Policy Statement, 2003)

- Increased patient and family adherence to treatment plans (King, King, and Rosenbaum, 1996; MacKean, Thurston, and Scot;, 2005)

- New learning for residents and students (Muething and Kotagal, 2007)

- More knowledgeable and empowered patients and families (American Academy of Pediatrics Policy Statement, 2003)

Health care organizations

- Improved quality of care
- Safer health care environments (Rose, 2005)
- Decreased patient/family complaints and litigation (American Academy of Pediatrics Policy Statement, 2003)
- Better management of chronic diseases (Lorig, 2003)
- Decreased length of stay (American Academy of Pediatrics Policy Statement, 2003; Johnston and others, 2006)

Changing the Concept of Families as Visitors

Planetree encourages the development of open visitation policies. Many patient-centered hospitals have relaxed their visiting policies, and others have eliminated visiting restrictions completely. The goal is to have families present and embraced as participants on the health care team. In the future, it is likely that the term *visitors* will no longer be used to describe patients' families. As we work toward this, many hospitals are starting by changing their views about visitors. Examples of this philosophy are summarized in Table 3.2.

A nurse manager of an intensive care unit in the Calgary Health Region shared this story about how she came to change her view of patients and families as visitors in the hospital. Her brother experienced a long illness and a prolonged hospital stay. Just before her brother's death, he indicated the hospital staff he most appreciated were "the housekeeping staff." Her brother explained that they routinely knocked

TABLE 3.2. Examples of Visiting Guidelines and Policies.

Hospital	Visiting Guideline or Policy
Sharp Coronado Hospital and Healthcare Center in California	"Visitors are welcome at any time of the day or night according to the needs and desires of the patient."
Griffin Hospital in Connecticut	"Patient visiting is allowed at any time unless there are medical reasons preventing it."
Alberta Children's Hospital, Calgary Health Region	"Parents/caregivers can visit their children anytime. You play a key role in your child's health and happiness while (s)he is in the hospital. We encourage you to visit your child as often as possible and to take an active part in his or her care."
Bayhealth Medical Center in Delaware	"It is our belief that the family plays a significant and positive force in the progress and recovery of patients. In order to facilitate this support for patients, families are welcome to visit at any time."

before entering his room, introduced themselves, and treated him with dignity and respect. In short, they behaved as if they were coming as guests into his home. In wrapping up her story, this ICU manager said, "For many patients and families, this [hospital unit] becomes their home for whatever period of time; we do go home at the end of the day and they do not. And yet we have this belief that the patient room is ours; we treat them like the visitor. . . . If we shifted our perspective and when entering the patient's room, viewed ourselves as visitors, we would demonstrate our respect for the patient as a person and for their privacy. This represents a philosophical shift."

Patients and Families are Members of the Care Team

Spectrum Health, in Grand Rapids, Michigan, provides a full continuum of care through its seven hospitals and more than 140 service sites and has garnered more than fifty national quality awards in the past ten years. Much of the organization's success is attributed to its focus on all aspects of the patient's experience—quality, safety, patient satisfaction, and efficiency. Using a patient-centric approach to enhance the care experience was a founding principle in establishing the Center for Exceptional Experiences, which has a small staff, dedicated to supporting patient-centered changes.

A basic tenet of Spectrum Health's patient-centric philosophy is that the family, along with the patient, is an essential component of the care team. To bring about the cultural change needed to help make this a reality, the Center for Exceptional Experiences engaged a multidisciplinary team of employees in designing a new patient experience. They were asked to look at care "through the eyes of the patients."

The result is a holistic approach that begins in admitting. Patients are asked about their expectations and concerns. They are asked about family—who is family to them, from relatives to friends to neighbors. What are the family's expectations? What else should the hospital know? This is encapsulated in a portion of the electronic health record specifically created so that there is one source for all providers for this information. Does a father work a second shift and need after-hours access? Are there other family stressors that we need to know about to help us deliver better care? Conversations like these are initiated in the earliest patient encounter and continue throughout the patient's stay.

FOR EXAMPLE

An organization-wide Family Presence Team was created to identify strategies for providing support to families so they can come and go as needed—day or night. In addition to helping family members feel comfortable, the team also considers everyone's privacy, security, and safety. Measures for achieving these ends include escorting family members to patients' rooms when they are called back to the hospital at night, and asking visitors who are in the hospital after 9 P.M. to wear badges to clearly identify them. Such measures ensure security for patients, families, and staff.

Encouraging family presence when the patient is not in a private room presents challenges that are dealt with by conversations with staff and the other patients in the room to negotiate a solution that works for everyone involved.

The fourteen-member Patient and Family Advisory Council guides the Spectrum Health program in its continuous improvement journey. The result is a growing national reputation for patient-centric excellence and innovation.

CONTRIBUTED BY KRIS WHITE, SPECTRUM HEALTH

Family Presence

Although there is still a gap between how much families would prefer to be involved and how much they are allowed to be involved (McGahey-Oakland, Lieder, Young, and Jefferson, 2007)—particularly in acute care settings—recent health care literature illustrates that this gap is narrowing. Increasingly, family presence is being described as current practice. This trend is most notable in child health care settings (Fulbrook, Latour, and Albarran, 2007), but it is also being frequently described in some adult health care settings. For example, family presence during resuscitation and other invasive procedures is becoming increasingly accepted by health care professionals as common practice in critical care and emergency departments (Davidson and others, 2007; Duran and others, 2007; Gold, Gorenflo, Schwenk, and Bratton, 2006; Halm, 2005; MacLean and others, 2003; Farah, Thomas, and Shaw, 2007). There is increasing acknowledgment that patients need access to the people they love, but tension still exists around the question of when families should be asked to leave and about the kinds of roles that they are "allowed" to play.

A guiding principle for all hospital policies should be never to separate family from the patient—unless the patient requests it. Rather than allowing family members to be present as an exception to the rules, excluding family members should be the exception. When patients are very ill, or for other reasons are unable to be involved in their own care and the decision making around their care, family members are likely to be increasingly involved. This requires a significant shift in thinking for many acute care environments, where providers bring highly specialized expertise to the patient encounter. A key aspect of this is listening to patients and family members.

A family member who has been with a hospitalized patient for the previous hours or days may be the first to notice a change in the patient's condition. Ignoring these concerns can be dangerous or even catastrophic, as described by John Lewis in his poignant account of his daughter's death (Hicock and Lewis, 2004). Recognizing the important role that family members can play in increasing the safety of health care, in some hospitals family members are able to call the rapid response team. The Sentara Williamsburg Regional Medical Center has such an initiative, the Family Initiated Rapid Response Safety Team (FIRRST). The FIRRST response team is an inpatient rapid response program designed to attend immediately to patients and families. Other hospitals have introduced a similar option for families to summon assistance with "Code H" or "Code Help." The importance of involving the patient and family as a means to improve patient safety is discussed in more depth in Chapter Thirteen.

Although health care professionals may initially be cautious about allowing families to witness resuscitation, many of the reasons identified for not allowing this practice, such as concerns that family members will interfere or will create increased stress for staff or medicolegal concerns, have been disproved (Nigrovic, McQueen, and Neuman, 2007; Tsai, 2002). In fact, a number of professional associations are in favor of offering families the option of being present during invasive procedures or resuscitation (Tsai, 2002) and recommend that a protocol be in place so that the family members are supported. The February 2007 clinical practice guidelines from the Society of Critical Care Medicine include endorsement of a shared decision-making model; early and repeated care conferencing; family presence at both rounds and resuscitation, open visiting, and family support before, during, and after death.

Other promising practices in enabling patient and family involvement include conducting rounds and nurse shift changes in the patient's room with patients and families; inviting family presence during induction and post-anesthesia care, as well as during invasive procedures and resuscitations; and encouraging patients and families to read and contribute to the patient's medical record. Facilitating patients' access to their medical record is discussed in more detail in Chapter Two.

Patients and Families as Partners in Health

In their 2001 article Dr. Tom Delbanco and colleagues challenge us to consider how we can put the philosophy of "nothing about me without me" into practice in our health care facilities. If we see patients and their families as part of health care teams, then it follows that we should be trying to include them in the process, to the extent that they wish to be included. At the very least, we should not exclude them. The following section highlights some promising practices for involving patients and their families across North America and internationally.

Chronic Diseases. Chronic diseases deserve special mention in a chapter on partnerships for a number of reasons: the burden of illness that chronic diseases impose on individuals and health systems, the expertise that patients and families develop as they deal with these diseases, and the improvement in health outcomes that follow from really engaging patients and families in care.

Chronic diseases are the leading cause of death in the United States and Canada, and it is estimated that about half the population is living with one chronic disease and a quarter are living with two or more (National Center for Chronic Disease Prevention and Health Promotion, 2008; Public Health Agency of Canada, 2008), meaning that large amounts of health care are taking place in the community.

When requiring inpatient or outpatient hospital services, most people want to continue to have some form of involvement if they are able. Many patients also appreciate having people they love with them and involved in their care. Optimally, this transition between community and hospital should feel smooth. Otherwise we risk giving confusing messages to patients and families, akin to Arthur Kleinman's description in his well-known book *The Illness Narratives: Suffering, Healing, and the Human Condition* (1988). In one passage, Kleinman describes the conflicting demands frequently placed on these individuals by health professionals. "First, be independent, not passive and dependent, and be active in your care; but when you have a serious exacerbation, place yourself submissively in our hands, and we will blame you for what you did or failed to do to worsen your disorder" (p. 170).

Efforts to support people in the community in managing chronic illness and to involve them while they are in the hospital are worth the investment. There is ample and growing evidence of the effectiveness of self-management education, designed to provide patients with the knowledge and skills they require to live an active and meaningful life with their chronic condition. Lorig (2003) emphasizes that effective, evidence-based self-management must begin with a partnership that incorporates the views of patients and health professionals into the content of a self-management program. Effective self-management programs complement traditional patient education programs, which offer information and technical skills (Bodenheimer, Lorig, Holman, and Grumbach, 2002) and enhance patients' confidence to manage their lives while living with a chronic disease. Peer-led classes on living with a chronic illness, such as the Calgary Health Region's Row Your Own Boat program, are increasingly recognized as a critical component of effective self-management programs. This is another example of partnering with patients and families to improve outcomes. The importance of support from health professionals, friends, family, and the community is emphasized (Lorig, 2003).

The Planetree Care Partner Program. Many Planetree hospitals have implemented a highly successful program called Care Partners (Edgman-Levitan, 2003). It is an effective strategy for supporting family and friends to be involved in caring for a loved one in the hospital. The Care Partner is a family member, friend, or volunteer selected by the patient to participate at various times in educational, physical, psychological, and spiritual support of the patient. Perhaps the most meaningful part of the program is that care partners are encouraged to be active participants in the care process. They are advised to speak up with questions, especially if something does not seem right, such as unexpected tests or procedures, unexplained medications, or adverse reactions. Good Samaritan Hospital in Nebraska has such a program in place.

FOR EXAMPLE

Care Partner Program

The purpose of the Care Partner Program at Good Samaritan Health System in Kearney, Nebraska, is to enhance the quality of patient care by involving a loved one who has been selected by the patient to participate in providing care while the patient is in the hospital. The level of Care Partner involvement is specific to the particular patient's needs and is flexible enough to accommodate the interests and abilities of the individual Care Partner, who may be a family member, a friend, or even a volunteer. Among the responsibilities that the Care Partner may assume are assisting with meals, baths, massage, and nail care; making simple dressing changes; assisting with walking or wheelchair trips; and managing the patient's comfort.

Care Partners Are Welcome program materials are on display in gathering areas and are distributed to patients upon admission—letting them and their loved ones know of their option to participate in the program. After a request from the patient, a nurse explains the program in more depth and provides the Care Partner with a badge to wear for identification. In addition to alerting staff to the loved one's involvement in the patient's care, the badge also entitles the Care Partner to discounts at the gift shop and cafeteria. The Care Partner is given a tour of the unit and provided with a journal in which to enter patient notes. Journal entries are then read by nurses at the beginning of each shift, along with a review of activities that the Care Partner will be participating in, and any education that may be required.

Involving loved ones to this extent in patient care was not a change that came about effortlessly. The Family Care Team that initiated the program at Good Samaritan was met with resistance from hospital staff who were concerned about the time demands of orienting Care Partners and from physicians who questioned what the program would mean for patient outcomes.

Experience, though, has demonstrated that these initial concerns were unfounded. In fact, the program has been a time-saver for staff. Call light requests formerly directed to nursing staff are now handled by the Care Partner, who can easily respond to the patient's requests for a blanket, water, or food. Rather than numerous loved ones calling the nurse or physician for an update on the patient's status, these inquiries are now directed to the Care Partner. The program has also been advantageous in preparing patients for discharge, because the Care Partner is informed about what care the patient will require at home. Since the program's launch, not one physician has expressed any concerns.

Approximately 20 percent of Good Samaritan Hospital's inpatients have participated in the Care Partner Program. In the four years since the program's introduction, measures of overall inpatient satisfaction have steadily increased, with notable gains in areas specifically affected by the program, including ratings of discharge instructions, responsiveness, and how well caregivers worked together as a team (see Figure 3.1). These quantitative data are substantiated by comments from participants on program evaluations, such as "we feel very prepared to care for our loved one at home" and "it was a comfort to us all to participate in this program."

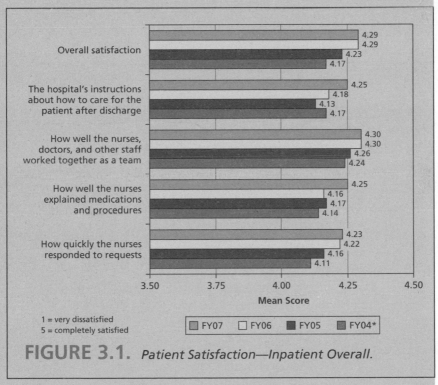

FIGURE 3.1. *Patient Satisfaction—Inpatient Overall.*

*The Care Partner Program was implemented in FY04.

CONTRIBUTED BY KATHLEEN SCHMITT, GOOD SAMARITAN HOSPITAL

Ways to Involve Patients and Families. As described in Chapter Two, the care conference brings together the physician, the nurse, and other professionals with the patient and the family to clarify goals and expectations of the treatment plan and to discuss discharge planning. These conferences encourage patient and family participation in decisions regarding care, and they identify the family's needs, so that they can be addressed before discharge.

Sharing clinical pathways with patients and families is another powerful patient-centered improvement strategy. Ideally, these guidelines are provided to patients and families upon admission or when they come in for preadmission workups. The pathway informs family members of the expected length of stay and enables them to begin preparing for the patient's discharge. When families use these guidelines to monitor the clinical course, they are often the first to identify problems. The guidelines often trigger questions and discussion that can help patients and their families become better managers of long-term chronic problems.

Griffin Hospital in Derby, Connecticut, has developed a series of patient pathways for more than twenty common diagnoses. These are provided to patients and their families during the collaborative care conference (Edgman-Levitan, 2003, p. 61).

Partners in Co-creating Better Health Care

People who have experience using health care services can also partner with us at an organizational level, bringing unique insights into organizational policy, planning, and quality improvement. They are experts on the experience of being a patient, so they are able to assist in designing services that are truly responsive to patients and their families. This integration of the patient/client and family voice into organizational planning and decision making is vital to advancing an organizational philosophy of patient-centered care.

The Calgary Health Region engages patients and families as patient experience advisers, who participate on region committees and teams, bringing the perspective of patients and families to this work. Experience as a health care user is all the experience that is required. They sit as members of patient/family advisory committees affiliated with a particular hospital, program, initiative, or geographical community. They are also involved on committees and work groups that consist mostly of health professionals, including ethics committees, quality improvement committees, and family-centered care committees, working together to design health care services that truly meet the needs of patients and families.

There are many ways to invite the patient and family perspective and their experience with us and incorporate it into our health care organizations (for example, comment cards, satisfaction surveys, and focus groups).

Having patient experience advisers working collaboratively on committees with health care professionals is not meant to replace these other mechanisms, but to complement them. There are benefits to working together over a period of time to shape health services delivery. These include the following:

- Shared meaning, shared understanding—both what it's like to be a patient or a family member and what it's like to be a health professional

- Better planning, decisions, policies, and practice—as seen through the eyes of the patient and family members

- Shared realization that only by working together will we create a better health care system for all—health care providers do not have all the answers, and neither do patients and families

- Inspired, energized, and engaged staff, patients, and families

Experience has shown that working with patient experience advisers on committees and teams is rewarding, but it also requires resources and support from staff and management. It is important to set the stage from the start by being clear about the underlying principles that support the work, the purpose of the committee, and the roles of all committee members. Once a positive stage has been set, finding and recruiting patient experience advisers, with the aim of achieving a mutually beneficial match, is a key step.

Preparing the team to work together and creating an environment that supports the development of a truly collaborative team are critical. Taking time to get to know one another, through sharing information openly and telling stories, will help the team members develop real connections (Jeppson and Thomas, 1994). Maintaining energy over time can be a challenge, particularly for standing committees. Group processes should be regularly revisited and the achievements of the committee routinely evaluated and celebrated.

"Informing all those who have been involved and may have been affected is also key. This is particularly important for patients. People will only give their time and energy if they can see that their efforts have resulted in some positive changes. Producing evidence that this has happened, and informing people of your findings and results, is a key part of the process" (National Health Service Modernisation Agency, 2005, p. 23).

VOLUNTEERS AS PARTNERS

As we continue to work toward transforming the health care system to create a patient-centered system of care, we must recognize a powerful and often untapped resource: community volunteers. Some examples of volunteer activities are briefly described in Table 3.3. In order for a volunteer program to be successful, it is important to match the needs of the hospital with the desire and skills of the volunteer. A thorough screening, including background checks, formalized orientation, and ongoing evaluation of the volunteer ensures the quality of the program.

The Changing Face of Volunteers

Health care organizations are becoming increasingly attractive places in which to volunteer, and the face of today's volunteer has changed. No longer "the pink lady" or "the candy striper," today's volunteers are male and female, youth and elder, retired and employed, physically fit and physically challenged, transient and permanent, and may or may not have a background in health care. The prospective volunteer arrives at the volunteer office for a variety of reasons: résumé building, internships, medical school acceptance, changing careers, community service, early retirement, physician ordered (to decrease isolation and loneliness), and more often than not with a strong desire to join a team committed to helping make the patient experience better.

Opportunities for Volunteers

Likewise, opportunities for the volunteer have expanded. Health care offers these individuals vast and dynamic opportunities to become involved. Volunteers are placed in clinical and nonclinical areas, on- and off-site. Flexible shifts are created to accommodate varying lifestyles: the golfers and the gardeners, the students and the servicemen, the crafters and the computer literate. Flexible locations are created for disabled volunteers. Everyone benefits from the flexibility; the adults prefer volunteering during daylight hours whereas the nocturnal college students appreciate being scheduled in the evening after classes. The servicemen appreciate the flexibility when they are on leave, and the disabled appreciate having opportunities to contribute from home.

Health care providers are increasingly seeing the value of including volunteers. Planetree promotes the family's and the loved one's roles as part of the care team for patients. For busy working families, it can sometimes be hard to be at the bedside of a loved one who is hospitalized.

TABLE 3.3. Volunteers as Partners.

Volunteer Program	Program Description
Hospital auxiliary*	The fundraising branch of the volunteer team strives to serve the health care needs of their communities by supporting their hospital's mission. In Williamsburg, funds raised from the auxiliary's Pineapple gift shop and other projects (for example, Festival of Lights, Mistletoe Market, book sales, jewelry sales, gently used computer and clothing sales), assist in the delivery of Sentara's patient-centered services and programs such as the auxiliary's Free Mammogram and Bone Density programs.
Finding Hope—support for families of children with life-limiting illnesses**	The Alberta Children's Hospital has a support group for families who have a child with a life-limiting illness. A volunteer works closely with professionals to support the work of this group, and all the families so appreciate her presence. Playing this role has also been an extremely rewarding experience for the volunteer involved.
Ball Hawks*	A group of golf enthusiasts collects lost golf balls on local golf courses, repackages them, and sells them in the hospital's gift shop. All proceeds from the ball sales have gone to support patient-centered initiatives, including the purchasing of two golf carts, driven by volunteers, to transport patients, staff, and visitors to and from the parking lot.

TABLE 3.3. *(Continued)*

Volunteer Program	Program Description
Travelling Tales Book Cart**	The book cart is not just about providing reading material, promoting health information, and encouraging literacy, but it is also about interacting with kids and their families. Although a staggering 364 books were signed out in the first two months of the program, it is the quality of the experience that stands out in the minds of patients, families, and volunteers.
ASSIST Program*	A Special Service Involving Stricken Travelers (ASSIST) is a humanitarian program staffed solely by volunteers that provides help and comfort to travelers, along with their families and traveling companions, who encounter medical problems while visiting in the Williamsburg area.
Wayfinder Program**	The volunteers involved in the Wayfinder program welcome patients, families, and visitors, helping to ease the stress and anxiety that people often experience. They can take the time to walk someone to a new appointment location or to sit down and chat with a patient or a family member while they are waiting.

*Sentara Williamsburg Regional Medical Center.
**Calgary Health Region.

Volunteers can provide that needed comfort and support in the absence of family and friends. In much the same way, trained volunteers can help serve as care partners. They can help implement programs and services that might otherwise be too difficult for paid staff to deliver, such as Calgary Health Region's Refreshment Program, which offers conversation, home baking, and tea or coffee, or Sentara Williamsburg Regional Medical Center's Inspiration Cart, which assists the chaplain by distributing spiritual materials and providing an opportunity to add a patient's name to a prayer list.

Volunteers can be instrumental in creating a more patient-centered environment of care by assisting the paid hospital staff to ensure that the needs of patients and families are met. This is not to suggest that they supplant the care provided by doctors, nurses, and other health care professionals, but rather to say that they enhance the care by supporting the patient, their families, and the professional staff. Volunteers are recognized by patients as goodwill ambassadors. When assisting with patient rounds, volunteers have a unique position that allows them to gather quality-of-care feedback, including patient safety and patient satisfaction data that might not be shared with paid hospital staff for fear of retribution.

Volunteers are trained to know the patient-centered programs and services that a hospital provides. They can be an excellent resource to educate patients and their families about the services that are available to them—whether it is after-hours dining options or where to go within the facility to take advantage of some quiet reflection areas, such as the chapel, the healing garden, or the labyrinth. In addition to contributing to a healing environment, the volunteers play a crucial role in safeguarding the environment as another pair of eyes and ears.

Volunteers can also help implement some complementary services in the health care setting. Sentara Virginia Beach General Hospital and Sentara Williamsburg Regional Medical Center partner with local massage schools, which offer staff massages by student massage therapists under the careful watch of licensed instructors. Certified Pet Therapy is another example of a volunteer service that can positively influence the patient care experience. The certified therapy dogs and their handlers visit those rooms that have a Certified Therapy Dog, Please Visit Me sign. This process does not interfere with the nurse's routine and ensures visits to only those patients requesting the dog's visit.

Some hospitals expand this program to include a Patient's Own Pet program, because for some patients, pets are a very important part of—or perhaps their only—family. Some hospitals allow pets to visit in the patients' rooms and have developed simple checklists to ensure that the pet has all necessary vaccinations and is kept on a leash when not in the patient's room. Others have developed special areas where patients can visit with pets outside their room.

QUO VADIS—THE FUTURE

A shift is occurring in the education and sophistication of our citizens. People's expectations regarding control over and involvement in all aspects of life are changing. The health care sector has lagged behind somewhat in recognizing this societal trend, but it is also experiencing a paradigm shift. It is no longer a question of *if* we should include patients and families as partners in our hospitals and health care systems, but rather *how* we do so.

"A fundamental shift is required in the distribution of power—so that our patients and families will have an active voice at the table. . . . a system that consistently includes patients and families will be safer and will provide a better experience—for patients, families and staff" (Jack Davis, CEO, Calgary Health Region, Institute for Family-Centered Care conference, Seattle, July 2007).

Patients and their families, and health care providers are recognizing that only by working together will we be able to achieve our common goals—a health system that provides a rich and rewarding work environment and a safe, high-quality experience for patients and their families. Health care will not achieve this promise if we do not value and use multiple types of expertise, including the expertise that patients and their families bring.

REFERENCES

Ahmann, E. "Examining Assumptions Underlying Nursing Practice with Children and Families." *Pediatric Nursing*, 1998, *23*, 467–469.

Ahmann, E., Abraham, M., and Johnson, B. *Changing the Concept of Families as Visitors: Supporting Family Presence and Participation.* Bethesda, Md.: Institute for Family-Centered Care, 2003.

American Academy of Pediatrics, Institute for Family-Centered Care. "Policy Statement: Family-Centered Care and the Pediatrician's Role." *Pediatrics*, 2003, *112*(3), 137–142.

Bodenheimer, T., Lorig, K., Holman, H., and Grumbach, K. "Patient Self-Management of Chronic Disease in Primary Care." *Journal of the American Medical Association*, 2002, *200*(19), 2469.

Botelho, R. J., Lue, B. H., and Fiscella, K. "Family Involvement in Routine Health Care: A Survey of Patients' Behaviours and Preferences." *Journal of Family Practice,* 1996, *42*(6), 572–576.

Bru, G., Carmody, S., Donohue-Sword, B., and Bookbinder, M. "Parental Visitation in the Post-Anesthesia Care Unit: A Means to Lessen Anxiety." *Children's Health Care,* 1993, *22*(3), 217–226.

Conlon, P. *No Need to Trouble the Heart: A Loving Journey Through Sickness and Health.* Vancouver: Raincoast Books, 2006.

Crocker, L., and Johnson, B. *Privileged Presence: Personal Stories of Connections in Health Care.* Boulder, Colo.: Bull Publishing, 2006.

Davidson, J. D., and others. "Clinical Practice Guidelines for the Support of the Family in the Patient-Centered Intensive Care Unit: American College of Critical Care Medicine Task Force 2004–2005." *Critical Care Medicine,* 2007, *35*(2), 605–622.

Delbanco, T., and others. "Healthcare in a Land Called PeoplePower: Nothing About Me Without Me." *Health Expectations,* 2001, *4,* 144–150.

Dunst, C. J., and Trivette, C. M. "Empowerment, Effective Helpgiving Practices and Family-Centered Care." *Pediatric Nursing,* 1996, *22,* 334–337, 343.

Duran, C. R., and others. "Attitudes Toward and Beliefs About Family Presence: A Survey of Healthcare Providers, Patients' Families, and Patients." *American Journal of Critical Care,* 2007, *16*(3), 270–282.

Edgman-Levitan, S. "Healing Partnerships: The Importance of Including Family and Friends." In S. B. Frampton, L. Gilpin, and P. A. Charmel (eds.), *Putting Patients First: Designing and Practicing Patient-Centered Care.* San Francisco: Jossey-Bass, 2003.

Farah, M. M., Thomas, C. A., and Shaw, K. N. "Evidence-Based Guidelines for Family Presence in the Resuscitation Room: A Step-by-Step Approach." *Pediatric Emergency Care,* 2007, *23*(8), 587–591.

Fulbrook, P., Latour, J. M., and Albarran, J. W. "Pediatric Critical Care Nurses' Attitudes and Experiences of Parental Presence During Cardiopulmonary Resuscitation: A European Survey." *International Journal of Nursing Studies,* 2007, *44*(7), 1238–1249.

Gerteis, M., Edgman-Levitan, S., Daley, J., and Delbanco, T. L. (eds.). *Through the Patient's Eyes: Understanding and Promoting Patient-Centered Care.* San Francisco: Jossey-Bass, 1993.

Gold, K. J., Gorenflo, D. W., Schwenk, T. L., and Bratton, S. L. "Physician Experience with Family Presence During Cardiopulmonary Resuscitation in Children." *Pediatric Critical Care Medicine,* 2006, *7*(5), 428–433.

Halm, M. A. "Family Presence During Resuscitation: A Critical Review of the Literature." *American Journal of Critical Care,* 2005, *14*(6), 494–511.

Harrison, A., and Verhoef, M. "Understanding Coordination of Care from the Consumer's Perspective in a Regional Health System." *Health Services Research,* Aug. 2002, *37,* 4.

Hicock, L., and Lewis, J. *Beware the Grieving Warrior.* Toronto: ECW Press, 2004.

Jeppson, E. S., and Thomas, J. *Essential Allies: Families as Advisors.* Bethesda, Md.: Institute for Family-Centered Care, 1994.

Jeppson, E. S. and Thomas, J. *Families as Advisors: A Training Guide for Collaboration.* Bethesda, Md.: Institute for Family Centered Care, 1997.

Johnston, A. M., and others. "Implementation and Case-Study Results of Potentially Better Practices for Family-Centered Care: The Family Centered Care Map." *Pediatrics,* 2006, *118*(Suppl. 2), S108–S114.

King, G. A., King, S. M., and Rosenbaum, P. L. "Interpersonal Aspects of Care-Giving and Client Outcomes: A Review of the Literature." *Ambulatory Child Health,* 1996, *2,* 151–160.

King, G., Law, M., King, S., and Rosenbaum, P. "Parents' and Service Providers' Perceptions of the Family-Centredness of Children's Rehabilitation Services." In M. Law (ed.), *Family-Centred Assessment and Intervention in Pediatric Rehabilitation* (pp. 21–40). New York: Hawkworth Press, 1998.

Kleinman, A. *The Illness Narratives: Suffering, Healing, and the Human Condition.* New York: Basic Books, 1988.

Lorig, K. "Self-Management Education, More Than a Nice Extra." *Medical Care,* 2003, *41*(6), 699–701.

MacKean, G. L., Thurston, W. E., and Scott, C. M. "Bridging the Divide Between Families and Health Professionals' Perspectives on Family Centered Care." *Health Expectations,* 2005, *8,* 74–85.

MacLean, S. L., and others. *American Journal of Critical Care,* 2003, *12*(3), 246–257.

McGahey-Oakland, P. R., Lieder, H. S., Young, A., and Jefferson, L. S. *Journal of Pediatric Health Care,* 2007, *21*(4), 217–225.

Muething, S. E., and Kotagal, U. R. "Family-Centered Bedside Rounds: A New Approach to Patient Care and Teaching." *Pediatrics,* 2007, *119*(4), 829–832.

National Center for Chronic Disease Prevention and Health Promotion. 2008. [www.cdc.gov].

National Health Service Modernisation Agency. *Improvement Leaders' Guide to Involving Patients and Carers.* Ipswich, U.K.: Ancient House, 2005.

Nigrovic, L. E., McQueen, A. A., and Neuman, M. I. "Lumbar Puncture Success Rate Is Not Influenced by Family-Member Presence." *Pediatrics,* 2007, *120*(4), E777–E782.

Public Health Agency of Canada. 2008. [www.publichealth.gc.ca].

Rose, J."Tearing Down the Walls." *Health Care Executive,* May 2005.

Rotman-Pikielny, P., and others. "Participation of Family Members in Ward Rounds: Attitude of Medical Staff, Patients and Relatives." *Patient Education and Counseling,* 2007, *65*(2), 166–70.

Sloper, P. "Models of Service Support for Parents of Disabled Children. What Do We Know? What Do We Need to Know?" *Child: Care, Health and Development,* 1999, *25,* 85–99.

Society of Critical Care Medicine. *Critical Care Medicine,* 2007, *35*(2), 605–622.

Thompson, A.G.H. "The Meaning of Patient Involvement and Participation in Health Care Consultations: A Taxonomy." *Social Science and Medicine,* 2007, *64,* 1297–1310.

Tsai, E. "Should Family Members Be Present During Cardiopulmonary Resuscitation?" *New England Journal of Medicine,* 2002, *346*(13), 1019–1021.

Tuller, S., and others. "Patient, Visitor and Nurse Evaluation of Visitation for Adult Postanesthesia Care Unit Patients." *Journal of Perianesthesia Nursing,* 1997, *12*(6), 402–412.

Vom Eigen, K. A., and others. "Carepartner Experiences with Hospital Care." *Medical Care,* 1999, *37*(1), 33–38.

Wetzels, R., and others. "Interventions for Improving Older Patients' Involvement in Primary Care Episodes." *Cochrane Database of Systematic Reviews,* 2007.

CHAPTER

4

NUTRITION: THE NURTURING AND HEALING ASPECTS OF FOOD

DAVID L. KATZ AND F. NICHOLAS JACOBS

This chapter does the following:

- Reviews the essential elements of a health-promoting diet
- Discusses the opportunity that hospitalization presents to promote better nutrition
- Presents strategies, through case studies, for patient-centered approaches to the presentation, preparation, and distribution of food for patients, families, and staff

Hippocrates, whose healing legacy is so fundamental to the Planetree philosophy, made a connection between food and health over two thousand years ago, when he advised, "Let food be your medicine." Food, of course, is an integral part of health. In addition to its nourishing aspects, food has the power to comfort and heal—or conversely to cause anxiety and aversion. Eating can be a powerful symbol of nurturing, love, and celebration. But which foods fit in the overall healing experience? How can they be incorporated into food service plans that work for the individual as well as for the hospital (modified from Reinke and Ryczek, 2003)?

This chapter explores food and diet as it pertains to creating a patient-centered, healing environment. It begins with an overview of the essential elements of a health-promoting diet and continues with a look at how one Planetree hospital revolutionized the way it approached food service in order to provide food that is both nurturing and nourishing, while also empowering individuals to achieve healthful eating habits in their daily lives.

FOOD, HEALTH, AND THE HEALING ENVIRONMENT

Food is the fuel on which the human body runs. It simply stands to reason that the quality of the diet has the potential to influence virtually every aspect of the quality of health.

And, yes, we truly are what we eat. The raw material used in the manufacture of a growing child comes from . . . food. How much tougher it becomes to be glib about "junk food" when one pauses to consider it is the source of material from which a child's body is being built! Would anyone willingly choose to build the heart, and nerve, and sinew of a growing child from the nutritional analogue of refuse?

Nor are we adults immune to this selfsame intimacy with food. Our bodies turn over billions of cells every day. Just as a river is never quite the same twice for its ceaseless flowing, so our bodies flow through a continuous process of remodeling and renewal. We, too, are what we eat. And while astronomer Carl Sagan was correct that at the level of our atoms, we humans are made up of star stuff (http://en.wikiquote.org/wiki/Carl_Sagan), referring to the heavier elements in our bodies that originate nowhere but in supernovas, at the level of our cells we might, alas, be more akin to Starburst fruit chews depending on the choices we make each day by the mouthful. What we eat matters for no lesser reason than what we eat becomes the very matter of ourselves.

Dietary pattern is thus unsurprisingly tied to almost any health outcome we know how to measure. The myriad effects of nutrition on health are documented in a vast scientific literature. In certain vital areas, consensus has yet to develop. Sufficient evidence has been gathered, however, to permit the generation of dietary recommendations for health promotion and disease prevention with considerable confidence.

The following list contains the steps that are needed to improve the typical Western diet, which are widely supported in the nutrition community.

Steps to Improve the Western Diet

- Reduce trans fat.

- Reduce saturated fat.

- Reduce sodium.

- Increase fruits and vegetables.

- Increase whole grains.

- Reduce refined starches and simple sugars.

- Replace "bad" fats with "good" fats.

- Increase fiber.

- Increase micronutrients.

- Control portion size and total calories (Katz, 2004).

Although the competing claims of popular diets might at times suggest otherwise, we are by no means clueless about the basic care and feeding of Homo sapiens! There is overwhelming consensus in support of a diet characterized by the following:

- A generous intake of vegetables and fruits, whole grains, beans, legumes, nuts, and seeds

- An emphasis on fish and skinless poultry or plant foods as protein sources

- Restriction of trans fat, saturated fat, refined starch, added sugar, and salt

- A shift from animal and other saturated fats to unsaturated plant oils

- Portion control conducive to energy balance and the maintenance of a healthy weight (see Tables 4.1 and 4.2)

TABLE 4.1. Dietary Pattern for Optimal Health and Weight Control.

Nutrient Class/Nutrient	Recommended Intake
Carbohydrate, predominately complex	Approximately **45 to 60%** of total calories
Fiber, both soluble and insoluble	At least **25 grams per day,** with additional potential benefit from up to 50 grams per day
Protein, predominantly plant-based sources	Up to **25%** of total calories
Total fat	Up to **30%,** and preferably approximately **25%,** of total calories
Types of fat	
Monounsaturated fat	**10 to 15%** of total calories
Polyunsaturated fat Omega-3 and omega-6 fat	Approximately **10%** of total calories 1:1 to 1:4 ratio
Saturated fat and trans fat (partially hydrogenated fat)	Ideally, less than **5%** of total calories; trans fat intake should be negligible

Sugar	Less than **10%** of total calories
Sodium	Up to 2,400 mg. per day
Cholesterol	Up to 300 mg. per day
Water	8 glasses a day/64 oz./2 liters, to vary with activity level, environmental conditions, and the fluid content of foods (for example, fruits)
Alcohol, moderate intake if desired	Up to one drink a day for women Up to two drinks a day for men
Calorie level	Adequate to achieve and maintain a healthy weight
Physical activity/exercise	Daily moderate activity for 30 minutes or more Strength training twice weekly

Source: Adapted from Katz and Gonzalez, 2002.

TABLE 4.2. Dietary Pattern for Meeting Nutritional Objectives.

Food Group	Foods to Choose
Whole grains	At least **7 to 8 servings** a day of whole grain breads, cereals, and grains, with **2 or more grams** of fiber per serving. Include oatmeal, oat bran, brown and wild rice varieties, semolina and whole wheat pasta, couscous, barley, and bulgur wheat.
Fruits	**4 to 5 servings** a day from a rainbow of colors, especially deep yellow, orange, and red: berries, apples, oranges, apricots, melons, mangos, and so forth. Select from fresh, frozen, canned packed in juice, and dried varieties. Buy locally grown in season whenever possible.
Vegetables	**4 to 5 servings** a day from a rainbow of colors, especially deep yellow, orange, red and leafy green: yellow, red, and green bell peppers, squash, carrots, tomatoes, spinach, sweet potatoes, broccoli, kale, Swiss chard, Brussels sprouts, eggplant, and so forth. Select from fresh, frozen, and canned varieties, but be mindful of the higher sodium content of canned. Buy locally grown in season whenever possible.
Beans and legumes	Include **3 to 4 times a week.** Beans and legumes make a good alternative to meat. Include a variety of beans and legumes in your diet: black, red, kidney, white, cannellini, garbanzo (chick pea), navy, pinto, lentils, split peas, black-eyed peas, and soy.
Fish (and seafood)*	Include as often as **3 to 4 times a week.** Fish is generally an excellent, lean source of high-quality protein, and several varieties (for example, tuna, salmon, mackerel, halibut, and cod) are excellent sources of omega-3 fatty acids. Seafood, such as shrimp and scallops, tends to be relatively high in cholesterol but is low in fat and is also a good source of omega-3 fatty acids.

Food category	Recommendation
Chicken and turkey*	Include **up to 1 to 2 times a week**. Skinless breast meat is preferred.
Lean beef, pork, and lamb*	**Moderate intake of meat**, working toward a goal of roughly 1 to 2 meat-based meals per week, or **4 to 8 per month**, if desired. Select lean meats; the loin and round cuts are the leanest.
Milk and cheese*	Choose at least **2 servings** a day from fat-free, skim, or low-fat versions.
Vegetable oils and other added fats	Choose monounsaturated and polyunsaturated sources daily; use in small amounts to avoid excessive calories: olive oil, canola oil, olives, avocados, almond butter, and peanut butter.
Nuts and seeds	Include **4 to 5 times a week** in small amounts of unsalted raw or dry roasted types: almonds, walnuts, pistachios, peanuts, pecans, cashews, soy nuts, sunflower seeds, pumpkin seeds, sesame seeds. Mix 1 tablespoon of ground flaxseed daily into other cooked foods.
Eggs*	Up to 1 egg per day on average (more egg white is fine). Preferably, choose an omega-3 fatty acid–enriched brand.
Sweets	In moderation. Choose low- or nonfat varieties whenever reasonable. Dark chocolate offers nutritional benefits.

*Optional items. Well-balanced vegetarian and vegan diets would omit these items. Note that fish is recommended for particular health benefits; flaxseeds or an omega-3 fatty acid supplement is especially recommended for those who do not eat fish.

Note: When absolute amounts are provided, they refer to a prototypical diet of 2,000 calories per day.

Source: Adapted from Katz and Gonzalez, 2002.

Recommendations to include nonfat dairy in the diet are less universal but nonetheless predominant.

The same dietary pattern is appropriate for the prevention of most diseases. This has not always been evident and is worthy of note. Patients with cardiovascular disease often have diabetes, also may have cerebrovascular disease, often have hypertension, may have renal insufficiency, may have had or have cancer, and are constantly vulnerable to infectious disease. If each disease required a different diet, consistent recommendations could not be made to an individual, let alone a population. A diet that is friendly to health is hostile to a long list of health threats.

In an age of epidemic obesity in the developed world, the maintenance of a healthy weight is a crucial if elusive goal of dietary health. Weight, ultimately, is about the balance between calories consumed and calories expended; therefore, portion control is fundamental (see Table 4.3). A dietary pattern consistent with recommendations for overall health facilitates portion control by offering satisfaction and satiety on fewer calories.

Food chosen well is a wellspring of health. Diets well constructed are pillars of disease prevention. In conjunction with a very short list of complementary behaviors—not smoking and being physically active, for instance—eating well offers enough promise to personal and public health to deserve the Nobel Prize many times over. An optimal diet could help reduce heart disease risk by 80 percent, diabetes risk by 90 percent, and cancer risk by 30 percent or more. Health care institutions therefore have an obligation to maintain high standards of nutrition or risk nothing less than hypocrisy. They have an opportunity to do so much more, showcasing healthful cuisine to patients, visitors, and staff alike.

Approximately forty million Americans are hospitalized at least once each year (www.ahrq.gov/data/hcup/factbk6/factbk6c.htm). When visits for all reasons are considered, the health care setting provides annual access to nearly the entire population. Why not leverage that contact to promote better nutrition for all? Perhaps chefs in training might spend a stint at a hospital, helping hospitals raise their culinary game, while gaining valuable work experience. Healthful dishes for patients and visitors alike might be accompanied by a laminated recipe card with nutrition facts. Imagine if visiting a loved one in the hospital created an opportunity for you to get healthier!

But of course food is not just about and generally not even mostly about health outcomes years down the line. Food is about gratification right now. Food is comfort and consolation; nourishment and nostalgia;

TABLE 4.3. Portion Size Guide.

Food Group	Standard Serving Size
Whole grains	• 1 slice bread • ¾ to 1 cup breakfast cereal • ½ cup cooked cereal, grains, or pasta
Fruits	• 1 medium piece of fresh fruit • 4 ounces of 100% fruit juice • ½ cup canned, cooked, or chopped fruit • ¼ cup dried fruit, about one small handful
Vegetables	• ½ cup cooked vegetables, about the size of a tennis ball • 1 cup raw vegetables or salad, about the size of your fist • 6 ounces vegetable juice
Vegetable oils and added fats	• 1 teaspoon oil • ⅛ avocado • 1 tablespoon salad dressing • 1 teaspoon soft margarine
Nuts and seeds	• 1 ounce or ¼ cup • 1 tablespoon peanut or almond butter, about the size of the tip of your thumb
Beans and legumes	• ½ cup cooked beans, lentils, or peas • ½ cup tofu • 1 cup soymilk
Fish, chicken, turkey, beef, pork, and lamb	• 3 ounces cooked, about the size of a deck of cards
Dairy	• 1 cup milk or yogurt • 1½ ounces low-fat cheese, about the size of four stacked dice • ½ cup ricotta cheese

Source: Adapted from Katz and Gonzalez, 2002.

satisfaction, solace, and solidarity. But the many roles of food in our lives are not mutually exclusive. The venerated Mediterranean diet stands out as a demonstration that food can be very good—and very good for us.

A healing environment must of course confer comfort. And of the many means for doing so, from gentle sound to kind touch, surely none delves quite so deeply into our very molecules or evokes such potent memory as food.

The healing environment committed to comfort has an obligation to respect our lifelong relationship with food. The comforting environment committed to health has an opportunity to foster nutritional well-being. Where better to showcase a whole new kind of fusion cuisine that offers pleasure in the pursuit of health and health in the pursuit of pleasure than a setting dedicated to a holistic vision of wellness? Combined, as is demonstrated in Nicholas Jacobs's description of Windber Medical Center's journey to transform the hospital food experience, the science of dietary health promotion and the art of human comfort may be blended into a recipe for food that we can love and that loves us back.

ONE HOSPITAL'S JOURNEY: WINDBER MEDICAL CENTER

Windber Medical Center's journey to transform the way patients and their loved ones eat has been defined by our total belief and commitment to the concept that the nurturing qualities of food are as important as the nutritional qualities of food. As a young executive in the tourism industry, I was invited to attend a meeting at a local chain restaurant with the director of marketing of this particular corporation. As we entered the main door of the restaurant, my olfactory nerves were overcome with the incredible smell of fresh baked goods: breads, rolls, cookies, pies, and cakes. I turned to the marketing executive and said, "What a wonderful smell," to which he replied, "Do you think this is an accident? We pipe these smells to the waiting area through a complex system of vents and ducts designed to bring them directly from the bakery to you. We do that to make you hungry!"

That was the beginning of my understanding of what this concept could mean to a hospital's patients and visiting families. Shortly after Windber Medical Center became a Planetree hospital, we began to bake bread every day on every floor, then later added popcorn in the lobby, not with the intention of making people hungry, but to release endorphins connected to wonderful memories of Grandma, Aunt Ruth, and everything good about life.

As a young trumpet player working in an 1890s-style entertainment center, I overheard the owner telling the food preparation employee, "Load it with salt! How do you expect us to sell beer?" This proves another point: food is and can be a manipulator in both a positive and a negative way. What is worse than melting green Jello beside a plate of unsalted, canned green beans, and a glob of mashed potatoes with canned gravy wrapped around chicken that would not be suitable for the fried-up nuggets that come in a kid's meal at a drive-through fast food restaurant?

Because it was never my goal to work in a hospital, and because it frankly was not a place that made me comfortable even as a visitor, my background allowed me to look at their world a little differently. It always struck me as obscene that our hospitals generally provided a selection of food that could be classified as somewhere between flavorless and nasty, sometimes unhealthy, and typically completely unappealing. It was all about the cost, the shelf life, and the requirements imposed by the state and The Joint Commission. Many times, short of road kill du jour, it is like institutional food. My first administrative journey into the hospital food world was the day my new chief operating officer said, "Dinners must never cost us more than $1.75 each."

Consequently, our goal as a Planetree hospital was to create a healing environment through the use of the environment, decorative fountains indoors and out, lighting, architectural design, live plants, sky lights, music, art, and especially food—good food, hotel-quality food. How do you create a healing environment through the presentation, preparation, and appropriate distribution of food? Our first decision was to hire a hotel manager, someone who was skilled in housekeeping, maintenance, and culinary services.

During his fifteen-minute orientation, it was explained very precisely that it was our vision to provide for our patients, staff, and families a healthful food selection. It is at this point that this writer must admit that this concept was as foreign to someone from the hospitality industry as it was to someone from among our culinary experts. Dining service and nutrition was its name, but fast, cheap, and long-lasting was the game. We determined that chefs were good and set out to hire two for basically the same monies as we had previously been paying cooks. Because we are located near a fairly substantial culinary training program, this was not impossible.

Serving healthy foods was also foreign to our chefs, so we imported healthy chefs to train our people from scratch. They learned about ingredients like spices, fresh herbs, and nonfat dairy. It was a fascinating journey as we encouraged them in a less-than-diplomatic fashion to have at least one dietary selection for each meal that was fat free, meatless, and healthy. We pushed for fresh vegetables from local organic farms, organic dairy, and numerous other healthy alternatives.

The decision to pursue this line of thinking was as controversial as any with which we have been involved. We would provide low-fat, vegetarian selections for all three meals, and the result was near panic. The decision could easily have been, "Bring your firstborn child to work for a sixty-year imprisonment." The organization reacted like the Green Bay Packers seeing their quarterback come into the lineup in a tutu.

The physicians and families reacted accordingly as well for at least three months of the nontrial. They mocked, joked, and bantered much like school kids in an uncomfortable situation. "Why do you eat that grass?" "Where's the beef?" "Are you having your tofu today? Be careful, there's plenty of estrogen in that stuff," were just a few of the comments. At an employee picnic, just one soy burger was consumed that first year and it was consumed by me. At our last picnic, 50 percent of the food consumed was healthful.

When Windber Medical Center's culture change implementation was considered—changing the colors of the walls, introducing 24/7 visiting hours, pajama bottoms, and care teams—it was all such a dramatic departure from the traditional that it must have felt like aliens had attacked. The push back was so intense and so complete at times that our dietary leadership began to question my sanity, but after it was determined that leadership was NOT going to discontinue the practice of providing healthy food, our customers began to try it, to try it and to like it. In fact, it became so popular that we were nudged into providing frozen entrees for purchase from our cafeteria.

After this phase of our vision was complete, we began to seek out a new world order for health care and hospitals, the complete elimination of all trans fats from food served to our patients. Once again, the reaction that we initially faced was, "Are you sure?" Our answer was not only "Yes," but "Definitely, yes." We are sure. Why should we poison our own patients? Cigarette machines were removed from our lobbies nearly forty years ago, yet we still made saturated and trans fat–packed foods available to our patients.

The logic behind trans fats is economics. They lengthen the shelf life of the food that contains them. They do not significantly alter the taste. They do not disrupt the digestive system. They only accelerate the severity of coronary artery disease. In response to our request, our food service purveyor, Cura, very actively began the pursuit of trans fat elimination company-wide.

As they explained to us, their cost would amount to about $150,000 annually company-wide per year to eliminate these man-altered molecules because of decreased shelf life, but they were eager to move forward with this project. So the "greening" of our food began. It took nearly nine months to eradicate trans fats, and when we announced this decision and the result of our work to the press as the only hospital in the United States that had successfully eliminated trans fats, we were inundated with a lack of response.

This may have been because of our size, under a thousand beds, or it may have been because it was during the same time period that Chicago and New York City both announced that they were banning the use of trans fat oils for cooking, a very different issue. The knowledge produced from the fact that we had successfully removed all trans fats from the foods presented for consumption at our facility produced a similar reaction as listening to my engine as I turn the key in my non-sound-producing hybrid automobile's electric ignition. It didn't make much noise, but I feel a lot better about our successful strides to make a better future for all of us.

As we continued to seek out alternatives to traditional institutional-type food service, it came to our attention that a neighboring hospital, once a competitor, now out of business, had introduced a wonderful concept as an alternative to traditional meal service. In fact, we discovered that while they were still operational, Planetree leadership had visited this site to determine the feasibility of reproducing their service concept to patients, family, and staff worldwide. Whether it was serendipity or just plain luck, we had—through our food service purveyor—secured the manager of their food service as our new director of dining services.

We held a meeting with her to determine the feasibility of instituting a similar service under the Windbercare banner. That service, in fact, would cost us some additional monies in the form of needed equipment, but it would be possible. The basic premise of this type of dietary service was on-floor dietary. Each patient care floor would be the recipient of a group of dietary employees. Food preparation would still take place in the kitchen, but actual distribution of the food would take place from a food service area established on each patient floor.

The hot food is now delivered to the floor via an electric-powered portable heating and mobile dining cart that is moved from floor to floor over a two-hour period for each meal. The servers either go from patient to patient and take orders, or if the patients are ambulatory, they are encouraged to come to the serving area to select their meal from the multiple dietary options from the heating trays.

For a nominal fee, employees, family members, and medical staff members are welcome to make a selection from the mobile dining cart as well. The impact of this type of service has been far reaching. Because we are not large enough to provide extensive cafeteria service 24/7, this service has helped to serve as a means of assisting our guests and their families to get a good, nutritional meal without developing carpal tunnel syndrome from working the handles of the vending machines.

Further, it gives patients the opportunity to actually choose their meals from a wholesome selection of entrees that are visually pleasing as well. Unlike the old system of lift the lid, determine the origin of the mystery meat, pray that it is not ice cold, and then eat the melted green Jello, in the new system, if the patients are ambulatory, they can get the satisfaction of actually walking to the food area and personally selecting the serving size and combination of foods that are most appealing to them.

The very crux of this philosophy is one of respect, choice, dignity, nurturing, love, and commitment to the patients and their families. Our patient satisfaction scores could not be higher. In ten years, we have paid out millions of dollars in premiums and have had less than $200,000 in settlement claims for slips, falls, or malpractice. When people are treated with dignity, there are no vendettas. Finally, as we watch the Pig move through the Python, remember that the seventy-eight million Boomers are not going to be as tolerant as their parents.

We are Boomers. We are, however, going to need tens of thousands of personal trainers, plastic surgeons, and medical liaison guides to help us find our way through the system. When we are older and grayer, we'll want gerontologists who understand the nuances of the aging body. You will very likely hear us request things like decaf lattes with soy milk or a nonfat grande chai tea rather than a packet of instant Sanka and a package of Nips as we continue to pamper our already sophisticated palates. We are especially not interested in excuses for vindictive workers, dirty rooms and hallways, restricted visiting hours, meager signage, and limited availability to complementary care.

FOOD AND HEALING

It is ironic that one of the most fundamental of human needs has been considered the domain of an *ancillary department* in hospitals—a service for the structure of the institution rather than for the healing of the patients. The Planetree adage that "everyone is a caregiver" is an apt reminder that every aspect of a patient's stay can contribute to his or her healing. Patients already know the importance of food. As hospitals explore the role that food can play, they will continue to discover ways to make nutrition an integral part of patient care and community health. Bringing a sense of community and caring to the hospital experience is a contribution well suited to nutrition services. Using the inherent symbolism of food to nurture, nourish, and comfort the body, mind, and spirit is an opportunity that exists in virtually all organizational settings. Recognizing the valuable role that dietary staff members can play in optimizing this opportunity and engaging them in enhancing the patient's experience is key to changing attitudes toward hospital food (modified from Reinke and Ryczek, 2003).

Providing Twenty-Four-Hour A La Carte Meal Service

In 1997, Kadlec Medical Center, a 172-bed hospital in Richland, Washington, began looking at ways to improve patient meal service. A then-new patient satisfaction report indicated that despite the resources invested in providing nutritious meals to patients, satisfaction with patient meal service was a mere 67 percent. Fully committed to enhancing patient meal satisfaction, Kadlec initiated a complete renovation of its Nutrition Services Department.

While exploring opportunities to improve this important component of the patient experience, the hospital found that 30 percent of patient meals were served outside of set tray line meal service times and after the kitchen was closed. These alternative meals included late trays, box meals, frozen meals, nourishments, and pantry supplies, with patients on oncology, pediatric, and birth center units the primary recipients of these alternative meals. As we talked with patients and staff, it became clear that even though traditional hospital meal service may have been efficient for the organization, it was not effectively fulfilling the hospital's goal of nourishing patients. This discovery paved the way for Kadlec's twenty-four-hour A La Carte Meal Service, which features a comfort food menu and allows patients to order "what they want when they want it."

FOR EXAMPLE

Recognizing that the new meal service program would affect daily patient care routines, a multidisciplinary Process Improvement Team worked out the details of implementing twenty-four-hour access to patient meals. The process improvement team focused on developing processes around diabetes care, medications and meal timing, diagnostic procedures, and physical therapy appointments as they related to meal service. An *A La Carte Meal Service Reference Book* was developed to educate staff.

When Kadlec's completely renovated kitchen opened in June 1998, the hospital was poised to empower patients and families with control over their mealtime preferences. The A La Carte menu book, including menus for pediatric patients and menus in Spanish and Russian, are now available in each patient room. Meal orders are made by phone to a call center, and meals are delivered within thirty minutes. The social aspect of mealtime is enhanced when family or friends also place an order and dine with the patient.

Patient meal satisfaction immediately improved and has been sustained over the years. Kadlec is currently in the 97th percentile for excellent ranking of patient meal service within its benchmarking group. Some patients actually request a discharge time that allows for "one last meal before I go home," and hospital staff report that twenty-four-hour patient meal service has allowed them to nourish patients on many levels that are not achievable in a traditional meal service program.

That the A La Carte meal volume capacity exceeded patient meal orders on night shift afforded the hospital the opportunity to create a "Night Shift Menu," from which staff can order meals after the café closes at 6:30 PM. This service consistently surprises new hires, who immediately take note of Kadlec's commitment not only to nourishing its patients but also to caring for its caregivers!

CONTRIBUTED BY CHELENE CAMPBELL, KADLEC MEDICAL CENTER

FOR EXAMPLE

International Menus

Swedish Covenant Hospital (SCH) is located in one of the North Side of Chicago's most ethnically diverse areas. Though the areas surrounding the hospital continue to be home to the descendants of the Swedish and German immigrants that first settled there, the neighborhoods are also home to many Korean, Hispanic, and Indian-Muslim residents. The area's population demographics are evidenced in the hospital's patient population.

Cognizant of every patient's cultural and religious identity, as well as of the impact that food can have on a patient's ability to heal, SCH administration tasked its Patient Food Services Department with developing recipes for the comfort foods of the hospital's Korean, Hispanic, and Indian-Muslim patients.

With many of these cuisines markedly different from traditional American cooking, the hospital's cooks were largely unfamiliar with the ingredients and cooking techniques that would be necessary to prepare these international menus. Nonetheless, it became obvious early on that using frozen or shelf-stable entrees were not viable options. Although they may have been effective in ensuring consistency, they were lacking in flavor. This first became evident in Korean maternity patients' reactions to the traditional seaweed soup they were served shortly after giving birth to regain their strength. Originally, Patient Food Services made this soup from a powdered mix; however, Korean patients expressed concern about the taste. Clearly, taste and authenticity could not be sacrificed for consistency and convenience.

In the development of all three menus—Korean, Hispanic, and Indian—authenticity was ensured by engaging hospital staff representing those cultures in sharing recipes and taste-testing every menu item. Today, thanks in large part to the input of SCH's Korean interpreter, the hospital's Korean menu features traditional specialties, like Korean barbeque beef, sticky rice, bi bim bap (pickled vegetables and rice with chili pepper seasoning and a fried egg), and of course, seaweed soup. Its Hispanic menu was informed in part by the Hispanic Nurse Liaison on staff and features regional cuisines on a seven-day rotation. One day might feature the Puerto Rican specialty lechon con gandules arroz (roast pork with rice and pigeon peas, seasoned with sofrito), and the next, stewed beef and plantains from the Dominican Republic. And with key leadership from a staff dietitian from Pakistan, cooks were taught to prepare authentic Indian dishes, like dal tadka (lentils seasoned with curry, green chili, garlic, and cumin, served with white rice or Indian flat bread), vegetable and chicken curry, chana masala (chickpeas seasoned with onion, tomatoes, and garam masala—a blend of Indian spices), and vegetable biryani (basmati rice, vegetables, and yogurt, seasoned with Indian spices).

The International Menu program at Swedish Covenant Hospital has been in place for over ten years, and it continues to be one of the hospital's most successful initiatives, with over eight hundred international dishes served a month. Most items on all three menus are prepared from scratch and use organic ingredients where possible. Menus are translated into the appropriate languages, and the response from patients has been overwhelmingly positive. Many state that "the food tastes like food from home."

CONTRIBUTED BY MARIA L. SIMMONS, SWEDISH COVENANT HOSPITAL

REFERENCES

Katz, D. L. Time Magazine/ABC News Summit on Obesity. Williamsburg, Va.: June 2004.

Katz, D. L., and Gonzalez, M. H. *The Way to Eat*. Naperville, Ill.: Sourcebooks, 2002.

Reinke, K., and Ryczek, C. "Nutrition: The Nurturing Aspects of Food." In S. B. Frampton, L. Gilpin, and P. A. Charmel (eds.), *Putting Patients First: Designing and Practicing Patient-Centered Care*. San Francisco: Jossey-Bass, 2003.

ADDITIONAL SOURCES

Albert, N. M. "We Are What We Eat: Women and Diet for Cardiovascular Health." *Journal of Cardiovascular Nursing,* Nov.–Dec. 2005, *20*(6), 451–460.

Alvarez-Leon, E. E., Roman-Vinas, B., and Serra-Majem, L. "Dairy Products and Health: A Review of the Epidemiological Evidence." *British Journal of Nutrition,* Aug. 2006, *96*(Suppl. 1), S94–S99.

Bazzano, L. A., Serdula, M. K., and Liu, S. "Dietary Intake of Fruits and Vegetables and Risk of Cardiovascular Disease." *Current Atherosclerosis Reports,* Nov. 2003, *5*(6), 492–499.

Bengmark, S. "Impact of Nutrition on Aging and Disease." *Current Opinion in Clinical Nutrition and Metabolic Care,* Jan. 2006, *9*(1), 2–7.

Chahoud, G., Aude, Y. W., and Mehta, J. L. "Dietary Recommendations in the Prevention and Treatment of Coronary Heart Disease: Do We Have the Ideal Diet Yet?" *American Journal of Cardiology,* Nov. 2004, *94*(10), 1260–1267.

Cordain, L., and others. "Origins and Evolution of the Western Diet: Health Implications for the Twenty-First Century." *American Journal of Clinical Nutrition,* Feb. 2005, *81*(2), 341–354.

"Diet, Nutrition and the Prevention of Chronic Diseases." *World Health Organization Technical Report Series,* 2003, *916,* i–viii, 1–149.

Ding, E. L., and Mozaffarian, D. "Optimal Dietary Habits for the Prevention of Stroke." *Seminars in Neurology,* Feb. 2006, *26*(1), 11–23.

Dwyer, J. "Starting Down the Right Path: Nutrition Connections with Chronic Diseases of Later Life." *American Journal of Clinical Nutrition,* Feb. 2006, *83*(2), 415s–420s.

Giugliano, D., Ceriello, A., Esposito, K. "The Effects of Diet on Inflammation: Emphasis on the Metabolic Syndrome." *Journal of the American College of Cardiology,* 2006, *48*(4), 677–685.

Holmes, S. "Nutrition and the Prevention of Cancer." *Journal of Family Health Care,* 2006, *16*(2), 43–46.

Howard, B. V., and others. "Low-Fat Dietary Pattern and Risk of Cardiovascular Disease: The Women's Health Initiative Randomized Controlled Dietary Modification Trial." *Journal of the American Medical Association,* 2006, *295*(6), 655–666.

Hu, F. B., and Willett, W. C. "Diet and Coronary Heart Disease: Findings from the Nurses' Health Study and Health Professionals' Follow-up Study." *Journal of Nutrition, Health and Aging,* 2001, *5*(3), 132–138.

Hu, F. B., and Willett, W. C. "Optimal Diets for Prevention of Coronary Heart Disease." *Journal of the American Medical Association,* 2002, *288*(20), 2569–2578.

Jolly, C. A. "Diet Manipulation and Prevention of Aging, Cancer and Autoimmune Disease." *Current Opinion in Clinical Nutrition and Metabolic Care,* 2005, *8*(4), 382–387.

Katz, D. L. "Pandemic Obesity and the Contagion of Nutritional Nonsense." *Public Health Review,* 2003, *31*(1), 33–44.

Katz, D. L. "Competing Dietary Claims for Weight Loss: Finding the Forest Through Truculent Trees." *Annual Review of Public Health,* 2005, *26,* 61–88.

Katz, D. L. *"Dietary Recommendations for Health Promotion and Disease Prevention."* In D. L. Katz with R.S.C. Friedman (eds.), *Nutrition in Clinical Practice.* (2nd ed.) Philadelphia: Lippincott, 2008.

Kennedy, E. T. "Evidence for Nutritional Benefits in Prolonging Wellness." *American Journal of Clinical Nutrition,* 2006, *83*(2), 410s–414s.

Knowler, W. C. "Optimal Diet for Glycemia and Lipids." *Nestle Nutrition Workshop Series: Clinical and Performance Programme,* 2006, *11,* 97–102.

Raatz, S. "Diet and Nutrition: What Should We Eat?" *Minnesota Medicine,* 2003, *86*(11), 28–33.

Reddy, K. S., and Katan, M. B. "Diet, Nutrition and the Prevention of Hypertension and Cardiovascular Diseases." *Public Health Nutrition,* 2004, *7*(1a), 167–186.

Schaefer, E. J. "Lipoproteins, Nutrition, and Heart Disease." *American Journal of Clinical Nutrition,* 2002, *75*(2), 191–212.

Uauy, R., and Solomons, N. "Diet, Nutrition, and the Life-Course Approach to Cancer Prevention." *Journal of Nutrition,* 2005, *135*(12 Suppl.), 2934s–2945s.

Walker, A. R., Walker, B. F., and Adam, F. "Nutrition, Diet, Physical Activity, Smoking, and Longevity: From Primitive Hunter-Gatherer to Present Passive Consumer—How Far Can We Go?" *Nutrition,* 2003, *19*(2), 169–173.

Willett, W. C. "Diet and Health: What Should We Eat?" *Science,* 1994, *264*(5158), 532–537.

Willett, W. C., and others. "Mediterranean Diet Pyramid: A Cultural Model for Healthy Eating." *American Journal of Clinical Nutrition,* 1995, *61,* 1402s–1406s.

Willett, W. C., and Stampfer, M. J. "Foundations of a Healthy Diet." In M. E. Shils and others (eds.), *Modern Nutrition in Health and Disease.* (10th ed.) Philadelphia: Lippincott, 2006.

Williams, M. T., and Hord, N. G. "The Role of Dietary Factors in Cancer Prevention: Beyond Fruits and Vegetables." *Nutrition in Clinical Practice,* 2005, *20*(4), 451–459.

CHAPTER

5

SPIRITUAL AND CULTURAL DIVERSITY: INNER RESOURCES FOR HEALING

STEVEN L. JEFFERS AND DENNIS KENNY

This chapter does the following:

- Presents a historical overview of the role of spirituality in medicine
- Distinguishes between the definitions of religion and spirituality and discusses the clinical relevance of each

This chapter's section on Planetree spirituality draws heavily from a chapter by G. Handzo and J. C. Wilson, "Spirituality: Inner Resources for Healing," in the first edition of *Putting Patients First* (2003).

- Describes specific patient-centered practices to integrate spirituality into patient care

- Identifies ways that caregivers can provide support and enhance spiritual growth for patients and families during end-of-life care

RELIGION, SPIRITUALITY, AND MEDICINE

I daresay that you have heard eminent physicians say to a patient who comes to them with bad eyes that they cannot cure the eyes by themselves, but if the eyes are to be cured the head must be treated. And again they say that to think of curing the head alone and not the rest of the body also is the height of folly. Arguing in this way, they apply their methods to the whole body and try to treat and heal the whole and the part together [quoted in Jowett, 1924].

These words were not written in modern times, but several hundred years Before the Common Era (BCE) by the renowned Greek philosopher Plato, who goes on to say:

I learned these lessons when serving with the army from one of the physicians of the Thracian King Zamolxis, who said, "As you ought not to attempt to cure the eyes without the head or the head without the body, so neither ought you to attempt to cure the body without the soul." And this is the reason why the cure of many diseases is unknown to the physicians of Greece, because they are ignorant of the whole which ought to be studied also, for the part can never be well unless the whole is well. Therefore, if the head and body are to be well, you must begin by curing the soul [quoted in Jowett, 1924].

Herophilus, a physician who lived in Alexandria, Egypt, in the third century BCE stated, "When health is absent, wisdom cannot reveal itself, art cannot become manifest, strength cannot be exerted, wealth is useless and reason is powerless" (Citation of Herophilus extracted from wall in Kansas City, Missouri, Department of Public Health Building) (Von Staden, 1989).

These notable figures from antiquity affirm that human well-being involves more than good physical health. It includes a number of dimensions, the physical being only one of them; one need also include mental, emotional, spiritual, professional, financial, and relational dimensions.

Numerous cultures, early in their history, have thought of illness, disease, and health as more than simply the physical aspect of humankind. Therefore, when "physicians" approached healing in distinct ways—some addressing the spiritual component and others dealing with the bodily features—their practices were not antithetical to each other. Illness and health were viewed in ways that encompassed the spiritual and the physical needs of those who were ill. Medicine and spirituality were linked as complementary avenues to healing rather than as separate entities.

Things began to change, though, when both early Greek dualistic philosophy (the viewpoint of seeing the mind and body as separate) and dualistic Christian thought (as found in some of the writings of the apostles Paul and John) interacted in such a way as to enable a split between bodily and spiritual spheres. (This viewpoint was later deemed heretical by the Christian Church through the statements generated by the Church Councils beginning in the fourth century CE.) As this rift between matters of the spirit and those of the body became more apparent in Western intellectual history, the spiritual and physical domains became further distinguished, opposed, isolated, and mutually exclusive.

One cannot underestimate the impact of the scientific revolution on views of illness, health, and the further separation of medicine and spirituality. With the inauguration of the biomedical model, physicians were trained first and foremost as scientists (Droege, 1991). In the nineteenth century, technological progress in medicine allied with scientific methodology and empowered medicine with heightened authority over matters of religion and spirituality, now increasingly viewed as abiding in the realm of *nonscience*. At the same time, stricter accreditation requirements enabled lay persons to achieve their medical licenses so that lay persons as degreed professionals, not clergy or nuns, soon became the healers. All of this caused a wall between faith and medicine to be erected that existed for hundreds of years, especially in Western medicine. This fissure between body and spirit, however, was less prominent in numerous other cultures and traditions. For instance, Asian cultures and traditions managed to preserve a perspective of the human as a unity of body and spirit, so that they generally did not and do not view illness and disease as the exclusive preoccupation of scientific medicine. Asian societies continued to endorse the compatibility of both traditional approaches to healing that assume the primacy of spirituality as a necessary ingredient in healing and medicine that tends to rely more on the physiological character of illness causation and healing. Whether it concerns the weight of *karma* (in Hindu and Buddhist traditions), *kami* (divine forces of nature in Japanese Shinto), or *shaman* as priest and healer, Asian worldviews continued to assume an integration of human, natural, and spiritual. However, the twentieth century began a renewed interest in the importance of religion and spirituality in medicine. This may well help explain the interest shown in Eastern spirituality late in that century and into the present. In many Eastern cultures, medical practices did not separate the care of the body, mind, and spirit as was done in the West. In the mid-1990s, at the Institute for Health and Healing at California Pacific Medical Center in San Francisco, a former physician to the Dalai Lama presented a several-week, sold-out course on Tibetan medicine. In a question-and-answer period, the doctor, also a Buddhist monk, was asked to explain how the body, mind, and spirit worked in caring for patients in Tibetan medicine. After a pause, the interpreter shared with the audience that the physician "did not understand the question." The question was clarified and asked again, but the response was the same. One could conclude from the conversation that the Tibetan physician did not see a distinction among the various aspects; he saw a harmonious whole. With this historical overview in mind, we shift our attention to defining terms and discussing their role in the health care setting.

DEFINITIONS OF RELIGION AND SPIRITUALITY

Why are definitions important? Are not *religion* and *spirituality* synonymous? Many would answer yes. Others make a distinction between the two words, which is reflected in the statement, "I am spiritual, but not religious," though the meaning of that quotation can vary from person to person. However, the point is that there is a difference. In the health care setting, it is important to make that distinction clear for several reasons: (1) to serve the needs of the *religious* and the *nonreligious,* (2) religious patients often have spiritual, not necessarily religious, needs (for instance, Scripture, ritual, and so forth), and (3) some patients are mad at God and equate God with religion.

One way of understanding religion is that it is the discovery of how to live in the world. Individuals order their lives based on the prescriptions and proscriptions of religious teachings. It is their responses to experiences of the holy as they seek to understand, honor, and share them. Religion can also be defined as a system of *symbols, beliefs, myths* and *rites* experienced as profoundly significant, primarily because it provides individuals, groups, and societies with a means of drawing close to and in oneness with God (material obtained in a personal communication with Dr. E. Taylor regarding her course Spiritual Dimensions in Healthcare, at University of Southern California, Department of Nursing, 2000).

Dale Matthews, MD, has described religion as being more focused on establishing community, more objective and measurable to the external observer, more formal in worship, more based in behavior, and more focused on outward practices; religion can be more authoritarian, with patterns of prescribed and proscribed behavior, more particularizing, distinguishing one group from another, and more orthodox and systematic in doctrine (Matthews, 1998, p. 183). Suffice it to say that religion is something one chooses.

In contrast, spirituality is broader in its import. It can be understood as that inner source that energizes people with significance, the capacity to discern meaning in anything they experience. Even if a person cannot walk physically, the metaphorical language of Edward Canda points the way: "Spirituality is the way to walk in a sacred manner, to walk in harmony with the beauty all around us and within us" (personal interview, November 2006). Dennis Kenny (2002) refers to spirituality as a "spiritual covenant or agreement with our higher power that is sustainable in crisis, abundance and investigation" (p. 30). He has seen *spiritual covenants* in his health care ministry as a primary factor in the health and illness of the patients he has served. Rigid spiritual covenants are not helpful and may be contributing factors in the development of illness, noncompliance with medical orders, and a negative influence on healing. Flexible, sustainable covenants can be major contributors to healing, helping the adjustment to the situation contribute to making meaning of the experience and helping the person participate in treatment.

As most people have developed some form of spirituality (whether they use this term or not), it is important to recognize that spirituality is a way of being that determines how people respond to what they experience in life. A person's spirituality assists the decision-making process to incorporate personal values and beliefs. Ian Mitroff (letter to the author, 1999) has identified several characteristics of spirituality through his interviews with many people in preparation for writing a book on spirituality, which he identified as:

- Universal and timeless

- Broadly inclusive

- Ultimate source and provider of meaning and purpose to life

- Sacredness of everything

- Integrally connected to inner peace and calm

- Expression of awe felt in the presence of the transcendent
- Provision for inexhaustible source of faith

Kenneth Pargament (2001) agrees with Kenny when he says, "Spirituality is not necessarily about God, and yet spirituality is a search for the sacred." Steve Jeffers (2005), who concurs with Pargament and Kenny, offers this definition:

> *Spirituality, often expressed in a cultural or religious tradition, is the constituent of people's being that provides the framework for their understanding of life's purpose and meaning, their sense of well-being and their relationships with humanity and the divine. It is a determining factor in how individuals explain and react to life events. Spirituality is an important element in patients' and families' ability to find answers to questions of meaning and purpose in life as well as enable them to cope with illness, dying and death. Spirituality is an indispensable component of quality, holistic healthcare. This is the definition of spirituality written and utilized by the Institute for Spirituality in Health of Shawnee Mission Medical Center, a regional medical center in the suburbs of Kansas City.*

It is important to notice in both definitions that there is no specific mention of God or religion, yet the definition can be embraced by any person, religious or nonreligious.

What is the relationship, if any, between religion and spirituality? One way to answer the question is to say that spirituality is not a religion, and yet it is Baha'i, Buddhist, Christian, Hindu, Islamic, Jewish, Sikh, in the sense that these are historically important ways in which it has been experienced and celebrated. Religion is one way in which people express their spirituality. Both spirituality, which pertains to healthy, spiritual covenants that foster ultimate purpose and meaning in life, and religion, which pertains to expressions of faith and belief, have clinical relevance.

FOR EXAMPLE

Banner Health—Page Hospital's Hogan

Located in Northern Arizona, Page Hospital is surrounded by the Navajo Nation and other Native American tribes. Native American medicine men have often visited Native American patients at the hospital, but they were unable to authentically perform traditional healing ceremonies because of their use of fire and smoke. Often patients would go outside or into their cars to complete the ceremony.

Understanding the importance of these ceremonies to Native American patients, staff at Page Hospital formed the Native American Cultural Committee (NACC) to investigate the potential for building a traditional hogan on-site. The Navajo family's traditional dwelling, the hogan, is constructed according to instructions found in the Navajo creation story. They are designated male or female according to their shape; have six or eight sides constructed of wooden poles, tree bark, and mud; have dome-shaped ceilings; and have a doorway that opens to the East so inhabitants can greet the morning sun. The earthen floor symbolizes Mother Earth and the round roof Father Sky. Hogans are considered sacred to those who live traditionally, and although most Navajos now live in modern homes, many still use hogans ceremonially.

With the support of physicians and the Native American community secured, the NACC set forth on its journey to construct a hogan on-site but faced a number of setbacks related to city codes and the use of fire inside buildings, a necessity for a traditional hogan. Hope for realizing the project ultimately came in the form of a gazebo that could easily be transformed into a hogan by enclosing the half-walls with custom-made tarps. By using a gazebo that was not a permanently enclosed structure, the NACC had hit upon a solution that satisfied the city codes while also incorporating the significant aspects of a traditional hogan, including the shape, use of wood, opening in the roof, and eastern-facing entrance. The fire issue was resolved by using a portable stove. Located in one of the hospital's beautiful healing gardens, the gazebo also serves as a serene space for the hospital's non-Native American patients and visitors.

Page Hospital's hogan was completed five years after the idea was first conceived and has affected the hospital in many ways. The number of Native Americans choosing to receive their health care at Page has increased, with many attributing their decision to having heard from family or another tribe member that the hospital honors Native American traditional practices. Beyond honoring the cultural diversity of patients, experiences suggest that such practices may also positively affect clinical outcomes. At Page, medicine men have had an approximate 80 percent success rate turning breech babies, averting the need for C-sections, and have been approximately 50 percent successful in advancing labor for women who have failed to progress, again eliminating the need for a C-section.

At Page, facilitating traditional ceremonies to be performed has been a way to provide personalized care that honors patients' beliefs. Patients and family members have consistently expressed their gratitude for the opportunity to practice these meaningful cultural traditions.

CONTRIBUTED BY MICHELE GRIM, PAGE HOSPITAL

IMPORTANCE OF RELIGION AND SPIRITUALITY IN HEALTH CARE

In order to lay a proper foundation for the clinical relevance of religion and spirituality, it seems prudent to return to the words of Plato found in the opening section: "And this is the reason why the cure of many diseases is unknown to the physicians of Greece, because they are ignorant of the whole which ought to be studied also, for the part can never be well unless the whole is well" (quoted in Jowett, 1924).

Study the whole? Cure the soul? What is meant by such questions?

The *head* and the *body* are studied routinely in the medical community. Psychiatry, internal medicine, and the various subspecialties are accepted as standard medical practice. But according to the ancient philosopher Plato and many modern people as well, the *whole* is composed of three constituent parts, not two. Spirit, or *soul,* as it is often called, is the completing element of the triad.

It seems logical to conclude, then, that the study of the whole should include the study of the soul in conjunction with the study of the mental and physical aspects of humankind. Is it even possible, though, to study the soul? If so, is it important to consider such a study?

Consider the following assertions: "Disease forges an especially close relationship between God and man; the Divine Presence Itself, as It were, rests on the head of the sickbed," said the late Immanuel Jakobovits, the former Chief Rabbi of the British Commonwealth of Nations (quoted in Post and others, 2000). Similarly, Ram Dass (2000), former professor at Harvard University and author of *Still Here,* among his other writings, stated that "Facing dread of the future is an excellent vehicle for entering into the spiritual dimension" (Dass, 2000, p. 133). From the medical community come these words of Christina Puchalski, MD: "Spirituality is the essence of what makes us human. It is important to recognize this dimension in healthcare" (personal communication, 2003).

According to these and many other individuals who would posit the indissoluble relationship among body, mind, and spirit, study of the soul seems of paramount importance, and attention to the spiritual dimension should be an integral component of a patient's assessment and plan of care and treatment.

Currently, the renewed interest in things of the spirit has a tendency to focus on the spiritual resources of the person being treated and how they might be a support in the healing or coping process. This is the emphasis of both diagnosis and treatment. This is a subtle way of keeping spirituality as a separate (but possibly not equal) component of the healing process. The harder and riskier work of integration is the task. This may require closer looks at the role spirituality plays in illness, as well as the role it plays in supporting the physical healing process. This is the major lesson other cultures have taught the West, as illustrated by the approach taken in Tibetan medicine, as discussed earlier. Illness is an illness of the whole person. Healing happens to the entire person, and if that is the case, then treating the spirit as adjunct or supportive misses the point of integration. "If we do not treat all of the person as we perform surgeries or give medications, then we will see that person again," said an internationally known cardiac surgeon when discussing the role of spirituality in healing.

In the mid-1900s *studying the whole,* to use Plato's nomenclature, became an academic exercise in prestigious university-based medical centers across the United States, in places like Duke (Koenig, 1999; 2001a; 2001b) and George Washington University (Puchalski, 2000, 2001). Similarly, the Cleveland Clinic, the Mayo Clinic (Koenig, 2001c), California Pacific Medical Center's Institute for Health and Healing, and Shawnee Mission Medical Center's Institute for Spirituality in Health also advocate for the importance of the role of spirituality in health. These and many other institutions engaged in research to determine, scientifically, the relationship between spirituality, physical health, and mental health.

The results were overwhelmingly conclusive in many of the scientific studies and clinical trials, showing that patient spirituality enhances the body's healing process, facilitates greater coping abilities, and contributes to one's overall sense of well-being. Examples of this are numerous. A meta-analysis of forty-two studies by McCullough and others (2000), involving over a hundred thousand individuals, indicated that deeply spiritual people have a 29 percent greater survival rate after hospitalization when compared with less-religious persons. One study showed that secular Jewish individuals had a greater propensity for a first myocardial infarction than Orthodox Jews (Friedlander, 1986), and another study of 157 hospitalized adults experiencing moderate to severe pain reported that prayer was second only to pain medications (76 percent versus 82 percent) in pain management (McNeil and others, 1998). Another study involving 1,620 people with cancer and HIV found that a sense of spiritual well-being in the patients was the single most important predictor of a health-related quality of life apart from physical, emotional, and social well-being (Brady and others, 1999). Another study consisting of 100 men with HIV demonstrated that an increase in spirituality slowed the progression of HIV over four years (Ironson, Stuetzie, and Fletcher, 2006). Spirituality has also been found to be significantly correlated to better physical health, mental health, sexual function, and fewer urinary problems in men with prostate cancer (Krupski and others, 2006). In a study with 309 cardiac patients, religion was demonstrated to reduce postoperative psychological distress through positive religious coping (Ai and others, 2007). Several studies demonstrate religion in helping patients cope with depression (Koenig, George, and Peterson, 1998; Koenig and others, 1992). People's religious beliefs do affect how they experience various maladies (Graber and Johnson, 2001; Mueller and others, 2001; Curlin, Lawrence, Chin, and Lantos, 2007; Conlon, 2006).

What, then, does all of this mean for physicians and other health care providers? Without question, illness, dying, and death raise the awareness of God and often cause crises of faith for many patients and their families. For this reason, being intentional in initiating appropriate spiritual interventions is a necessity in providing quality holistic care. Therefore, the *journey to excellence* in patient care must not only include evidence-based medical practices but also evidence-based spiritual care practices.

But the research must not be an end unto itself. In order to provide optimal care for patients and their families, there needs to be an increase in the number of clinically trained clergy and lay people. In addition, physicians and other health care providers must become cognizant of the importance of spirituality in reducing morbidity and mortality and be willing to receive training in the art of identifying and addressing the spiritual concerns of patients. Discussing advance care planning, utilizing a spiritual history assessment tool, and having a heart-to-heart conversation are examples of ways to initiate dialogue with a patient about spiritual matters (Jeffers and others, 2005; Puchalski and Romer, 2000; Lo and others, 1999; Kuhn, 1988; Maugans, 1996; Anandarajah and Hight, 2001). As we increase our abilities and scrutiny of our practices along with engagement in research, the medical community will increasingly come to view spiritual care providers as partners in the healing process.

Centre de réadaptation Estrie

At the Centre de réadaptation Estrie (CRE), a rehabilitation hospital in Sherbrooke, Quebec, spirituality plays a vital role in the rehabilitation process, as is evidenced by one patient's story.

Antoine, a courier, loved his work, especially the endless challenges to meet customer expectations. No matter how short the deadline, he always found a way to deliver his parcel on time. One day, he hit a tree head-on while attempting a risky passing. He woke up in a hospital bed, hooked up to sophisticated machines, unable to comprehend why and how his life had changed so drastically. Antoine began his rehabilitation in the Neuro-traumatology Program of the Centre de réadaptation Estrie. Like many other victims of craniocerebral trauma, he had little understanding of his cognitive losses. He expected to return to work as soon as the injuries to his feet were healed and firmly believed that he would be able to take up where he had left off. Antoine's broken bones did heal, but despite his progress he still was not allowed to drive. After several unsuccessful attempts, he finally understood that never again would he be able to do the work that had meant so much to him.

As part of the CRE rehabilitation process, Antoine completed a questionnaire called Ariadne's Thread, through which he shared his past experiences, his beliefs and values, dreams, and aspirations. Once all of these elements were considered collectively, his social worker identified the *thread* of his life. "Look Antoine," he was told, "ever since childhood, what has mattered most to you is making other people happy. You want to be of service, a bit like your grandfather whom you admire for his work with disaster victims. This is the 'thread' that has always guided your life."

From this experience, Antoine became aware that over all those years, the desire to help others and to excel had been his deepest motivations. His work as a courier had allowed him to be of service to people. This understanding did not happen overnight. Antoine spent many hours

FOR EXAMPLE

mulling things over in the Inukshuk room, sometimes alone, sometimes in the company of his *guides,* as he called his therapists. The CRE's Inukshuk room is a place of spirituality, named after the stone constructions that guide the Inuit through unfamiliar territory. The Inukshuk room is a refuge, a beacon, a landmark for anyone on the journey into self.

Today, Antoine has taken control of his life. It is no longer speed and last-minute challenges that bring him satisfaction, but the gratitude shown by his customers. Like his grandfather, he has chosen to become an insurance adjuster. Antoine's story is only one among many of CRE patients who in the aftermath of misfortune have lost the meaning of life but have found it again on the path to rehabilitation. Recognizing the importance of the spiritual dimension to rehabilitation, CRE offers employee workshops that allow them to reflect on their own search for meaning and then explore spirituality as a resource in the rehabilitation process.

CONTRIBUTED BY JOCELYN CHOUINARD AND JOHANNE TARDIF,
CENTRE DE RÉADAPTATION ESTRIE

SPIRITUALITY IN THE CARE OF THE DYING

Your world has been shattered. You have been told by your physician that you have an incurable, life-limiting illness. As a result, multiple and persisting emotions arise: disbelief, shock, anger, sadness, fear. Questions begin to flood your thoughts. What does all of this mean? Why is this happening to me? How long do I have? Is there any hope for a cure? Will dying be painful? Who will take care of my family? How long will I be able to work? What will my friends and work colleagues think? Will I ever see any of them again? Will people miss me when I am gone? Is God trying to tell me something in all of this? God, why are you doing this to me?

These and many other questions are not uncommon when people are confronted with their own mortality. The last two in the litany indicate that spiritual concerns are one of the many concerns that people have during times of critical illness, in the dying process, and about the aftermath of death. Spirituality significantly influences the mental and physical aspects of both living and dying. Spirituality, though, is not static, but rather dynamic. It has multiple facets, and they are expressed in a variety of ways during the course of the dying process. These spiritual needs that can arise at any time provide opportunities for spiritual growth, which can be and often is stimulated in times of critical illness and dying. Professional caregivers interested in providing holistic, patient-centered care to patients and families should be looking for ways to enhance spiritual growth made possible by the onset of serious illnesses and the prospect of dying. One way to accomplish this is to facilitate a process for dialogue among patients and families of the four common concerns of the terminally ill: (1) regrets, (2) unfinished business, (3) celebration of life, and (4) spiritual and religious matters.

It is also helpful to incorporate Dr. Ira Byock's five elements of relationship completion into that conversation: (1) I forgive you, (2) you forgive me, (3) I love you, (4) thank you, and (5) good-bye (1997, p. 140). Helping the dying and their families verbalize these issues is a priceless gift to them during a dark time in their lives.

Finally, many people simply fear bad dying, which includes not saying good-bye, not planning ahead, not arranging personal affairs, and not decreasing family burden. In fact, these things are often feared more than death itself. The professional caregiver can help the patient and family avoid a bad dying experience by attending to the multifaceted spiritual needs that arise during end of life. This can usually be accomplished by facilitating dialogue to include the four common concerns, five elements of relationship completion, and any other relevant concerns. Spiritual care is about helping the dying and their families work through religious and spiritual issues, as well as other issues and questions, in order to help facilitate a *good death,* which can be described as follows:

- Death without pain

- Death with family present

- Death at home or in familiar surroundings

- Death without prolongation of dying

- Death without financial burden

- Death with reconciled relationships

- Death having made a difference in life

The period between the diagnosis and death can be one of chaos, fear, and bewilderment. It can also be a time of restful peace, encouraging hope, and overpowering love. Individuals can forgive and be forgiven, give and receive thanks, address any regrets, take care of unfinished business, discuss spiritual issues, and take advantage of the opportunity to express sincere, heartfelt, gentle good-byes. This is the ultimate goal of patient-centered care.

PLANETREE SPIRITUALITY

All Planetree affiliates start with an understanding that patient care encompasses mind, body, and spirit, but each affiliate addresses spiritual care differently. Most have an interfaith chapel, sanctuary, or meditation space that provides a sacred and quiet space for patients, families, and employees. To acknowledge the important role of caregivers, many Planetree affiliates have established a ritual for the Blessing of Hands, which is provided by going throughout the hospital to include all the staff. For some affiliates, this is part of the Planetree retreat.

The chaplain at Columbia Memorial Hospital developed a series of classes for interested staff members, to help them become more aware of the impact that spirituality has on health and well-being. The three one-hour sessions include experiential exercises, discussions on the difference between spirituality and religion, and an overview of world religions. The purpose of the classes is to give staff members greater insight into their own spirituality so that they can be more attentive to the spiritual needs of the patients.

Banner Health System, which includes health care facilities in Arizona and Colorado, has developed a variety of creative means for addressing spiritual care. A portable labyrinth, used for meditation, can be taken to various sites. In one setting within Banner, the Clinical Pastoral Education program obtained grant monies to create a pastoral and spiritual training program for bilingual Hispanic chaplains. This special initiative enabled the program to better meet the spiritual needs of the third of its patients who are Spanish-speaking.

In another Banner facility, a chaplain (who is of the Sikh tradition) created a beautiful banner with the words "Let us pray" in the twenty different languages spoken by the staff members. People were invited to a ritual where they were asked to write "Let us pray" in their native language. The banner was hung in the chapel, and a photograph of it was made into a bookmark to be given to all patients.

The hospice at Wellmont Bristol Regional Medical Center in Bristol, Tennessee, has linked with local churches to provide support for hospice families and caregivers. Each month, a different church stocks the family kitchen with snack foods and staples and provides care packages for all patients in the hospice program—both inpatients and outpatients. Prayer cards are provided for patients as well as for the hospice staff, often with the name of the church member who is praying for them. At Wellmont Holston Valley Medical Center in Kingsport, Tennessee, patients who choose to be admitted to an *intensive prayer unit* can include prayer in their plan of care.

Many Planetree members have implemented a White Rose program to honor patients who have died. After a death, a white silk rose is placed on the patient's pillow, privacy curtain, or door, out of respect for the patient and as a means of communicating to other caregivers that a death has occurred. The rose is then given to the family as a keepsake. Other sites provide spiritual care twenty-four hours a day, seven days a week, through a volunteer chaplain service. Local pastors rotate as the on-call chaplain and also provide Sunday and holiday services for those who may be unable to attend regular services.

Patient care is by its very nature spiritual. Although Planetree hospitals differ in how they address the spiritual needs of patients, families, and staff members, being sensitive to traditions and cultures, as well as to religious and spiritual practices, is a primary goal.

ORGANIZATIONS AND THEIR SPIRITUALITY

Individuals have functional spirituality that defines meaning for them, acts as a major influence in decision making, and defines failures and successes. In their own way, organizations also have spiritual principles by which they live (Kenny, 2002), and these principles (developed by leaders, by history, or critical events in the life of the organization) are often so much a part of the fabric of the organization that they are not identified or evaluated in the context of the vision, mission, and goals of the organization. When these spiritual principles, though, are not identified or communicated or are not in sync with the stated mission and goals of the organization, it may become a significant source of conflict for employees, patients, and families and can thus inhibit the growth and success of an organization.

For instance, a health care organization in the South often confounded both the community and its employees by communicating that its core value was compassionate, people-centered care. Its business practices, however, were often described as "cutthroat." The health center's functional core value was to control the regional market, eliminate all competition, and put profitability as the highest value in the organization. These are not necessarily bad practices, in and of themselves, but they caused practices that were antithetical to the stated core values of the hospital.

Health care professionals and the organizations to which they belong can put effort into identifying the spiritual principles that guide them. If they do that and match them with mission and goals and their functional decision making, then they may create an organization that has been aptly described by Graber and Johnson (2001, p. 48): "with proper consideration and caution by clinicians and managers, a truly 'spiritual' health care organization can be developed: one that supports patients' expressions of faith; provides guidance and direction to staff on how to discuss faith, health and meaning in illness; encourages staff and clinicians to be warm, caring and sensitive; and supports individuals' (patients, families, physicians and hospital employees) search for meaning and fulfillment."

Their words are consistent with the root passions and goals of Planetree in calling on organizations to match their care of patients with their stated values and mission. This commitment has helped make Planetree successful and struck a chord with many who work in health care organizations.

An important element of Planetree, throughout its history, has been issuing a clarion call to health care organizations to match their practices with their core spirituality. The desired result of such a call would be compassionate caring, patient-centered values, and *meaning-making* practices that influence the life of the organization in how it conducts business.

In conclusion, it may well be that a major task in health care in the West in the twenty-first century is a *rekindling* of an understanding of people (analogous to that of the Tibetan physician) and what makes them sick and what helps them live as fully as they can for as long as they can (Weil, 2005). This would entail a modification in the overall care of patients to incorporate the holistic approach to healing.

REFERENCES

Ai, A. L., and others. "Psychosocial Mediation of Religious Coping Styles: A Study of Short-Term Psychological Distress Following Cardiac Surgery." *Personality and Social Psychology Bulletin,* 2007, *33*(6), 867–882.

Anandarajah, G., and Hight, E. "Spirituality and Medical Practice: Using the Hope Questions as a Practical Tool for Spiritual Assessment." *American Family Physician,* 2001, *63*(1), 81–88.

Brady, M., and others. "A Case for Including Spirituality in Quality of Life Measurement in Oncology." *Oncology,* 1999, *8*, 417–428.

Byock, I. *Dying Well: The Prospect for Growth at the End of Life.* New York: Riverhead Books, 1997.

Conlon, M. "When Faith and Medicine Collide." *Reuters,* Dec. 24, 2006.

Curlin, F., Lawrence, R., Chin, M., and Lantos, J. "Religion, Conscience, and Controversial Clinical Practices." *New England Journal of Medicine,* 2007, *356*(6), 593–600.

Dass, R. *Still Here: Embracing Aging, Changing and Dying.* New York: Riverhead Books, 2000.

Droege, T. *The Faith Factor in Healing.* Philadelphia: Trinity Press, 1991.

Friedlander, Y. "Religious Orthodoxy and Myocardial Infarction in Jerusalem: A Case Control Study." *International Journal of Cardiology,* 1986, *10*, 33–41.

Graber, D., and Johnson, J. "Spirituality and Healthcare Organizations." *Journal of Healthcare Management,* 2001, *46*(1), 39–50.

Handzo, G., and Wilson, J. C. "Spirituality: Inner Resources for Healing." In S. B. Frampton, L. Gilpin, and P. A. Charmel (eds.), *Putting Patients First: Designing and Practicing Patient-Centered Care.* San Francisco: Jossey-Bass, 2003.

Ironson, G., Stuetzie, R., and Fletcher, M. A. "An Increase in Religiousness/Spirituality Occurs After HIV Diagnosis and Predicts Slower Disease Progression Over 4 Years in People with HIV." *Journal of General Internal Medicine,* 2006, *2*, S62–S68.

Jakobovits, I. *Jewish Medical Ethics: A Comparative and Historical Study of the Jewish Religious Attitude to Medicine and Its Practice.* New York: Block, 1975.

Jeffers, S., and others. "Patients and Spirituality." *The Leading Edge,* winter 2005, *2*(1). [www.acpe.org/publications/PEJ/index.aspx].

Jowett, B. "Charmides." *The Dialogues of Plato.* Vol. 1. New York: Oxford University Press, 1924.

Kenny, D. *Promise of the Soul.* New York: Wiley, 2002.

Koenig, H. *The Healing Power of Faith.* New York: Simon & Schuster, 1999.

Koenig, H. "Religion and Medicine IV: Religion, Physical Health and Clinical Implications." *International Journal of Psychiatry in Medicine,* 2001a, *31*(3), 321–336.

Koenig, H. *Spirituality in Patient Care.* Pennsylvania: Templeton Foundation Press, 2001b.

Koenig, H. "Religion, Spirituality and Medicine: How Are They Related and What Does It Mean?" *Mayo Clinic Proceedings,* 2001c, *76*(12), 1189–1191.

Koenig, H. G., George, L., and Peterson, B. "Religiosity and Remission from Depression in Medically Ill Older Patients." *American Journal of Psychiatry,* 1998, *155*, 536–542.

Koenig, H. G., and others. "Religious Coping and Depression in Elderly Hospitalized Medically Ill Men." *American Journal of Psychiatry,* 1992, *149*, 1693–1700.

Krupski, T., and others. "Spirituality Influences Health Related Quality of Life in Men with Prostate Cancer." *Psychooncology,* 2006, *15*, 121–131.

Kuhn, C. "A Spiritual Inventory of the Medically Ill Patient." *Psychiatric Medicine,* 1988, *6*(2), 87–100.

Lo, B., and others. "Discussing Palliative Care with Patients." *Annals of Internal Medicine,* 1999, *130*(9), 744–749.

Matthews, D. *The Faith Factor.* New York: Penguin Group, 1998.

Maugans, T. "The SPIRITual History." *Archives of Family Medicine,* 1996, *5,* 11–16.

McCullough, M., and others. "Religious Involvement and Mortality: A Meta-Analytic Review." *Health Psychology,* 2000, *19,* 211–222.

McNeil, J., and others. "Assessing Clinical Outcomes: Patient Satisfaction with Pain Management." *Journal of Pain and Symptom Management,* 1998, *16,* 29–40.

Mitroff, I. *A Spiritual Audit of Corporate America.* San Francisco: Jossey-Bass, 1999.

Mueller, P., and others. "Religious Involvement, Spirituality and Medicine: Implications for Clinical Practice." *Mayo Clinic Proceedings,* 2001, *76,* 1225–1235.

Pargament, K. "God Help Me: Spirituality as a Resource in Self-Care." Care for the Caregiver Bioethics Conference, Loma Linda University, Loma Linda, California, 2001.

Post, S., Puchalski, C., and Larson, D. "Physicians and Patient Spirituality: Professional Boundaries, Competency and Ethics." *Annals of Internal Medicine,* 2000, *132*(7), 578–583.

Puchalski, C. "Physicians and Patient Spirituality: Professional Boundaries, Competency and Ethics." *Annals of Internal Medicine,* 2000, *132*(7), 578–583.

Puchalski, C. "Spirituality and Health: The Art of Compassionate Medicine." *Hospital Physician,* 2001, *37*(3), 30–36.

Puchalski, C., and Romer, A. "Taking a Spiritual History Allows Clinicians to Understand Patients More Fully." *Journal of Palliative Medicine,* 2000, *3*(1), 129–137.

Puchalski, C. "Institute for Spirituality in Health" [brochure]. Shawnee Mission, Kan.: Shawnee Mission Medical Center, 2003.

Von Staden, H. (ed.). *The Art of Medicine in Early Alexandria.* London: Cambridge University Press, 1989.

Weil, A. *Healthy Aging: A Lifelong Guide to Your Physical and Spiritual Well-Being.* New York: Knopf, 2005.

CHAPTER

6

INTEGRATING COMPLEMENTARY AND ALTERNATIVE PRACTICES INTO CONVENTIONAL CARE

DAVID L. KATZ AND ATHER ALI

This chapter does the following:

- Defines complementary and alternative (CAM) medicine
- Asserts that access to CAM treatments is an important means of patient empowerment

- Addresses the implications of the increasing use of CAM modalities
- Discusses the value of an integrative approach to care
- Presents examples of CAM modalities being integrated into inpatient and outpatient care at Planetree sites

Historically, the Planetree model has advocated for patient choice and the availability of time-honored approaches to health care in combination with the best practices offered by conventional Western medicine. Over the last two decades, many Planetree hospitals have incorporated a variety of treatment modalities in response to patient interest. This interest has continued to grow throughout the Western world, fueling a multibillion-dollar complementary and alternative medicine movement (Tindle, Davis, Phillips, Eisenberg, 2005; Eisenberg and others, 1998), both within and outside the mainstream health care industry.

DEFINITION OF CAM

Complementary and Alternative Medicine (CAM) is one among the numerous designations for diverse medical practices not routinely taught to MD candidates in medical school, and not incorporated into conventional medical practice (National Center for Complementary and Alternative Medicine, Publication No. D347). Each of the terms applied to such practices is limited or objectionable in some way. *Alternative* implies both that such practices are defined by what they are not and that they are exclusive of conventional medical care. *Complementary* implies that such practices are supplemental to mainstream medicine. The inconsistency in suggesting that such practices are both alternative and complementary to conventional care has been noted (Druss and Rosenheck, 1999; Katz, 1999). Despite its shortcomings, CAM is the most widely used appellation.

Whatever term is applied, CAM practices encompass a broad range of approaches to health care that include whole medical systems, such as naturopathic medicine, chiropractic, traditional Chinese medicine, and homeopathy, as well as specific techniques, such as acupuncture, mind-body medicine, massage, and many others. Traits widely shared by CAM approaches include an emphasis on the individualization of care, the devotion of time and attention to each patient, a reliance on or faith in the healing powers of the body, and a preference for natural remedies. Other than these prevailing characteristics, CAM is in fact an extremely heterogeneous array of practices, ranging from those well supported by scientific evidence to those that defy any plausible scientific explanation, and it is delivered by providers of widely diverse training and credentials (Katz and others, 2003a). Some self-professed CAM practitioners have no formal training and are subject to no formal credentialing. At the other extreme, naturopathic physicians require the same four years of postgraduate training for their ND degree as MDs do for theirs. The naturopathic scope of practice is regulated by the states (Hough, Dower, and O'Neil, 2001).

Some of the distinctions among medical disciplines are captured in their names. Conventional medicine is known as *allopathic* medicine, in which *allo* means different from and *path* refers to disease. The mainstay of allopathic therapy is to *attack* disease states with therapies that are unrelated to the condition being treated: treating by "the other." In contrast, *homeopathic* medicine relies on treatments that supposedly cause (*homeo*) the symptoms being addressed, with the belief that the body will eradicate the disease by responding to minute doses of the remedy. Of note, the term *allopathy* was coined as a pejorative term by Samuel Hahnemann, the nineteenth-century German physician credited for founding homeopathy. *Naturopathic* medicine obviously relies on *natural* treatments in its approach to treatment and healing.

EPIDEMIOLOGY AND POPULATION SIGNIFICANCE

Interest in and use of CAM has experienced a dramatic increase in recent years. The majority of the United States populace (75 percent of the adult population) have reported the use of at least one alternative therapy (Barnes, Powell-Griner, McFann, and Nahin, 2004). Visits to alternative therapy practitioners in 1997 exceeded visits to all primary care physicians by 243 million, with the majority seeking alternative treatment for chronic diseases, syndromes, or pain (Eisenberg 1998; Barnes, Powell-Griner, McFann, and Nahin, 2004). An increasing percentage of people seek help from an alternative practitioner while being concurrently treated by an allopathic physician—a rise from 8.3 percent in 1990 to 13.7 percent in 1997 (Eisenberg and others, 1998).

Particularly revealing about the popularity of alternative treatments is the fact that the magnitude of the demand for these therapies continues to rise despite the lack of insurance coverage for such services. Americans spent an estimated $21.2 billion out of pocket for visits to alternative providers in 1997, an increase of 45 percent from 1990. The majority—58 percent—of those surveyed who used alternative therapies did so for disease prevention, whereas 42 percent used such services for actual medical problems. The use of alternative therapies is more prevalent among white, female, better-educated, higher-income (over $50,000 per year) populations (Eisenberg and others, 1998). Although the use of CAM is greatest among people aged thirty to forty-nine years, use among elderly patients—those over sixty-five years of age—is on the rise (currently reported at 39.1 percent) and is likely to increase with the growing incidence of chronic illnesses as populations age. The use of CAM has been found to be especially high in patients with Alzheimer's disease, multiple sclerosis, rheumatic diseases, cancer, AIDS, back problems, anxiety, depression, headaches, head colds, and chronic pain (Barnes, Powell-Griner, McFann, and Nahin, 2004; Astin and others, 1998).

Predictors of alternative health care use include poorer health status, a holistic philosophical orientation to health and life, a chronic health condition, classification in a cultural group identifiable by its commitment to environmentalism or its commitment to feminism, and an interest in spirituality and personal growth psychology (Astin and others, 1998). Although research findings vary somewhat, common reasons that people choose CAM include: an interest in combining conventional medicine with CAM, dissatisfaction with the ability of conventional medicine to adequately treat chronic illnesses, a desire to avoid the harmful side effects of conventional medicine and treatments, an interest in and greater knowledge of how nutritional, emotional, and lifestyle factors affect health, and a broader focus on disease prevention and overall health (Barnes, Powell-Griner, McFann, and Nahin, 2004; Eisenberg and others, 1998; Astin and others, 1998).

Thus, access to CAM modalities affords patients a greater opportunity to obtain care that is consistent with their beliefs and preferences. The availability of CAM treatments may therefore be considered an important means of patient empowerment. In this way, the provision of CAM options and a patient-centered approach to care may be seen as fundamentally interrelated. Given the popularity of CAM in the United States today, one might argue that most patients cannot be fully empowered in their health care decision making without having reasonable access to certain CAM therapies.

Despite the significant increase in the use of alternative therapies over recent years, fewer than 40 percent of alternative medicine users disclose such information to their primary care provider, which reveals an important disconnect between the preferences of patients and their willingness to share these views with their doctors (Eisenberg and others, 1993, 1998; Astin and others, 1998; Elder, Gillchrist, and Minz, 1997; Feldman, 1990; McKee, 1988; Mitchell, 1993; Perelson, 1996). This important deficiency in physician-patient communication (Elder, Gillchrist, and Minz, 1997; Feldman, 1990; McKee, 1988; Rao and others, 1999) may reflect patient dissatisfaction with the conventional medical system (Astin and others, 1998; Perelson, 1996), distrust, or simply an accurate assessment of their physician's level of interest.

There is widespread reticence about (if not outright opposition to) CAM practices among conventional physicians. Those most opposed to the use of CAM argue that alternative therapists do not have the extensive knowledge that is required to diagnose an illness properly, and they often cite the lack of evidence of the efficacy of CAM (Astin and others, 1998). The latter is the most heatedly debated among proponents of conventional medicine. But the claim that conventional medicine is science that is supported by evidence is not always accurate. The Office of Technology Assessment of the U.S. Congress has estimated that fewer than 30 percent of the procedures currently used in mainstream medicine have been rigorously tested (Relman and Weil, 1999). One reason why most alternative therapies are not evidence based is that the majority were introduced prior to the advent of the randomized controlled clinical trial (RCT). Such limitations are evident in conventional medicine as well; however, they are often overlooked because of the apparent or established effectiveness of a particular treatment. The common and accepted use of antithrombotic agents for cardiovascular diseases and their complications (myocardial infarction, stroke, and pulmonary embolism) supports this contention. Three of the agents prescribed by conventional physicians for millions of patients every day—warfarin, aspirin, and heparin—were introduced prior to the era of randomized clinical trials and therefore had not been exposed to the rigorous research standards in effect today (Dalen, 1998). Few physicians would consider these drugs unconventional treatments, despite the fact that they were not put through RCTs at the time they were introduced. Conversely, many CAM interventions are indeed supported by methodologically rigorous trials (Ornish and others, 1998; Perlman and others, 2006; Katz and others, 2003a). Disparities in evidence between conventional and CAM practices do exist—and are likely to persist—because of great discrepancies in the availability of funds to support definitive clinical trials (Tufts Center for the Study of Drug Development, 2001).

With patients increasingly interested in CAM and conventional practitioners widely reticent, a system of unintegrated or, worse, disintegrated health care prevails in the United States. Many conventional physicians actively discourage the use of CAM wholesale, without considering the differences in modalities or practitioners— or the potential value of CAM treatments. Practitioners of CAM may be just as apt to discourage the use of conventional medicine, citing its reliance on dangerous drugs and invasive procedures, its failure to respect the healing powers of nature, and its lack of compassion and patient-centeredness.

The patient under such conditions is left in a precarious position. Those seeking both conventional care and CAM are likely to receive conflicting advice and to lack the expertise required to make prudent reconciliation between the two. Those choosing to follow both sets of advice may be subject to dangerous interactions that neither half of the care system knows about. Those avoiding a possible conflict by limiting their selection to just one medical discipline may be losing important benefits offered by others, with resultant deficiencies in care. The patient with a chronic health problem for which conventional treatment is ineffective may be left to seek aimlessly among a wide array of therapies, with no place to go for expert guidance that considers all of the options. The costs of such possibly aimless care are likely to be high in both human suffering and dollars, with patients choosing therapies that may be futile, causing them to potentially lose hope and causing insurers to continue to resist including CAM modalities among covered benefits.

Thus, even as CAM in the United States health care system is known to be widely and increasingly popular among the public (Tindle, Davis, Phillips, and Eisenberg, 2005; Harris and Rees, 2000; Kessler and others, 2001), resistance to the proliferation of CAM among conventionally trained practitioners persists (Marcus, 2001; Beyerstein, 2001; Sampson, 2001; Angell and Kassirer, 1998). Health insurers, although uncertain as to the potential costs and benefits, are subject to increasing pressures to reimburse for various CAM practices (Pelletier, Marie, Krasner, and Haskell, 1997; Pelletier, Astin, and Haskell, 1999). These tensions and incompatibilities constitute a challenge and a threat to patient-centered, holistic approaches to care.

INTEGRATIVE MEDICINE

Patient empowerment is one of the dominant principles and trends in modern health care, but there are others. The popularity of CAM is itself an important trend, as is interest in natural therapies and holism. The importance of evidence as the basis for therapies and decisions is an increasingly salient feature in medical education and practice. Finally, the advent of managed care has resulted in increasing attention to the cost-effectiveness of medical interventions.

The confluence of these trends represents the context in which CAM and conventional medicine must coexist. To date, the outpatient setting, where patient autonomy is far greater and regulation of practice is less strict, is where CAM has flourished. With few but noteworthy exceptions, such as the cardiac surgery program at Columbia Presbyterian Medical Center in New York City (Oz, 2002; Okvat, Oz, Ting, and Namerow, 2002), the inpatient setting has been largely inhospitable to CAM thus far. Hospital care is particularly dominated by concerns for evidence-based practice, as well as the stipulations of insurers. Despite this, hospitals are increasingly tempted to address the public's interest in CAM by making some of the most clearly benign therapies, such as massage, available (Hemphill and Kemp, 2000). Such gestures may enhance patient satisfaction, and they are laudable. However, they generally leave control over fundamental aspects of care entirely in the hands of the conventional medical staff.

Efforts to align the interest patients have in alternative care with the practices and procedures of allopathic medicine have resulted in the emergence of *integrative medicine.* As the name implies, this approach to care encompasses both conventional medicine and CAM. However, beyond the name, much of what integrative medicine is—or should be—about is open to interpretation. Andrew Weil, at the University of Arizona, is widely credited with coining the term *integrative medicine,* and he runs a program in which conventional physicians receive supplemental training in CAM disciplines and natural medicine. At other sites, centers are developed in which CAM and conventional practitioners occupy adjacent offices and refer patients back and forth.

Perhaps the ultimate expression of integrative care is when practitioners from both CAM and conventional medicine make their recommendations available to patients, who can then choose, with expert guidance and support, from a wider array of options. Although few and far between thus far, such models do exist, and they appear likely to proliferate.

The advantages of integrative care, in which diverse practitioners collaborate, are compelling. The traditional wall of silence between CAM and conventional practice is overcome, thereby avoiding the risk of adverse interactions or gaps in care. Interaction in the care of a patient can help practitioners learn about one another in a manner conducive to more productive collaborations over time. Rather than relying on the limited expertise in all of medicine that any one individual can attain, physicians can take a collaborative approach to care, which provides the patient with access to practitioners who have complementary knowledge and expertise. Because training, credentials, and legitimacy of practice vary widely across the expanse of CAM, and because proficiency varies among conventionally trained physicians, direct communication among practitioners can also help patients identify the most competent, credible, and suitable providers.

As one example of an integrative care model that embraces these principles, the Integrative Medicine Center (IMC) at Griffin Hospital in Derby, Connecticut, offers outpatient care that is fully consensus based (Katz and others, 2003b). The IMC is codirected by a conventional physician and a naturopathic physician. Patients, either self- or physician referred, are evaluated sequentially by a conventionally trained medical provider and by a naturopathic physician. Each such evaluation terminates with a consensus conference, in which the providers from both disciplines review with the patient the array of treatment options. The IMC is supported by a panel of CAM providers throughout the state of Connecticut, to whom patients may be referred for specialized therapies. Among the services the IMC provides is an evaluation of the credentials and practice history of these practitioners, thereby helping patients find the most reputable practitioners.

Other models of integrative medicine around the country have addressed integration in a variety of ways. At Celilo, the cancer treatment facility at Mid-Columbia Medical Center in The Dalles, Oregon, radiation therapy and chemotherapy are offered in conjunction with an array of CAM services. The spa-like setting includes a meditation garden, saunas, Jacuzzi tubs, and steam rooms. Staff massage therapists provide pre- and post-treatment massages to both patients and their waiting family members. Acupuncture is an important tool that is used to assist in nausea and pain control. Visualization instruction is provided to elicit the power of the patient's mind to combat his or her cancer. Humorous videotapes are available for viewing during treatment sessions.

This truly integrative center has far exceeded the initial volume projections, drawing patients from as far away as Portland, Oregon, despite Portland's larger medical centers. Clearly, patients are willing to travel in order to access care in a more holistic setting.

The case for integrative medicine at this juncture in the evolution of health care is compelling. Given the clear and growing interest of patients in CAM, a system of care that fails to address CAM simply cannot be truly patient-centered. Patient-centeredness in care, the very principle to which the Planetree model is dedicated, can and should guide medical practices. Patient empowerment and autonomy, however, should not be at the expense of science and evidence, and thus wholesale endorsement of CAM in conventional medical institutions is equally inappropriate.

Integrative medicine offers the promise of reconciliation between patient autonomy and interest in CAM within the prevailing conventions of health care. The ultimate goal of integrative care should be to make the widest array of appropriate options available to patients so that they may choose care that feels right for them. Appropriateness should be predicated on fundamental considerations that pertain equally to conventional and CAM practice: treatment safety and treatment effectiveness. Treatment safety and treatment effectiveness must, in turn, be interpreted in light of the available evidence.

The ultimate goal in the evolution of integrative care should be the blurring of boundaries between conventional care and CAM. Both disciplines should be subject to rigorous scientific inquiry so that interventions that work are systematically distinguished from those that do not (Vickers, 2001). Safety should not be assumed in either case but should similarly be derived from rigorous evaluation.

Although the importance of scientific evidence in modern medicine is indisputable, its application is often questionable. Evidence simply does not exist to indicate the best treatments for many chronic conditions and syndromes. Under such circumstances, practitioners who choose to view evidence as the sole basis for medical decisions have nothing to offer. However, evidence could be a tool at the clinician's disposal rather than the bars of a cage (Katz, 2001). Where strong evidence in support of a particular therapy exists, that therapy should be recommended in preference to others. The less clear it is as to which might be the "right" treatment choice, the more important it is to work down a hierarchy of evidence, considering safety, effectiveness, alternatives, and the evidence supporting each. For many conditions, such as chronic fatigue syndrome or fibromyalgia, a definitive therapy does not exist, and the best available treatments are those likely to be safe—and possibly effective. Access to CAM modalities greatly broadens patient options at this end of the evidence hierarchy, where options are generally most needed.

Many CAM modalities are now well-established aspects of the outpatient health care landscape in the United States. Among these are chiropractic, acupuncture, massage therapy, nutritional supplements, and mind-body interventions such as meditation (Kessler and others, 2001). Some of these same modalities are available in the hospital setting, although this trend is as yet nascent. Any effort to incorporate CAM practices into conventional care will likely proceed from the more evidence based, or at least time-honored, CAM modalities, expanding from the outpatient to the inpatient setting.

FOR EXAMPLE

CAM at Sharp Coronado Hospital

For Sharp Coronado Hospital in Coronado, California, integrating complementary therapies throughout the entire hospital was an important part of its strategy to foster a culture of patient-centered care. The opening of a new hospice unit shortly after the hospital adopted the Planetree model offered the opportunity to begin introducing a variety of complementary therapies. An education plan was developed that would require all licensed team members to be trained in healing touch, clinical aromatherapy, and massage. This plan was presented to the Medical Staff Leadership with the goal not of competing with the medical treatment plan, but rather as additional nursing interventions to relieve pain, stress, anxiety, nausea, insomnia, and other such symptoms that are frequently experienced by hospice patients. The Medical Executive Leadership unanimously supported the plan.

Initially, the Complementary Therapies Program at Sharp Coronado Hospital was limited to this one unit. Not long after the hospice unit opened, though, a hospice patient was admitted to the acute care area of the hospital. The patient's family requested that team members continue to provide healing touch, clinical aromatherapy, and massage treatments, as they considered these treatments and the compassionate nature of the caregiving team instrumental in easing their mother's pain. Following this event, the family wrote a letter attesting to the outstanding care and treatment their mother received. This letter and a request to expand the Complementary Therapies Program throughout the entire hospital were presented to Medical Executive Leadership and received immediate, unanimous approval.

Since that time, over seventy team members have been trained with competency validation in healing touch, clinical aromatherapy, and massage. In addition, these unique competencies are a part of the annual education for all nursing personnel. The hospital now employs two massage therapists, two acupuncturists, and a healing touch practitioner, who treat outpatients in addition to spending time treating inpatients and training new staff members. In a 2006 pilot study, sixty healing touch treatments were evaluated. Pre- and post-treatment anxiety and pain scales were administered, and in each case the patients experienced reduced anxiety and pain.

Although a traditional hospital environment might not be viewed as a relaxing arena for complementary therapies, Sharp Coronado's holistic team was able to break through that stigma by transforming a hospital room into an integrative wellness room. Relaxing music, a water fountain, plants, and artistic furnishings all contribute to creating a serene environment that feels far from clinical.

Today, the Complementary Therapies Program at Sharp Coronado Hospital is flourishing. The program has even expanded beyond treatments for patients and now includes services available to a growing clientele throughout the entire community. Lectures on CAM modalities are offered, and a marketing campaign has been implemented. Most recently, a partnership with the local College for Alternative Therapies has begun. Sharp's patients, physicians, staff, and community have fully embraced these unique programs.

CONTRIBUTED BY SUSAN STONE, SHARP CORONADO HOSPITAL

The ultimate advantages of integrative medicine pertain to both settings. Although inpatient applications are more challenging, many Planetree hospitals have found innovative ways to incorporate these options. For example, at Longmont United Hospital in Longmont, Colorado, every new mother on the maternity unit receives a therapeutic massage following delivery. In order to cover the expense without charging patients, the staff has scrutinized expenditures on the unit, cutting out such things as the traditional "goodie bags" of diapers, powder, and other items, in favor of the massage sessions. Patient satisfaction on the unit has soared, with many patients citing the massage as the most positive aspect of their stay.

Aromatherapy has also made its way into a growing number of inpatient settings, particularly on behavioral health units. Nursing staff members on Griffin Hospital's inpatient psychiatric unit who are trained in aromatherapy employ a variety of scents, distributed via atomizers, to enhance the moods of patients. Studies conducted by the staff on the unit have found that in 90 percent of patients with insomnia, the aroma of lavender has been effective in improving sleep. Sage oil, used for patients with anxiety, effected a 48 percent decrease in scores on the Hamilton Scale, and bergamot oil, used for depressed patients, effected a 45 percent decrease in scores on the Beck Depression scale (M. Schwartz, personal communication, 2002).

CONCLUSIONS

For Planetree's principles of patient empowerment to be fully and meaningfully honored, CAM modalities simply must be made accessible to patients. If this occurs independently of conventional practice, it will result in disconnected systems of care that have the potential for dangerous incompatibilities and regrettable gaps. Much is to be gained by overcoming the historical distinction between conventional and complementary care and instead thinking of care as properly involving all reasonable treatment options. The reasonableness of such options should be based on the thoughtful application of a hierarchy of evidence that pertains to safety, effectiveness, and alternatives as well as the beliefs and preferences of the patient.

Advances in integrative care have thus far occurred predominantly in the outpatient setting, and this trend will likely continue for some time. However, this approach to the incorporation of CAM modalities among treatment options is no less reasonable in the hospital setting. In the inpatient setting, the credentialing requirements for CAM practitioners would likely be more stringent, and the scope of practice would be more limited. Even so, the options available to patients could be meaningfully enhanced. Progress toward more integrative inpatient care could very reasonably begin with the most accepted and evidence-based

CAM modalities, including acupuncture, chiropractic, nutritional therapies, massage, and meditation, to name a few.

The challenges of achieving integrative medicine as the prevailing norm in modern health care are great. The reticence of the conventional medical establishment must be overcome. CAM practitioners must be prepared to find common ground and common language with their conventional colleagues. All practitioners must embrace the importance and value of scientific evidence yet be willing to acknowledge its limits. Insurers will need to reimburse for those CAM modalities sanctioned by practitioners of integrative medicine before the public can realize the full benefit. In support of this goal, cost-effective models will need to be developed.

Integrative care should continue its evolution in outpatient settings. As CAM and conventional modalities are successfully aligned for outpatients, these experiences should inform a gradual transformation of inpatient care, where the barriers are greater and the stakes are perhaps somewhat higher. Emphasis should be placed on CAM modalities that are best supported by evidence, for which credentialing and training are most stringent and for which the need is greatest, including naturopathic medicine, acupuncture, chiropractic, nutritional and herbal medicine, mind-body interventions, and therapeutic massage.

We are perhaps quite a long way from integrative care as the standard of practice in the conventional medical system. Yet the very trends that are reshaping modern health care—patient empowerment among them—may propel us in that direction. One can envision a day when the compatibility of treatment options with a patient's beliefs and values is a universal priority. One can envision a day when practitioners with varied training and expertise collaborate in a spirit of mutual respect. One can envision a day when evidence is universally valued and every practitioner acknowledges that patients should not be abandoned if their needs take them past evidence's leading edge.

It has been said that the single best way to predict the future is to create it. Perhaps, then, envisioning the advantages of integrative care is the first best step toward realizing them. Like conventional medicine, CAM includes therapies that are safe and effective, therapies that are either safe or effective, and therapies that are neither. Caution must therefore be exercised as CAM is integrated into established systems of inpatient and outpatient care. But the need to be cautious and thoughtful is no reason not to proceed. We should all aim for the day when there is no "alternative" or "conventional" care but rather just good options predicated on science, evidence, safety, effectiveness, and patient preferences and beliefs. When all of medicine is available to all patients, when responsibility and responsiveness are universally aligned, the center of care and the interests of the patient will truly coincide. Patient empowerment and the best achievable outcomes in health care will be realized when expert guidance to one continuous spectrum of treatment options is routinely available.

REFERENCES

Angell, M., and Kassirer, J. "Alternative Medicine: The Risks of Untested and Unregulated Remedies." *New England Journal of Medicine,* 1998, *39,* 839–841.

Astin, J., and others. "A Review of the Incorporation of Complementary and Alternative Medicine by Mainstream Physicians." *Archives of Internal Medicine,* 1998, *58,* 2303–2310.

Barnes, P., Powell-Griner, E., McFann, K., and Nahin, R. "Complementary and Alternative Medicine Use Among Adults: United States, 2002." CDC Advance Data Report #343. May 27, 2004.

Beyerstein, B. "Alternative Medicine and Common Errors of Reasoning." *Academic Medicine,* 2001, *76,* 230–237.

Dalen, J. "'Conventional' and 'Unconventional' Medicine." *Archives of Internal Medicine,* 1998, *158,* 2179–2181.

Druss, B., and Rosenheck, R. "Association Between Use of Unconventional Therapies and Conventional Medical Services." *Journal of the American Medical Association,* 1999, *282,* 651–656.

Eisenberg, D., and others. "Unconventional Medicine in the United States." *New England Journal of Medicine,* 1993, *328,* 246–252.

Eisenberg, D. M., and others. "Trends in Alternative Medicine Use in the United States, 1990–1997." *Journal of the American Medical Association,* 1998, *280,* 1569–1575.

Elder, N., Gillchrist, A., and Minz, R. "Use of Alternative Health Care by Family Practice Patients." *Archives of Family Medicine,* 1997, *6,* 181–184.

Feldman, M. "Patients Who Seek Unorthodox Medical Treatment." *Minnesota Medicine,* 1990, *73,* 19–25.

Harris, P., and Rees, R. "The Prevalence of Complementary and Alternative Medicine Use Among the General Population: A Systematic Review of the Literature." *Complementary Therapies in Medicine,* 2000, *8,* 88–96.

Hemphill, L., and Kemp, J. "Implementing a Therapeutic Massage Program in a Tertiary and Ambulatory Care VA Setting: The Healing Power of Touch." *Nursing Clinics of North America,* 2000, *35,* 489–497.

Hough, H., Dower, C., and O'Neil, E. *Profile of a Profession: Naturopathic Practice.* San Francisco: Center for the Health Professions, University of California, 2001.

Katz, D. "Conventional Medical Care and Unconventional Therapies." *Journal of the American Medical Association,* 1999, *281,* 56.

Katz, D. *Clinical Epidemiology and Evidence-Based Medicine.* Thousand Oaks, Calif.: Sage, 2001.

Katz, D. L., and others. "Evidence Mapping: Introduction of Methods with Application to Complementary and Alternative Medicine Research." *Alternative Therapies in Health and Medicine,* 2003a, *9*(4), 22–30.

Katz, D. L., and others. "Teaching Evidence-Based Integrative Medicine: Description of a Model Programme." *Evidence-Based Integrative Medicine,* 2003b, *1*(1), 77–82.

Kessler, R., and others. "Long-Term Trends in the Use of Complementary and Alternative Medical Therapies in the United States." *Annals of Internal Medicine,* 2001, *135,* 262–268.

Marcus, D. "How Should Alternative Medicine Be Taught to Medical Students and Physicians?" *Academic Medicine,* 2001, *76,* 224–229.

McKee, J. "Holistic Health and the Critique of Western Medicine." *Social Science Medicine,* 1988, *26,* 775–784.

Mitchell, S. "Healing Without Doctors." *American Demographics,* 1993, *15,* 46–49.

National Center for Complementary and Alternative Medicine (NCCAM), National Institutes of Health. NCCAM Publication No. D347.

Okvat, H., Oz, M., Ting, W., and Namerow, P. "Massage Therapy for Patients Undergoing Cardiac Catheterization." *Alternative Therapies in Health & Medicine,* 2002, *8,* 68–70, 72, 74–75.

Ornish, D., and others. "Intensive Lifestyle Changes for Reversal of Coronary Heart Disease." *Journal of the American Medical Association,* Dec. 16, 1998, *280*(23), 2001–2007.

Oz, M. "Emerging Role of Complementary Medicine in Valvular Surgery." *Advances in Cardiology,* 2002, *39,* 184–188.

Pelletier, K., Astin, J., and Haskell, W. "Current Trends in the Integration and Reimbursement of Complementary and Alternative Medicine by Managed Care Organizations (MCOs) and Insurance Providers: 1998 Update and Cohort Analysis." *American Journal of Health Promotion,* 1999, *14,* 125–133.

Pelletier, K., Marie, A., Krasner, M., and Haskell, W. "Current Trends in the Integration and Reimbursement of Complementary and Alternative Medicine by Managed Care, Insurance Carriers, and Hospital Providers." *American Journal of Health Promotion,* 1997, *12,* 112–122.

Perelson, G. "Alternative Medicine: What Role in Managed Care?" *Journal of Clinical Residency,* 1996, *5,* 32–38.

Perlman, A. I., and others. "Massage Therapy for Osteoarthritis of the Knee: A Randomized Controlled Trial." *Archives of Internal Medicine,* Dec. 11–25, 2006, *166*(22), 2533–2538.

Rao, J., and others. "Use of Complementary Therapies for Arthritis Among Patients of Rheumatologists." *Annals of Internal Medicine,* 1999, *131,* 409–416.

Relman, A., and Weil, A. "Is Integrative Medicine the Medicine of the Future?" *Archives of Internal Medicine,* 1999, *159,* 2122–2126.

Sampson, W. "The Need for Educational Reform in Teaching About Alternative Therapies." *Academic Medicine,* 2001, *76,* 248–250.

Tindle, H. A., Davis, R. B., Phillips, R. S., and Eisenberg, D. M. "Trends in Use of Complementary and Alternative Medicine by U.S. Adults: 1997–2002." *Alternative Therapies in Health and Medicine,* 2005, *11,* 42–49.

Tufts Center for the Study of Drug Development. "A Methodology for Counting Costs for Pharmaceutical R&D." Nov. 1, 2001. [http://csdd.tufts.edu/NewsEvents/RecentNews.asp?newsid=5].

Vickers, A. J. "Message to Complementary and Alternative Medicine: Evidence Is a Better Friend Than Power." *BMC Complementary and Alternative Medicine,* 2001, *1,* 1.

CHAPTER

7

EFFECTS OF VIEWING ART ON HEALTH OUTCOMES

ROGER S. ULRICH

This chapter does the following:

- Provides an overview of current research that demonstrates the effects of viewing art on medical outcomes
- Underscores that the decisive criterion for health care art is whether it improves patient outcomes
- Provides evidence-based guidelines for the selection of health care art
- Describes why special care should be taken in considering the incorporation of abstract art into a health care setting
- Provides examples of arts programs in Planetree hospitals

Portions of this chapter draw heavily on the arts and health research discussed by Ulrich and Gilpin in the first edition of *Putting Patients First* (2003).

Long before science was synonymous with medicine, the arts and healing were closely intertwined. In the years before Hippocrates, the healing temples of ancient Greece surrounded patients with paintings, sculpture, gardens, fountains, music, poetry, and storytelling. An environment rich with art was seen as therapeutic, providing a means to alleviate physical discomfort and emotional distress. With the advent of scientific medicine, the therapeutic uses of the arts diminished in importance but were still perceived intuitively to enhance healing. Florence Nightingale, in her book *Notes on Nursing* ([1860] 1969), described the patient's need for beauty, even to look out a window or gaze at a vase of flowers: "People say the effect is only on the mind. It is no such thing. The effect is on the body, too" (p. 59).

But medical science does not preclude the arts. The Planetree model was founded on the belief that science-based care is best delivered in an environment that reduces stress and is conducive to healing. The first Planetree unit provided patients with a wide variety of arts, including painting, music, storytelling, movies, and clowns.

Somewhat ironically, the science that once overshadowed the arts is now verifying their importance in medicine. Researchers are finding evidence for what was believed intuitively centuries ago: that art can play an important role in improving medical outcomes. The effect of viewing art (paintings, prints, photographs) on stress reduction, pain relief, and other outcomes has been a growing area of investigation and is the focus of this chapter.

WHAT ARE HEALTH OUTCOMES?

An important term relevant to research on the arts as related to health is *health outcome,* which serves as a measure of a patient's condition and an indicator of health care quality (Ulrich, 1999). There are different types of health or medical outcomes, including the following:

- Clinical indicators that are observable signs and symptoms relating to patients' conditions (examples: length of hospital stay, blood pressure, intake of pain medication)

- Satisfaction and other reported outcomes (examples: patient satisfaction, health-related quality of life, staff satisfaction)

- Economic outcomes (examples: cost of patient care, recruitment costs due to staff turnover, revenue from patients choosing a hospital, philanthropy)

Different combinations of outcomes are used for studying patients with different types of diagnoses. If the objective is to research the effects of artwork on patients recovering from surgery, for example, relevant medical outcomes could include recovery indicators such as reported pain, intake of pain medication, how soon the patient can move or walk, and length of hospital stay. By contrast, the selection of outcomes would be different for gauging the influences of art, for instance, on terminally ill persons in a hospice, and might focus on evaluating whether exposure to art increases reported quality of life and reduces depression, pain, and family stress (Ulrich, 2008).

Outcome studies have major importance in medicine because they provide the most sound and widely accepted basis for judging whether particular treatments or interventions (art, here) are medically effective and cost-efficient. They are also important for helping medical professionals evaluate whether treatments or interventions are ethical. The ethics of displaying a given artwork in a museum or workplace is only occasionally an important consideration. Ethics become an imperative consideration, however, when art is displayed to a captive population of vulnerable patients who are stressed, fearful, in pain, and may be unable to choose the art displayed to them. A key dictum that medical students and nurses learn is "First do no harm." The obligation ethically and professionally in the case of art, therefore, is to provide evidence, or at least a chain of plausible reasoning, that the art intervention will cause little or no harm and will have positive effects on the great majority of patients (Ulrich and Gilpin, 2003). Adverse reactions to the art should be mild and should occur at acceptably low rates, as virtually any medical treatment may trigger some adverse reactions (Martin, 1999).

Although some artists and designers may assume that nearly any type of visual art or painting is "good" and will beneficially affect patients, it must be kept in mind that artwork varies enormously, and the content and styles of much art are challenging or strongly emotional (Ulrich, 1991). Accordingly, it is reasonable to expect that certain types of art will be positive for patients, whereas other types could be stressful and worsen outcomes (Ulrich, 1991). The decisive criterion for health care art is whether it improves patient outcomes, not whether it receives praise from art critics and artists or approaches museum standards for quality (Ulrich, 1991, 1999; Martin, 1999; Friedrich, 1999).

THEORIES: ART THAT CAN IMPROVE OUTCOMES

Two different theoretical perspectives, *biophilia* and *emotional congruence,* are helpful in understanding why certain types of art have been found effective in improving health outcomes.

Biophilia Theory

Nature art can reduce stress. The intuitively based belief that viewing nature can be calming, reduce stress, and promote health dates back many centuries and appears across Asian and Western cultures (Ulrich and others, 1991). Writers traditionally attributed this belief to culture and learning, arguing that societies teach or condition their populations to revere nature but perceive cities and built areas as stressful and negative (Ulrich and others, 1991). Cultural explanations, though, have failed to adequately explain the mounting scientific evidence that a wide variety of diverse cultures and socioeconomic groups exhibits striking agreement in responding positively to nature views (Ulrich, 1993). *Biophilia* or evolutionary theory readily accounts for this similarity by proposing that millions of years of evolution have left modern humans with a partly genetic proneness to respond positively to nature settings that fostered well-being and survival for early humans (Wilson, 1984; Appleton, 1975; Orians, 1986; Ulrich, 1983, 1993, 2008; Kaplan and Kaplan, 1989).

Biophilia theory predicts that nature art will promote restoration across diverse groups of people if it contains these features and properties: calm or slowly moving water, verdant foliage, flowers, foreground spatial openness, park-like or savannah-like properties (scattered trees, grassy understory), and birds, deer, or other nondangerous wildlife (Ulrich, 1993, 1999, 2008). Furthermore, biophilia theory proposes that in addition to such nature art, humans are genetically predisposed to pay attention to and be positively affected by images of smiling or caring human faces (Ekman, Friesen, and Ellsworth, 1972).

Also, biophilia theory is very useful for identifying features and subject matter that should be *avoided* when selecting art for stressed patients. Speaking generally, a biophilic/evolutionary perspective holds that humans also have a partly innate proneness to respond negatively (with stress, fear, avoidance behavior) to natural elements and situations that have signaled threats or dangers throughout evolution (Coss, 1968; Ulrich, 1993; Ulrich and others, 1991). These disturbing and often stressful stimuli include snakes and spiders, reptilian-like tessellated scale patterns, nearby large mammals staring directly at the viewer, pointed or piercing forms, shadowy enclosed spaces, and angry human faces (Öhman, 1986; Coss, 1968, 2003; Ulrich, 1993). Findings from several studies of identical twins have left no doubt that genetic factors play a major role in stressful fear responses to certain visual stimuli, such as snakes and angry faces (for example, Kendler, Karkowski, and Prescott, 1999). This partly genetic underpinning underscores the importance of excluding art containing such phenomena from health care spaces where stress is a problem.

Emotional Congruence Theory

Patient feelings influence art perceptions. In addition to biophilia theory, another perspective that is quite useful for understanding patient responses to health care art is that of *emotional congruence* theory. Research in the behavioral sciences has shown that emotions or feelings have important effects on perception and thinking. From this work has emerged emotional congruence theory—the notion that our emotional states bias our perception of environmental stimuli in ways that match our feelings (Bower, 1981; Singer and Salovey, 1988; Niedenthal, Setterlund, and Jones, 1994). Other research suggests that emotional states also enhance recall of emotionally similar memories but inhibit recall of emotionally dissimilar information (for example, Isen, 1987). Happy or pleasant feelings are accordingly likely to promote happy or positive associations and memories, whereas fearful feelings will cue fearful or anxious associations. Given the focus here on health care art, an important implication of emotional congruence theory is that patients should tend to perceive, interpret, and have associations with art in ways that match their emotional states or feelings (Ulrich, 1999).

Here, the point cannot be overemphasized that patients experience stress and negatively toned feelings (fear, anxiety, anger, and sadness) and that many suffer acute emotional distress. Therefore it can be predicted on the basis of emotional congruence theory that such negative feelings could dispose patients to perceive and interpret certain art styles and subject matter in emotionally matching negatively stressful ways (Ulrich, 1999; Ulrich and Gilpin, 2003). A related prediction is that acutely stressed patients are especially vulnerable to interpreting art as stressful or even frightening when the styles and subject matter are ambiguous or abstract and can be readily interpreted in widely different ways (Ulrich, 1999). According to emotional congruence theory, a healthy person in good spirits may tend to interpret an abstract or ambiguous painting in an emotionally matching positive manner. The same person could be more prone to reacting negatively to the identical painting, however, when he or she is hospitalized and experiencing strongly negative feelings. The important message from emotional congruence theory is that caution should be exercised when considering ambiguous or abstract art for patient spaces or high-stress waiting and treatment areas.

PREFERENCES FOR VISUAL IMAGES

Much research has examined people's responses to art and other types of visual images, but the vast majority of studies have measured preferences or aesthetic liking rather than effects on stress recovery (restoration) and other medical outcomes. Although the relationship between visual preference responses and restoration/health effects is not well understood scientifically, preference studies are still useful for providing insights about what types of art are most liked by diverse groups of people. Limited research suggests that restorative responses strongly influence preferences, raising the possibility that art preferences reflect and are linked to restorative responses (Van den Berg, Koole, and Van der Wulp, 2003; Ulrich, 2008).

General Public Preferences

Consistent with biophilia theory, a clear-cut conclusion supported by well over a hundred published preference studies on real visual environments—such as urban settings, building facades, room interiors, forests, and gardens—is that adult populations from different areas of the world evidence strong similarity in preferring nature scenes over urban or built environments, especially when the latter lack nature content such as foliage and water (Ulrich, 1983, 1993).

These environmental preference findings are closely paralleled by art studies showing that the great majority of adults across different cultures prefer realistic or representational nature art over art with other subject matter (Kettlewell, 1988; Winston and Cupchik, 1992; Wypijewski, 1997; Ulrich, 1991). A considerable majority of adults internationally also evidences striking similarity in *disliking* abstract art (Wypijewski, 1997). Another research finding that should be emphasized for its health care implications is that the greater part of the public considers art aesthetically pleasing if it fosters positive feelings such as happiness. In this regard, a study of a national random sample of adult

Americans found that most people strongly agreed with statements such as, "I only want to look at art that makes me happy" and "art should be relaxing to look at" (Wypijewski, 1997). By contrast, most of the general public *disagreed* with statements such as, "I like to look at art that is challenging or provocative."

Patient Preferences

A limited amount of research on hospital patient art preferences has yielded findings consistent with those for the nonpatient public. Carpman and Grant (1993) showed a varied collection of pictures to three hundred randomly selected inpatients and asked them to rate each picture for how much they would like to have it hanging in their hospital rooms. Results indicated that the hospital inpatients consistently preferred representational nature scenes but disliked or rejected abstract art.

Hathorn and Ulrich (2001) carried out small-scale preliminary studies at a large urban hospital to assess the health care art preferences of groups of African Americans and whites. Participants were given binders containing a highly diverse collection of 676 color pictures of paintings and asked to rate how appropriate or inappropriate each picture was for display in patient areas. Consistent with biophilia theory, both blacks and whites rated as very appropriate and preferred representational paintings of nature landscapes and rural areas (Hathorn and Ulrich, 2001). Irrespective of race or ethnicity, participants gave highly positive ratings to nature paintings showing spatially open settings in clear, sunny weather, with water features and verdant or healthy green vegetation. As well, paintings of gardens with flowers were rated as highly appropriate and preferred.

The same preliminary studies further suggested that both blacks and whites judged as appropriate figurative artworks that depicted people with clearly positive facial expressions and who displayed body language and gestures that were caring or friendly (Hathorn and Ulrich, 2001).

Nanda, Hathorn, and Neuman (2007) displayed a diverse collection of seventeen paintings to patients in their hospital rooms in a large Texas medical center and asked patients to rate each painting for the following questions: (1) How does the picture make you feel? and (2) Would you like to hang this picture in your hospital room? The picture collection included seven best-selling images from three independent art-vendors (for instance, "The Kiss" by Gustav Klimt), seven pictures chosen on the basis of evidence-based guidelines for selecting health care art developed by Ulrich and Gilpin (2003), and three other images. Findings indicated that patients were significantly more positive about the paintings selected according to evidence-based criteria than they were about best-selling pictures or even works by masters such as Chagall and Van Gogh (Nanda, Hathorn, and Neuman, 2007). The highest scoring positive painting depicted a gentle waterfall with vegetation. Also, realistic pictures of nature settings containing human figures and harmless animals such as deer were preferred over counterparts that were stylized or somewhat abstract (Nanda, Hathorn, and Neuman, 2007).

Eisen (2006) carried out one of the first scientific studies of the art preferences of school children and hospitalized pediatric patients. The art preferences of children were compared across four age groups: five to seven years of age, eight to ten years of age, eleven to thirteen years of age, and fourteen to seventeen years. Findings suggested that across all age groups and both genders, the great majority of hospitalized pediatric patients and school children were similar in preferring nature art over abstract images that varied in complexity, color brightness, and presence versus absence of a cartoon-like image. For example, consistent with biophilia theory, nearly 75 percent of school children, irrespective of age or gender, accorded highest preference either to a representational nature painting (forest with lake and deer) or an impressionistic nature painting (beach with waves) (Eisen, 2006). It should be noted that these findings run counter to traditional intuition-based design guidelines that have often recommended abstract or cartoon-like images for health care spaces for children.

Artist and Designer Preferences

The art preferences of artists, environmental designers, and people seriously interested in art, however, differ greatly from those of the general public and the subset of the public who are patients (Ulrich, 1999). In complete contrast with the great majority of the public, artists and experienced art viewers like artworks that are challenging or emotionally provocative (Winston and Cupchik, 1992). Moreover, they *disagree* with the notion that art should produce positive feelings in a broad audience. They further differ from the general public in that they tend to like artwork that ranges across a diversity of styles—abstract as well as representational. In sum, this implies that if artists and designers follow their personal aesthetic tastes when selecting art for health care settings and fail to involve patient representatives or consult research evidence, they may unwittingly specify art that widely misses the mark of patient preferences and provokes negative reactions (Ulrich, 1999).

STRESS-REDUCING EFFECTS OF VIEWING ART

Several studies of nonpatient groups (university students, for example) indicate that even briefly viewing nature can produce substantial restoration from stress. (For surveys of studies, see Ulrich, 1999, 2008; Parsons and Hartig, 2000; Joye, 2007.) These research results are in harmony with biophilia writings described earlier. Considerable evidence shows that the restorative effects of viewing nature are manifested within minutes as a combination of beneficial physiological and emotional or psychological changes. Concerning the first, physiological indications of stress recovery, scientific studies have consistently found that viewing nature can quickly promote substantial restoration as is evident, for instance, in blood pressure, heart activity, muscle tension, and brain electrical activity (for example, Ulrich and others, 1991; Parsons and Hartig, 2000; Parsons and others, 1998). Fredrickson and Levenson (1998) exposed participants to a fear-producing film and reported that persons assigned randomly to watch a nature film (water) afterwards exhibited substantial recovery from cardiovascular stress in only twenty seconds.

Regarding emotional/psychological effects, looking at most nature views elevates positive feelings such as pleasantness and calm and lessens negatively toned emotions such as anxiety, anger, and dejection (Ulrich, 1979; Ulrich and others, 1991). Furthermore, many nature scenes effectively sustain positive interest and thus function as pleasant distractions that may block worrisome, stressful thoughts.

Evidence also indicates that nature scenes dominated by vegetation, flowers, or water are considerably more effective in restoration than the great majority of built scenes lacking nature. Pictures of outstanding architecture can be liked aesthetically, but they appear not to produce restoration as effectively as nature scenes. Research in Sweden by Hartig and his colleagues (1996) found that looking at nature promoted more relaxation and greater overall emotional well-being than did the viewing of an exceptionally attractive built district lacking nature.

The discussion up to this point has used restoration or stress recovery in reference to recuperation from excessively high physiological excitement or activity levels, accompanied by negative feelings and thoughts. But restoration is a broader concept that also is relevant to recovery from excessively low excitement or arousal linked with understimulation and boredom (Ulrich and others, 1991). For groups suffering from understimulation, the capacity of visual images to be positively interesting and mildly stimulating over long time periods becomes a key therapeutic issue. Evidence suggests that representational landscape pictures outperform other categories of visual subject matter when installed for extended periods in isolated and confined work environments where boredom is a problem.

One investigation by Clearwater and Coss (1991) focused on scientists who worked for one year in isolated and confined circumstances in Antarctic research stations. The researchers found that nature landscape pictures, both with and without water features, were more effective than other types of subject matter in sustaining interest, preference, and relaxation throughout the year of isolated work. Spatially open nature landscapes proved superior to such pictures as those depicting humans in action or wild animals. In a second study, the investigators displayed a collection of ninety-five pictures of sixteenth- to twentieth-century paintings to volunteers confined in a realistic mock-up of a module for the International Space Station (Clearwater and Coss, 1991). Findings suggested that in the confined setting of the space station mock-up, people responded most positively to paintings of natural landscapes with high depth of field.

Similar to findings for stressed nonpatients, a limited amount of research focusing on patients has found that looking at nature images for only a few minutes can promote significant restoration, even in acutely stressed individuals. An investigation by Heerwagen (1990), for example, suggested that stress in a dental clinic was appreciably lower on days when a large nature mural was hung on a wall of the waiting room, in contrast with days when the wall was blank. Coss (1990) displayed ceiling-mounted pictures to highly stressed patients lying on gurneys in a presurgical holding room and reported patients had lower blood pressure when exposed to serene nature photographs than when assigned either a control condition of no picture or beautiful but stimulating pictures, such as a seascape with brisk wind conditions. A study focusing on stressed blood donors found that participants had lower pulse rates and blood pressure when a television in the clinic waiting room displayed a nature videotape, compared with when the television showed either daytime television programs or a videotape of urban areas and buildings (Ulrich, Simons, and Miles, 2003). Research on patients with dementia, including Alzheimer's disease, suggested that adding large color nature images and a nature sound track (birds, brook) to a shower room diminished stress and reduced incidents of aggressive agitated behavior, such as hitting and kicking (Whall and others, 1997).

EFFECTS OF VIEWING NATURE ON PAIN

Several strong scientific studies have shown convincingly that looking at nature can produce substantial and clinically important pain mitigation. In explaining why viewing nature should reduce pain, most investigators have referred to *distraction theory*. According to distraction theory, if patients become engrossed in or are diverted by a pleasant distraction such as a nature painting, they will have less conscious attention to allocate to their pain and accordingly will experience less pain (McCaul and Malott, 1984).

Ulrich (1984) found that patients recovering from abdominal surgery needed far fewer potent narcotic pain doses, had shorter hospital stays, had fewer minor postsurgery complications, and had better emotional well-being if they had bedside windows with a nature view (trees) than if their windows overlooked a brick wall. A study of burn patients suffering intense pain revealed that distracting the persons with a videotape of scenic nature (forest, flowers, ocean) during burn dressing changes lowered pain intensity, anxiety, and stress (Miller, Hickman and Lemasters 1992). Research by Diette and colleagues (2003) on patients undergoing a painful bronchoscopy procedure found that those assigned to look at a ceiling-mounted nature scene experienced less pain than a control group who viewed a blank ceiling in the bronchoscopy procedure room. Another well-controlled study showed that volunteers in a hospital had a higher threshold for detecting pain and much greater pain tolerance when they viewed a nature videotape in contrast to looking at a blank screen (Tse and others, 2002).

In addition, Lee and others (2004) studied the effects of nature distraction on pain and patient-controlled sedation during colonoscopy and reported that viewing nature alone reduced pain but not intake of sedative medication. However, a more engrossing audiovisual distraction (nature scenery with classical music) during colonoscopy reduced both pain and self-administered sedative medication (Lee and others, 2004). This finding is in accord with the prediction from distraction theory that the more engrossing and diverting a distraction, the greater the pain reduction (McCaul and Malott, 1984; Ulrich, 2008). If nature art is combined with sound or music, it may tend to be more engrossing and hence effective for alleviating severe pain (Ulrich, 2008).

EFFECTS OF NATURE VERSUS ABSTRACT IMAGES ON OUTCOMES

A study at a university hospital in Sweden investigated whether displaying different types of pictures, including abstracts and realistic nature scenes, improved outcomes following heart surgery (Ulrich, Lundén, and Eltinge, 1993). Heart surgery patients in intensive care units were each assigned to view one of six picture interventions: two representational nature scenes (one dominated by water and trees, the other a forest), two types of abstract pictures (one having straight or rectilinear contours, the other curvilinear forms), or two control conditions (either no picture or a white panel). Results suggested that patients exposed to the landscape picture with water, trees, and high depth of field experienced less anxiety and suffered less intense pain than patients assigned to any of the other five picture conditions (Ulrich, Lundén, and Eltinge, 1993). An unexpected finding was that the abstract picture dominated by straight-edged forms worsened outcomes, compared with having no picture at all (Ulrich, Lundén, and Eltinge, 1993; Ulrich, 1999). Several patients assigned this abstract picture had strongly negative reactions when looking at it, necessitating immediate removal of the picture. The ambiguity of the straight-edged abstract evoked stressful, frightening emotional reactions and associations.

An earlier small-scale study of psychiatric patients in a Swedish hospital similarly found that patients responded positively to representational nature paintings and prints but reacted negatively to several abstract artworks (Ulrich, 1991, 1999). The ward was extensively furnished with wall-mounted paintings and prints. Patients reported having positive feelings and associations with respect to the great majority of nature pictures. By contrast, several individuals expressed negative reactions to abstract artworks in which the content was ambiguous and could be interpreted in multiple ways. Moreover, archival data revealed that patients had physically attacked seven of the paintings and prints, all displaying abstract styles and ambiguous content (Ulrich, 1991).

Further evidence of the potential for ambiguous or abstract art to have unintended negative impacts comes from the example of a large-scale sculpture installation created as a window view for cancer patients in a large university medical center (Ulrich, 1999). The purpose of the sculpture was to create a pleasant and restorative visual distraction for patients. This "Bird Garden" installation contained many bird figures executed in abstract and representational styles. (Although called a *garden,* the installation contained no flowers or other nature.) Prominent in the installation were several tall metal sculptures dominated by straight-edged and abstract forms, many having pointed or piercing features.

Shortly after the abstract sculpture garden was installed, hospital administrators began to receive anecdotal reports of strong negative reactions by some patients (McLaughlin and others, 1996). In response to these concerns, a questionnaire study was conducted to make possible an evidence-based assessment of the effects of the artworks. Twenty-two percent of the cancer patients reported having an overall negative emotional response to the sculpture garden (Hefferman, Morstatt, Saltzman, and Strunc, 1995). Many found the art installation ambiguous ("doesn't make any sense"), and in a manner consistent with emotional congruence theory, certain patients interpreted the sculptures, for instance, as frightening predators (Ulrich, 1999). Administrators and medical staff members decided that the rate and intensity of negative reactions was too high, and the art installation therefore was removed for medical reasons.

GUIDELINES FOR SELECTING HEALTH CARE ART

On the basis of the foregoing discussion of theory and research, this section lists evidence-based guidelines intended to increase the likelihood that the health care art (paintings, prints, and photographs) selected will improve outcomes for stressed patients (Ulrich, 1991; Ulrich and Gilpin, 2003; Hathorn and Ulrich, 2001). These guidelines do not necessarily encompass a complete set of all art selection considerations that might affect patient well-being and health.

It is recommended that *all* the visual art (paintings, prints, and photographs) displayed in patient areas have unambiguously positive subject matter and convey a sense of security or safety. In addition, priority should be given to selecting representational art that depicts the following categories of subject matter:

Waterscapes

■ Calm or nonturbulent water, not stormy conditions

Landscapes

■ Visual depth or openness in immediate foreground

■ Landscapes depicted during warmer seasons, when vegetation is verdant and flowers are visible; landscapes conveying bleakness should be avoided

■ Scenes with positive cultural artifacts, such as barns and older houses

■ Presence of nonthreatening wildlife, such as birds or deer

■ Landscapes with low hills and distant mountains

Flowers and Gardens

■ Flowers that appear healthy and fresh, not wilted or dead

■ Types of flowers that are generally familiar to patients, not novel or strange

■ Garden scenes with some openness in the immediate foreground

Figurative Art

■ People at leisure in places with prominent nature

■ Emotionally positive facial expressions, gestures, and body language that are caring or friendly

■ Relationships among people that are friendly, nurturing, or caring

■ Generational and cultural diversity

The following characteristics should be avoided when selecting art for stressed patients (Ulrich, 1991; Ulrich and Gilpin, 2003; Hathorn and Ulrich, 2001):

■ Ambiguity or uncertainty

■ Emotionally negative or provocative subject matter

■ Surreal qualities

■ Closely spaced repeating edges or forms that are optically unstable or appear to move

■ Restricted depth or claustrophobic-like qualities

- Close-up, potentially threatening animals staring directly at the viewer

- Outdoor scenes with overcast or foreboding weather

In conclusion, the research discussed in this chapter implies that visual artwork in health care facilities is no mere luxury or unimportant embellishment. To the contrary, findings increasingly support the notion that the evidence-based selection of emotionally appropriate art contributes an important environmental dimension to patient care—one that lessens patient stress and pain and improves other medical outcomes.

PLANETREE ARTS PROGRAMS

In the Planetree model, the arts have been described as inspiration for the mind, language for the emotions, and balm for the soul. In addition to visual art, addressed earlier in this chapter, music, storytelling, poetry, humor, and other expressive arts can all play a vital role in creating a healing environment for patients and their families, as well as providing a positive working environment for staff.

Numerous studies have documented the efficacy of incorporating a variety of art forms, beyond the visual arts, into health care environments. Nilsson and colleagues (2001) found that women undergoing hysterectomies who listened to calming music and sounds of ocean waves while under general anesthesia experienced less pain, were less fatigued, and were able to sit up sooner following surgery than patients who had not listened to music. Music has also been shown to mitigate the effects of nausea and emesis among patients undergoing chemotherapy (Standley, 1992) and has been found to calm agitated patients. Researchers (Ragneskog and others, 1996) observed the reaction of patients with dementia to three different types of music played during dinner time, finding that patients were particularly affected by soothing music. At times when music was played, patients spent more time at dinner and ate more calmly (Ragneskog and others, 1996).

Evidence further suggests that incorporating opportunities for involvement in the arts can help reduce stress levels of patients' loved ones as well as health care staff. In one study (Walsh, Martin, and Schmidt, 2004), one hour of involvement in a simple art-making exercise reduced depression symptoms, anxiety, and stress for family caregivers of cancer patients. Another study (Bittman and others, 2003) documented the effects of a six-week recreational music-making opportunity at a Pennsylvania nursing home. The organization implemented weekly drumming sessions for its staff, and outcomes included a 46 percent improvement in mood, which was translated by an independent consulting group as the potential to reduce turnover by 18.3 percent (Bittman and others, 2003).

Studies such as these document the physiological effects of the arts on health and healing, but many patient-centered care providers choose to include a variety of arts simply for their usefulness as *positive distractions,* offering a diversion from anxiety, discomfort, and loneliness. Whereas art therapy uses the arts, in conjunction with counseling skills, as a therapeutic technique, the purpose of Planetree arts programs is to bring the experience of the arts to patients and their families. This experience can offer a respite from the intensity of illness and the anxiety of hospitalization. The arts can also diminish boredom and provide a space for reflection and inspiration.

An arts program need not be expensive. Many operate primarily with volunteers and donated equipment. Many hospitals find that community groups, local art associations, and volunteers are willing to donate time and resources to create and maintain an active arts program. The arts program at the first Planetree site began with a weekly movie night and a few donated audiotapes and cassette players for patients. After its initial success, the program was expanded.

Arts programs vary at Planetree sites. Many schedule performances by local musicians. Others have introduced clown programs and humor carts. Poetry corners, art carts (where patients select their own art), roving magicians, and portable CD and DVD players are among the ways that patient-centered providers have introduced the arts as part of the healing environment.

Healing arts programs can also be participatory, engaging patients and residents in activities that can ease their minds and serve as positive diversions. The VA New Jersey Health Care System's Healing Arts Program is composed of a wide range of activities that help create a warm and welcoming environment, stimulate patients' creativity, ease their minds, and aid in the healing process. Painting classes engage veterans in the arts and provide an avenue for self-expression, and craft kits are provided to any interested veteran who is hospitalized. Project Healing Waters aids wounded vets in their physical and emotional recovery by introducing the skills of fly-fishing. A scrapbook-making activity provides the opportunity for hospitalized veterans to create a project, and the pages themselves shed light on the interests and experiences of individual patients, and thus have been useful tools for new staff looking to connect with a patient. The Healing Arts Program has also been an effective way to calm agitated patients. A harp therapist makes regular visits, which have been relaxing and calming for veterans in the nursing home, mental health, oncology, and spinal cord injury units.

The arts are an integral part of peoples' lives. The following case study demonstrates the profound power of the arts in the health care setting.

Music-Thanatology

Music-thanatology is a professional field that unites music and medicine in end-of-life care. During a music vigil, a music-thanatologist employs harp and voice at the bedside to serve the physical, emotional, and spiritual needs of the dying and their loved ones. The warmth of this *prescriptive music* can help ease physical and emotional symptoms while offering a space of intimacy and serenity. It affords families a chance to be with their loved one in a soothing atmosphere, where words are not necessary, yet the words that are said often come from a deep place, aided by the music. Such was the case for one couple struggling with a crisis of faith, anger, and fear, as the wife approached the end of life.

Rose was a fifty-six-year-old woman diagnosed with metastatic parotid cancer. Her husband, Ray, was twenty years older than she and coping with health challenges of his own, which limited his ability to care for her. Even so, he insisted on keeping her at home, contrary to medical recommenda-tion. Rose and Ray were active in their church, and even when all treatment options were exhausted, they were counting on a miraculous cure. Ray especially resisted conversations around end-of-life planning.

During the terminal phase of Rose's disease, the couple received eleven vigils from a certified music-thanatologist. In the early vigils, Rose expressed that the music lifted her out of her fear and pain, taking her to a peaceful place. During these vigils, Ray consistently left the room, until the sixth visit, when a significant shift occurred. Rose had broken her hip and was admit-ted to the hospital. Surgery was attempted but failed, due to bone metas-tases. By this time, she had been trying to discuss her final wishes with Ray, but he clung to hope for a miracle and refused to speak about it.

FOR EXAMPLE

Rose was groggy and somewhat agitated from sedatives, when the music-thanatologist arrived for the sixth vigil, and Ray sat beside her, studying the room service menu. Uncharacteristically, though, Ray remained seated as the music began. Opening with minor tonalities and unmetered rhythms, the music offered Rose release into an interior space of rest. Soon she slept. Meanwhile, Ray, who had struggled to maintain composure, began shaking with sobs. The musical focus turned to him to hold him in his grief. With warm harmonies and rocking rhythms, the music enfolded him as he wept. In the silence afterward he confessed to the music-thanatologist, "This is so hard." He explained that while listening to the music, he realized he was no longer able to care for Rose, and she would have to be admitted to a care facility. Then he asked, "You know what's happening, don't you? She's going home." His face crumpled in sorrow, and it was clear he meant Home with a capital "H."

Rose then awoke, later sharing that Ray's heart had been opened by the music, and they were finally able to have that talk. From that point on, Ray stayed for the music vigils and gradually made his peace with his wife dying. Rose fought valiantly until the end but always found a measure of solace and relief in the gentle beauty of the music.

CONTRIBUTED BY ANNA FIASCA, CERTIFIED MUSIC-THANATOLOGIST

REFERENCES

Appleton, J. *The Experience of Landscape.* Hoboken, N.J.: Wiley, 1975.

Bittman, M. D., and others. "Recreational Music-Making: A Cost-Effective Group Interdisciplinary Strategy for Reducing Burnout and Improving Mood States in Long-Term Care Workers." *Advances in Mind-Body Medicine,* 2003, *19*(3/4).

Bower, G. "Mood and Memory." *American Psychologist,* 1981, *36,* 129–148.

Carpman, J. R., and Grant, M. A. *Design That Cares: Planning Health Facilities for Patients and Visitors.* (2nd ed.) Chicago: American Hospital, 1993.

Clearwater, Y. A., and Coss, R. G. "Functional Aesthetics to Enhance Well-Being in Isolated and Confined Settings." In A. A. Harrison, Y. A. Clearwater, and C. McKay (eds.), *From Antarctica to Outer Space: Life in Isolation and Confinement.* New York: Springer-Verlag, 1991.

Coss, R. G. "The Ethological Command in Art." *Leonardo,* 1968, *1,* 273–287.

Coss, R. G. "Picture Perception and Patient Stress: A Study of Anxiety Reduction and Postoperative Stability." Unpublished paper, Department of Psychology, University of California, Davis, 1990.

Coss, R. G. "The Role of Evolved Perceptual Biases in Art and Design." In E. Voland, K. Grammer, and A. Heschl (eds.), *Evolutionary Aesthetics*. Cambridge, Mass.: MIT Press, 2003.

Diette, G. B., and others. "Distraction Therapy with Nature Sights and Sounds Reduces Pain During Flexible Bronchoscopy: A Complementary Approach to Routine Analgesia." *Chest,* 2003, *123*(3), 941–948.

Eisen, S. "Effects of Art in Pediatric Healthcare." Unpublished doctoral dissertation, Department of Architecture, Texas A&M University, 2006.

Ekman, P., Friesen, W. V., and Ellsworth, P. C. *Emotion in the Human Face.* New York: Pergamon Press, 1972.

Fredrickson, B. L., and Levenson, R. W. "Positive Emotions Speed Recovery from the Cardiovascular Sequelae of Negative Emotions." *Cognition and Emotion,* 1998, *12,* 191–220.

Friedrich, M. J. "The Arts of Healing." *Journal of the American Medical Association,* 1999, *281*(19), 1779–1781.

Gilpin, L. "Healing Arts: Nutrition for the Soul." In *Putting Patients First* (1st ed.). San Francisco: Jossey Bass, 2003.

Hartig, T., and others. "Environmental Influences on Psychological Restoration." *Scandinavian Journal of Psychology,* 1996, *37,* 378–393.

Hathorn, K., and Ulrich, R. S. "The Therapeutic Art Program of Northwestern Memorial Hospital." In *Creating Environments That Heal: Proceedings of the Symposium on Healthcare Design* (CD-ROM). Imark Communications and Center for Health Design, 2001. [www.healthcaredesign.com].

Heerwagen, J. "The Psychological Aspects of Windows and Window Design." In K. H. Anthony, J. Choi, and B. Orland (eds.), *Proceedings of the Twenty-First Annual Conference of the Environmental Design Research Association.* Oklahoma City: Environmental Design Research Association, 1990.

Hefferman, M. L., Morstatt, M., Saltzman, K., and Strunc, L. "A Room with a View Art Survey: The Bird Garden at Duke University Hospital." Unpublished research report, Cultural Services Program and Management Fellows Program, Duke University Medical Center, Durham, N.C., 1995.

Isen, A. "Positive Affect, Cognitive Processes, and Social Behavior." In L. Berkowitz (ed.), *Advances in Experimental Social Psychology.* Orlando: Academic Press, 1987.

Joye, Y. "Architectural Lessons from Environmental Psychology: The Case of Biophilic Architecture." *Review of General Psychology,* 2007, *11*(4), 305–328.

Kaplan, R., and Kaplan, S. *The Experience of Nature.* New York: Cambridge University Press, 1989.

Kendler, K. S., Karkowski, L. M., and Prescott, C. A. "Fears and Phobias: Reliability and Heritability." *Psychological Medicine,* 1999, *29,* 539–553.

Kettlewell, N. "An Examination of Preferences for Subject Matter in Art." *Empirical Studies of the Arts,* 1988, *6,* 59–65.

Lee, D.W.H., and others. "Can Visual Distraction Decrease the Dose of Patient-Controlled Sedation Required During Colonoscopy? A Prospective Randomized Controlled Trial." *Endoscopy,* 2004, *36*(3), 197–201.

Martin, C. "Let Me Through: I'm an Arts Practitioner!" *Lancet,* 1999, *353*(9162), 1451.

McCaul, K. D., and Malott, J. M. "Distraction and Coping with Pain." *Psychological Bulletin,* 1984, *95*(3), 516–533.

McLaughlin, J., and others. "Duke University's Bird Garden." In *Proceedings of the 1996 Annual Conference of the Society for the Arts in Healthcare.* Durham, N.C.: Durham Arts Council and Duke University Medical Center, 1996.

Miller, A. C., Hickman, L. C., and Lemasters, G. K. "A Distraction Technique for Control of Burn Pain." *Journal of Burn Care and Rehabilitation,* 1992, *13,* 576–580.

Nanda, U., Hathorn, K., and Neumann, T. "The Art-Cart Program at St. Luke's Episcopal Hospital, Houston." *Healthcare Design,* 2007, *7*(7), 10–12.

Niedenthal, P. M., Setterlund, M. B., and Jones, D. E. "Emotional Organization of Perceptual Memory." In P. M. Niedenthal and S. Kitayama (eds.), *The Heart's Eye: Emotional Influences in Perception and Attention.* Orlando, Fla.: Academic Press, 1994.

Nightingale, F. *Notes on Nursing.* New York: Dover, 1969. (Originally published 1860.)

Nilsson, U., and others. "Improved Recovery After Music and Therapeutic Suggestions During General Anaesthesia: A Double-Blind Randomised Controlled Trial." *Acta Anaesthesiologica Scandinavica,* 2001, *45*(7), 812–817.

Öhman, A. "Face the Beast and Fear the Face: Animal and Social Fears as Prototypes for Evolutionary Analyses of Emotion." *Psychophysiology,* 1986, *23,* 123–145.

Orians, G. H. "An Ecological and Evolutionary Approach to Landscape Aesthetics." In E. C. Penning-Rowsell and D. Lowenthal (eds.), *Meanings and Values in Landscape.* London: Allen and Unwin, 1986.

Parsons, R., and Hartig, T. "Environmental Psychophysiology." In J. T. Caccioppo, L. G. Tassinary, and G. Berntson (eds.), *Handbook of Psychophysiology.* New York: Cambridge University Press, 2000.

Parsons, R., and others. "The View from the Road: Implications for Stress Recovery and Immunization." *Journal of Environmental Psychology,* 1998, *18,* 113–140.

Ragneskog, H., and others. "Dinner Music for Demented Patients: Analysis of Video-Recorded Observations." *Clinical Nursing Research,* 1996, *5*(3), 262–277.

Singer, J. A., and Salovey, P. "Mood and Memory: Evaluating the Network Theory of Affect." *Clinical Psychology Review,* 1988, *8,* 211–251.

Standley, J. "Clinical Applications of Music and Chemotherapy: The Effects on Nausea and Emesis." *Music Therapy Perspectives,* 1992, *10,* 27–35.

Tse, M.M.Y., and others. "The Effect of Visual Stimuli on Pain Threshold and Tolerance." *Journal of Clinical Nursing,* 2002, *11*(4), 462–469.

Ulrich, R. S. "Visual Landscapes and Psychological Well-Being." *Landscape Research,* 1979, *4*(1), 17–23.

Ulrich, R. S. *"Aesthetic and Affective Response to Natural Environment."* In I. Altman and J. F. Wohlwill (eds.), *Human Behavior and the Environment. Vol. 6: Behavior and the Natural Environment.* New York: Plenum, 1983.

Ulrich, R. S. "View Through a Window May Influence Recovery from Surgery." *Science,* 1984, *224,* 420–421.

Ulrich, R. S. "Effects of Health Facility Interior Design on Wellness: Theory and Recent Scientific Research." *Journal of Health Care Design,* 1991, *3,* 97–109.

Ulrich, R. S. "Biophilia, Biophobia, and Natural Landscapes." In S. A. Kellert and E. O. Wilson (eds.), *The Biophilia Hypothesis.* Washington, D.C.: Island Press, 1993.

Ulrich, R. S. "Effects of Gardens on Health Outcomes: Theory and Research." In C. C. Marcus and M. Barnes (eds.), *Healing Gardens: Therapeutic Benefits and Design Recommendations.* New York: Wiley, 1999.

Ulrich, R. S. "Biophilic Theory and Research for Health Design." In S. Kellert, J. Heerwagen, and M. Mador (eds.), *Biophilic Design: Theory, Science, and Practice.* New York: Wiley, 2008.

Ulrich, R. S., and Gilpin, L. "Healing Arts: Nutrition for the Soul." In S. B. Frampton, L. Gilpin, and P. A. Charmel (eds.), *Putting Patients First: Designing and Practicing Patient-Centered Care.* San Francisco: Jossey-Bass, 2003.

Ulrich, R. S., Lundén, O., and Eltinge, J. L. "Effects of Exposure to Nature and Abstract Pictures on Patients Recovering from Heart Surgery." Paper presented at the 33rd meeting of the Society for Psychophysiological Research, Rottach-Egern, Germany, 1993. (Abstract published in *Psychophysiology,* 1993, *30*(supp. 1), 7.)

Ulrich, R. S., Simons, R. F., and Miles, M. A. "Effects of Environmental Simulations and Television on Blood Donor Stress. *Journal of Architectural and Planning Research,* 2003, *20*(1), 38–47.

Ulrich, R. S., and others. "Stress Recovery During Exposure to Natural and Urban Environments." *Journal of Environmental Psychology,* 1991, *11*, 201–230.

Van den Berg, A., Koole, S. L., and Van der Wulp, N. Y. "Environmental Preference and Restoration: How Are They Related?" *Journal of Environmental Psychology,* 2003, *23*, 135–146.

Walsh, S. M., Martin, S. C., and Schmidt, L. A. "Testing the Efficacy of a Creative-Arts Intervention with Family Caregivers of Patients with Cancer." *Journal of Nursing Scholarship,* 2004, *36*, 214–219.

Whall, A. L., and others. "The Effect of Natural Environments upon Agitation and Aggression in Late Stage Dementia Patients." *American Journal of Alzheimer's Disease and Other Dementias,* 1997, *12*(5), 216–220.

Wilson, E. O. *Biophilia.* Cambridge, Mass.: Harvard University Press, 1984.

Winston, A. S., and Cupchik, G. C. "The Evaluation of High Art and Popular Art by Naive and Experienced Viewers." *Visual Arts Research,* 1992, *18*, 1–14.

Wypijewski, J. (ed.). *Painting by the Numbers: Komar and Melamid's Scientific Guide to Art.* New York: Farrar Straus & Giroux, 1997.

CHAPTER

8

HEALING ENVIRONMENTS: CREATING A NURTURING AND HEALTHY ENVIRONMENT

KIMBERLY NELSON MONTAGUE AND ROBERT F. SHARROW

This chapter does the following:

- Identifies core elements for consideration in the design and development of a patient-centered, healing environment that engages the five senses

- Demonstrates how architecture and design can promote patient privacy and patient safety

- Presents strategies for reducing noise levels in health care settings

- Presents strategies for providing appropriate lighting that meets the needs of health care providers and the preferences of patients and loved ones

- Introduces ways to empower patients with a sense of control over their own environment

- Discusses ways to enhance *wayfinding* throughout a facility

- Addresses how to incorporate healing design principles into staff support areas and work stations.

It was once said that we design our buildings and they forever after shape the way we use them. If this is true, then the design of a Planetree environment is also shaped by the patients, visitors, family members, volunteers, and staff members who circulate through it on a daily basis. To create a nurturing and healthy Planetree environment then, we must examine the attributes that provide the greatest opportunity for affecting the spiritual, emotional, and physical needs of all those who are affected by the facility.

Just as a home is a reflection of one's personality, a Planetree environment mirrors the values, beliefs, and cultures represented by the community it serves. This unique concept of altering the physical and intangible elements of a building to create an environment of healing, however, is not new. Thirty years ago, Angelica Thieriot envisioned a healing environment that was warm, comfortable, and less institutional than the conventional environments of the time. Her desire was to create a space that appealed to all five senses and that personalized, humanized, and demystified the health care experience.

Here, though, it must be reiterated that the Planetree philosophy is not defined by a specific type of architecture or interior design. A beautiful health care unit is not necessarily one in which patients feel empowered and supported. A patient who is frightened, lonely, and isolated from family and friends is not likely to notice the meticulously decorated surroundings. It is only when architecture and interior design work in concert with the other Planetree components that the physical surroundings can achieve Thieriot's vision of a healing environment.

To facilitate this goal, Roslyn Lindheim, a founding board member of Planetree and professor of architecture at the University of California at Berkeley, developed several design principles that are at the core of every Planetree facility. These qualities are vital to the Planetree model, not simply for their architectural and aesthetic aspects but also because they have been shown to influence behaviors, interactions, and emotional responses. Lindheim emphasized that the design of health care settings should accomplish the following (Arneill and Frasca-Beaulieu, 2003):

- Welcome the patient's family and friends

- Value human beings over technology

- Enable patients to fully participate as partners in their care

- Provide flexibility to personalize the care of each patient

- Encourage caregivers to be responsive to patients

- Foster a connection to nature and beauty

These principles have evolved over time and have developed into the core elements for consideration in the design and development of a Planetree facility. And while new construction or extensive renovation provides optimal opportunities for incorporating healing design principles, in the absence of construction, there are also simple, low-cost ways to create a more patient-centered, healing environment in existing facilities.

PRIVACY

Privacy is a basic human need, and it is the most important factor in the design of a Planetree environment. One of the simplest ways to preserve a patient's sense of privacy is to provide individuals with personal, unshared rooms for changing, examinations, treatment, and sleeping. See Figure 8.1. For times when patients are not in their bedrooms, consider creating discrete, secluded areas where they and family members may wait for their appointments or procedures.

In addition to the expressed desires of patients for increased privacy in health care environments, the Health Insurance Portability and Accountability Act of 1996 also requires that treatment providers maintain patient confidentiality relative to all forms of medical information. Consequently, the law has significantly influenced the design of new health care facilities, whereby the provision of private patient rooms,

Midwest Medical Center

In 2004, Galena-Stauss Hospital and Healthcare Center, a forty-two-year-old eighteen-bed critical access facility located in the northwest corner of Illinois, became the first Planetree affiliate hospital in the state. During this same period, the hospital's leadership cast a vision for what they believed health care should be in their rural community. While the hospital underwent many changes to update and upgrade the existing facility, Galena-Stauss remained an antiquated, landlocked space with a myriad of facility challenges.

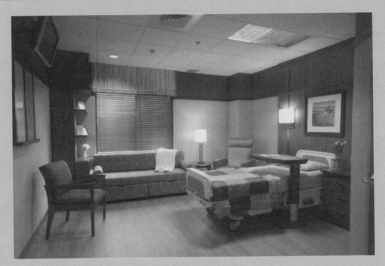

FIGURE 8.1. *Private Patient Room, Midwest Medical Center.*

It was at this time that CEO Jeff Hill and Board President Dan Mennenoh assembled a team of experts to help design, finance, build, and open the first replacement critical access hospital in Illinois. Every detail of what is now Midwest Medical Center incorporates the Planetree tenets. Upon entering the front doors, you are immediately taken in by the warm colors, rich woods, soothing sconce lighting, vaulted ceilings, and life-size windows that point to the blue Midwestern sky. From the water feature that keeps children entertained and gives parents a needed diversion, to the bubbling copper fountain in the healing garden, you immediately feel that you are in a place where you will be cared for. The mahogany baby grand player piano provides mood-elevating audio, while the majestic ceramic-tiled staircase that leads to the family room encourages visitors and staff to take the stairs rather than ride the elevators. Patient suites are private, warm, and comforting, with windows that offer a magnificent view and a place for family to rest. In-room dining, flat screen televisions, and carefully designed panels to hide medical gas controls are just a few of the features that help transform the patient experience.

In the design phase of the project, physicians, nurses, and allied health professionals were invited to provide their ideas for making Midwest Medical Center the optimal environment in which to practice medicine. Some of the outcomes from this collaboration include operating suites with windows to offer natural light, a sound system to which surgeons can connect their MP3 players, an alternative paging method to the traditional overhead system, a comfortable and spacious physician room in close proximity to medical records, and an emergency physicians' suite that promotes rest and comfort when breaks are well-deserved and needed.

Features such as the state-of-the-art Fitness Center, Resource Library, Meditation Suite, Whispering Willow Gifts, and Vista Café attract community members to visit the facility for reasons other than illness.

From a hospital that required patients to walk a long, dark corridor to use the bathing facilities to a truly beautiful, compassionate, patient-focused, and medically advanced facility, Midwest Medical Center has transformed health care in its community, the most significant evidence of which lies in the words of a mother who brought her son in for care a week after the doors opened, "I'll never pass you by and drive out of state for health care again."

CONTRIBUTED BY K. JEFFREY HILL, MIDWEST MEDICAL CENTER, AND MICHELLE M. RATHMAN, IMPACT! COMMUNICATIONS, INC.

charting, and conference areas for staff is the only way to ensure that confidentiality is maintained. Older health care facilities that were not designed to accommodate individual privacy face challenges in meeting this basic human need. Careful attention to the protocol used during a patient consultation in a semiprivate patient room situation needs to be considered, and if possible, relocating the patient to a private consultation room is preferred.

PATIENT SAFETY

The shift to private inpatient rooms brings many additional benefits. For instance, it practically eliminates the need to transfer patients to different rooms due to gender or roommate incompatibility issues. Private patient bedrooms have also been shown to reduce hospital-acquired infections and increase patient satisfaction (Ulrich and others, 2004). Research further demonstrates that single-bed rooms result in improved patient safety. In an effort to increase observation, improve assistance for patients, and reduce falls, Methodist Hospital in Indianapolis, Indiana, changed its coronary critical care unit from operating with a centralized nurse station and two-bed rooms to having decentralized nurse stations and large single-bed rooms (Hendrich, Fay, and Sorrells, 2002). Comparison of data from two years prior and three years after the unit redesign showed that falls were cut by two-thirds, from six per thousand to two per thousand (Ulrich and others, 2004).

When designing new inpatient units, another consideration should be the location and sizing of the patient's bathroom. Research has indicated that there is a high incidence of patient falls for those attempting to use the bathroom unassisted by staff (Alcee, 2000). In order to minimize such hazards, the bathroom should be located such that the door opens next to the patient's bed, with handrails mounted along walls or countertops to give patients a firm grip to steady themselves on the way to the toilet.

At Elmhurst Memorial Hospital in Elmhurst, Illinois, a new Planetree replacement hospital is being designed with privacy and safety as two of the primary considerations for inpatient bedroom and toilet room design. During review of mock-up rooms, nursing staff pointed out that sides of a patient toilet must be placed approximately twenty-four inches away from the side walls of the bathroom to allow for a "two-sided–patient-assist" of a heavier patient. In this maneuver, a patient is assisted by two staff members, one at each side of the toilet, thus necessitating substantial clearance at both sides of the toilet. For added patient safety, a folding grab bar was installed at each side of the toilet.

NOISE CONTROL

The World Health Organization standards for background noise in hospital patient rooms are 35 dB, with nighttime peaks in patient care areas not to exceed 40 dB (Berglund, Lindvall, and Schwela, 1999).

Many studies have shown that these maximums are often exceeded, with levels typically ranging from 48 to 68 dB, and peaks often exceeding 85 dB (Berglund, Lindvall, and Schwela, 1999). This level is equivalent to the noise level perceived while walking next to a busy highway.

Reducing the amount of noise is an important factor to be considered in the creation of a healing environment. Sound can be negative if it is perceived as noise and cannot be controlled; in fact, noise is one of the most significantly detrimental environmental factors known to cause physiological changes in the body and affect healing. From the reverberation of intercoms to the beeping of cardiac machines, hospital sounds can be discomforting and disturbing for patients.

Designers can reduce the noise levels in a healing environment by specifying carpeting or soft resilient floor covering in corridors, thus diminishing the noise from footsteps, rolling equipment, and voices. Other strategies to significantly reduce ambient noise in a patient unit include the use of high-quality supply carts with large rubber wheels and bearings, the installation of high-performance ceiling tiles in lieu of hard reflective ceiling surfaces, utilization of noiseless pagers, and the reduction of overhead paging systems.

In a recent study (Hagerman and others, 2005), ceiling tiles were exchanged in an occupied ICU on a random basis and data were collected for both patients and staff. The highest-performance sound-absorbing material used for ceiling tiles was demonstrated to reduce noise levels dramatically in the ICU, and the reduced noise levels were linked to lower levels of physiological stress in both patients and staff, lowered levels of medication errors, and improved patient recovery, as evidenced by a lowered level of readmission after discharge from the ICU. Based on this study, only high performance acoustical ceiling tiles should be used in noisy staff and patient care areas.

VIEWS OF AND ACCESS TO NATURE

It has been researched and well documented that views of nature can help reduce stress and aid in the healing process, and most of us have likely experienced the sense of calm and release of tension associated with either viewing our favorite nature scene, or better yet, experiencing it firsthand. As Angelica Thieriot describes in the Prologue to this book, it was an orchid that provided her with a positive distraction during a bleak time. One recent study noted that in order to provide for a restorative experience, four factors must be in place: fascination, coherence, sense of being away, and compatibility with inclinations and goals. Kaplan and Kaplan (1989) theorized that the objective is to provide coherent stimuli and not random or incomprehensible objects. In fact, there is strong evidence that even fairly brief encounters with real or simulated nature scenes can elicit significant recovery from stress within three to five minutes, at most (Parsons and Hartig, 2000; Ulrich, 1999).

While patients are infirm, it goes without saying that their stress level is elevated, and in many instances, stress levels are also elevated for visitors and staff. Providing a view to the out-of-doors—or at a minimum, artwork with nature scenes—can aid in relieving some of this anxiety. In some cases, views from patients' rooms are limited because of location. Simply changing the view of either a roof or adjacent building by providing a foreground view of a rooftop garden or trellis can have a positive effect on the environment. Even small changes can have a big impact, as at Aurora Medical Center Oshkosh in Oshkosh, Wisconsin, where an otherwise drab rooftop view was enhanced for the pediatrics unit by adding animal sculptures to the roof for children and their visitors to view.

At Alliance Community Hospital in Alliance, Ohio, an unsightly rooftop was converted to a garden for use by patients and visitors. Located near the surgery and obstetrics departments, it took the place of an unattractive gravel rooftop and transformed it to a garden that provides fresh air and respite from an otherwise hectic experience. See Figure 8.2.

If the opportunity exists to do it, the incorporation of outdoor patios or balconies can allow patients and visitors access to the outdoors during their stay at the facility. Even in northern climates, access to the outdoors and exposure to sunlight has been shown to have a positive effect on those who are susceptible to seasonal affective disorder (SAD). In fact, two studies in which people were asked what kind of place they went to when feeling troubled, upset, or in grief revealed that natural settings were predominantly cited (Francis and Cooper Marcus, 1991, 1992, 1995).

When the view of nature is not available, a clerestory or skylights can also allow daylight into the interior of a hospital department that might otherwise be lifeless. The addition of water features, ponds, and landscaping that is indigenous and appropriate for the climate and culture of the community can add a sense of life to a facility. Even when the courtyard is not accessible, adding low-maintenance plant material can change the view for patients. The healing garden at Aurora Medical

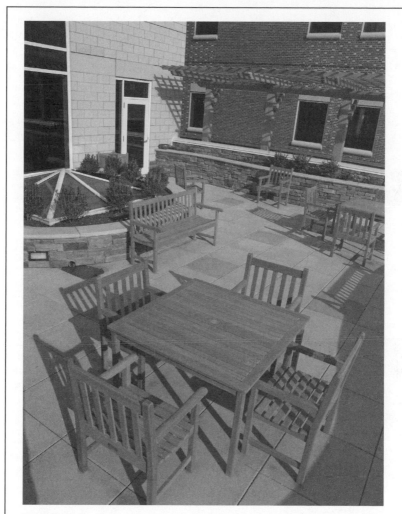

FIGURE 8.2. *Rooftop Garden, Alliance Community Hospital.*

Center Oshkosh is a wonderful example of the integration of landscaping into the facility design. Designed around the concept of a Zen garden, the courtyard provides quiet contemplative nooks throughout and a small gazebo for reflection and quiet. See Figure 8.3.

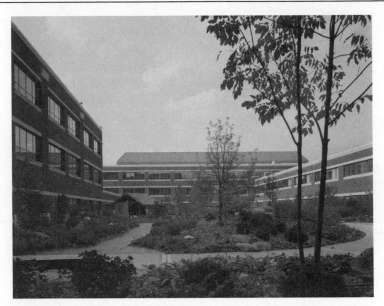

FIGURE 8.3. *Healing Garden, Aurora Medical Center Oshkosh.*

Source: Photo courtesy of Kahn; photograph by Justin Maconochie.

Many hospitals are also incorporating outdoor spaces as part of their spirituality component, constructing labyrinths within the healing gardens as a spiritual support. See Figure 8.4.

LIGHTING

Most hospitals provide general illumination in corridors through the use of two-by-four-foot fluorescent fixtures mounted in the ceiling. Although this provides a light level that is appropriate for cleaning and general patient care, in most instances, the amount of light is excessive and may be a major source of psychological and physical stress on patients. Bright lights can cause headaches and nausea, whereas lack of lighting has been known to cause fatigue and depression.

It is equally important for visitor areas to have appropriate lighting. Typically, these areas include overhead fluorescent fixtures that are

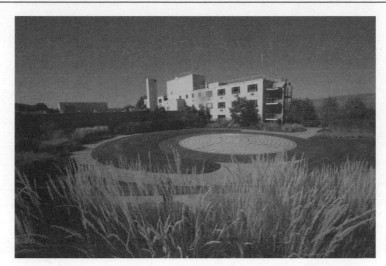

FIGURE 8.4. *Labyrinth, Mid-Columbia Medical Center.*

Source: Jim Semlor, Semlor Images.

stressful and not conducive to relaxation. By using a combination of different types of lighting, such as recessed fluorescent down-lighting for general illumination, accent wall washing fixtures to highlight artwork, and floor and table lamps for reading, designers can create a residential atmosphere that feels more comfortable, supportive, and nurturing.

In addition to considerations for artificial lighting, the provision of windows, clerestories, and skylights can have a profound effect on patients, staff, and visitors to the facility. In fact, it has been shown that patients in brightly lit rooms have a shorter length of stay compared with patients in dull rooms. In addition, exposure to morning light may be more effective than exposure to evening light in reducing depression (Ulrich and others, 2004). When designing a new facility or considering renovations, it is advisable to seek out opportunities for patients, staff, and visitors to have access to windows facing south, east, or west to maximize sunlight exposure. As depicted in Figure 8.5, at Sentara Williamsburg in Williamsburg, Virginia, the entrance lobby utilizes skylights and plenty of glazing to allow natural light to filter into the center of the space, creating a welcoming and light-filled environment.

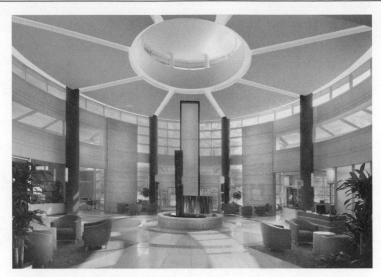

FIGURE 8.5. *Entrance Lobby, Sentara Williamsburg Regional Medical Center.*

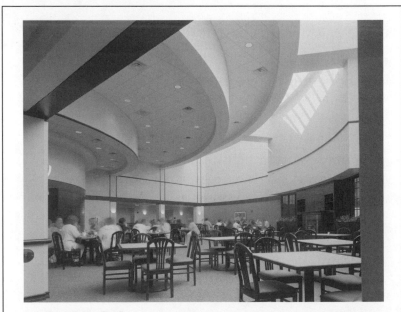

FIGURE 8.6. *Café, Aurora Medical Center Oshkosh.*

The café at Aurora Medical Center Oshkosh depicted in Figure 8.6 demonstrates how the incorporation of clerestory skylights allows light to filter into an interior space, making it feel more open and welcoming than it might otherwise be without windows.

THERAPEUTIC ENHANCEMENTS

The Planetree philosophy celebrates the importance of the five senses. This attention to sensory input should begin at the edge of the building site and seamlessly continue into the facility itself. In progressing from parking to entry to lobby and then on to one's destination in the health facility, what one sees, hears, smells, touches, and tastes is vital to the experience of being in a holistic, patient-centered environment.

One of the more unusual aspects of many Planetree facilities is a pleasant, small family galley, located on the nursing unit or in the ambulatory care and maternity center. This space is made available for families to prepare special meals or snacks for patients. Staff members and volunteers also use these kitchens to prepare treats for patients and visitors, including coffee, tea, and sometimes even freshly baked chocolate chip cookies. The aroma of baked goods not only creates a pleasant, homey feel, but it also helps to mask the "institutional" odors common to health care facilities.

Music has also been recognized as playing an integral part in the healing process, providing a positive distraction to patients' perception of noise. As patients tune in to the music, it becomes easier to disregard other unpleasant sounds commonly found in healing environments. If possible, consider placing a player piano in the lobby or schedule music performances by local musicians.

The concept of personalized space is also important to patients, and Planetree facilities should enable patients to transform an area of their room into a place that conveys a sense of personal harmony and individuality. Special shelves, bulletin boards, and niches enable the patient to display flowers, cards, and gifts, and they offer a way to view these items from their own bed.

GATHERING SPACES

In the Planetree model of care, family, friends, and community play vital roles in the healing process. Research has indicated that strong social support can reduce stress and accelerate healing, and the inclusion of a variety of different kinds of gathering spaces will foster the positive interaction and communication that is so vital to healing. The lobby presents the first opportunity to create a welcoming environment that comforts patients and their families with pleasantly unexpected sights, sounds and aromas. Comfortable seating allows patients and their families to feel at home as they gather or wait, while pleasing aromas wafting from a coffeehouse or bakeshop enhance that feeling. A fireplace can create a warm ambience, and fish tanks or water features delight people of all ages. These elements, coupled with the sounds of soft piano music, work in harmony to create a comfortable environment of care.

Another important gathering area for families is the dining center. Ideally, a variety of food options will be available for staff and patients, ranging from a conveniently located coffee shop with baked goods, to a full service dining area with comfortable tables and booths for families who wish to enjoy an unhurried dining experience.

The reception and lounge areas of each major hospital department, when designed with a patient-centered approach, will also provide gathering spaces for patients and their families. Family lounges should be divided into separate areas for quiet waiting or reading, with a distinct area for watching television. If children are present, a discrete family area with toys, games, and smaller seating groups is helpful. The main furniture groups (sofas and lounge chairs) should be arranged to foster social interaction, and other seating can be arranged for private conversations.

Likewise, patient rooms should have comfortable seating to accommodate a family of five to seven visitors, as well as a convertible bed or couch for a family member to spend the night if desired.

ICUs are high-energy work environments that quickly create stress in both patients and family members. The ICU design of Griffin Hospital separates the high-tech staff area from the visitor area by adding a separate entrance to each patient room through a corridor along the perimeter of the unit. In this way, family members can remain close to patients without undue stress or disrupting the medical staff. Along this corridor are lounges, small kitchenettes, bathrooms, and terraces for family members and friends to use while visiting their loved ones.

Spaces for spiritual support should also be conveniently located throughout a patient-centered facility. An ecumenical chapel or serenity room will support both private meditation and prayer as well as group services. Private quiet rooms should be located close to the Emergency Department, Surgery, and ICU units to support families during periods of great emotional need. Healing gardens can provide solace and should have private benches for use by patients, family members, and staff.

ENVIRONMENTAL CONTROL

In a hospital, patients often have a feeling of loss of control over many physical aspects of their own lives. Providing patients with the ability to control the comfort of their personal space can provide some psychological relief. In each patient room, it should be the goal to provide individual control of the room temperature. This can be done in a variety of ways, the most common of which is to include individual thermostatic control at the bedside or at a minimum located such that a family member or the staff can adjust it according to the patient's request.

Similarly, lights should be alterable by patients. Using a variety of lights and lighting levels can accommodate the clinical tasks at hand while providing flexibility, control, and comfort. For example, in patient rooms it may be necessary to have bright overhead examination lights, but patients should be able to shut them off when they are not in use. It is also recommended that reading lamps be made available on each bedside table. Another important consideration is the provision of low-level lighting to be utilized by staff in the middle of the night, so as not to disturb the patient. Designers should also acknowledge the need for control over the window coverings in the room, either through electronic means or simple pull cords that are easily reachable by the patient.

Most patient rooms have a television. This should be considered as a main form of education and communication for the patient and family, including the capability for music channels; educational channels; or relaxing, meditative nature scenes. The television could also be used for Internet access by those wanting to keep in touch with their family members and friends who perhaps are located far away.

Finally, not to be overlooked is the patient's bedside table. Furniture placement, size, and configuration should take into account the ability of a patient with limited mobility to reach for personal items, such as glasses, facial tissue, the television remote, or reading material.

GETTING AROUND THE FACILITY: WAYFINDING

The faster that patients are oriented to their environment and are able to find their destination, the greater their sense of control and reduction of stress. Simply traveling to a health facility can build fear and anxiety, so a patient's initial impression may depend on something as basic as being able to easily see and distinguish the correct entrance. Because most health care centers have several entrances, including emergency, main lobby, ambulatory services, birthing centers, and other support services, access to the desired destination should be clear and easily comprehended.

Parking can also be a major frustration for health facility users, particularly when combined with the anxieties and infirmities of a health- or age-related problem. Immediate, well-marked parking, combined with a covered drop-off, helps ensure a positive impression and minimizes frustration. A valet parking system can provide an effective resolution to parking frustrations for facilities where parking spaces are limited.

The lobby of a Planetree facility must provide access to clear, comprehensible circulation pathways. Some hospitals are replacing information desks with a roving greeter during busy morning hours. The greeter can quickly assess the destination of a visitor or patient and can give necessary directions without the need for waiting in line at a reception desk.

When a new facility is being constructed, many wayfinding issues can be eliminated with the careful design of corridor passages and lobbies that make it easy for a visitor to find his or her way throughout a facility. A few key points to consider are these:

- Minimize the number of entrances.

- Locate major departments and patient units with direct access from lobbies or public corridors.

- Locate public corridors along outside windows so that people are always oriented to the site and especially to parking lot areas.

- Design each entrance to open into a memorable interior lobby.

- Create *landmarks* to make unique lobbies and corridor intersections. Landmarks need to be memorable architectural elements (such as skylights, windows, atria), artwork, sculpture, seating, gathering spaces, and special accent lighting. See Figure 8.7.

- Locate elevator lobbies to the outside with windows to orient visitors and patients.

- Differentiate public spaces from private spaces with glass doors and sidelights. Rooms that are off-limits to the public can have painted doors that blend into the corridors, limiting the need for negative signage.

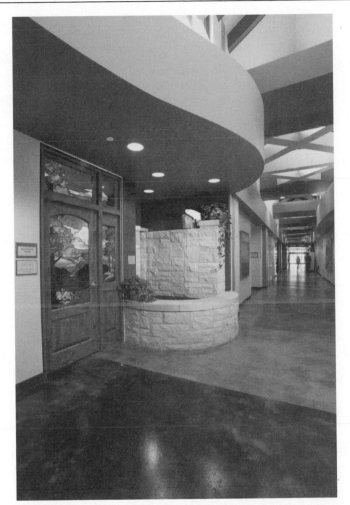

FIGURE 8.7. *Entrance to Meditation Room, North Valley Hospital.*

Source: Trevon Baker Photography.

■ Avoid negative verbiage on signage and include text that provides positive responses, such as, "Thank you for keeping our campus smoke-free."

Signage is best kept to a minimum and should be located at key turning points and corridor intersections. In busy corridor areas, ceiling-mounted signage is easiest to see. In less-crowded areas, wall-mounted signage will suffice. Directional signs should be limited to three or four destinations if possible to improve readability. Room signage should assist with wayfinding whenever possible, with room numbers progressing sequentially.

SEPARATION OF TRAFFIC TYPES

To create a Planetree experience, it is important to isolate *on-stage* public movement of patients and visitors from the movement of acutely ill patients and supply carts. This is exemplified at Walt Disney World in Orlando, Florida, which is designed with underground passage for use by support staff, actors, and for the delivery or removal of materials and supplies. These hidden passages ensure that the experience of amusement park customers is not affected by seeing support activities that are best kept behind the scenes.

Similarly, healing environments can be designed with on-stage areas, including public corridors linking lobbies and department entrances. These public spaces should be designed to be separated from purely back-of-house areas, including corridors and elevators, which are necessary to support the movement of staff, food, clean supplies, trash, soiled linen, and inpatients on carts.

STAFF SUPPORT AREAS

Research shows that there is a direct relationship between staff satisfaction and patient satisfaction (Press Ganey Associates, 2005). Clearly, it is important for Planetree hospitals to focus on the needs of their staff, especially the need to nurture and support their staff to be *present* as inspired healers for their patients. The positive support of staff members, therefore, is key to creating a positive healing environment in a Planetree facility.

An innovative idea incorporated into the design of the new replacement hospital for Planetree affiliate Elmhurst Memorial Hospital in

Elmhurst, Illinois, is a staff restorative/meditation room in each of the inpatient units and in the Emergency Department. This is a small private room with subdued lighting, relaxing music, and a comfortable recliner chair where a staff member can rest or meditate privately for a few minutes to recover from an emotionally trying experience or situation.

Staff lounges should be accessible from each department or unit, and these lounges should support the staff during breaks and lunch periods with a small kitchenette containing a microwave and refrigerator and comfortable lounge chairs and tables suitable for eating.

Lounges should provide acoustic isolation so that social chatting and laughter cannot be overheard by patients or their families and should be positioned adjacent to lockers and toilets for the staff so that break periods are most convenient. The best location for a staff lounge is along an outside wall with ample windows to allow access to natural daylight and views of nature if those are available.

STAFF WORKSTATIONS

In a hospital setting, it is extremely important for patients to feel connected with the staff if they are to feel less anxious and more supported in their health care experience. Nevertheless, it is not unusual to see large nursing stations on a typical patient unit set apart from patients by half-walls or glass partitions. These elements send a clear message that staff members are busy and inaccessible. Conversely, at the original Planetree facilities, the nursing stations were completely accessible to patients and consisted simply of tables and chairs in the center of an open space. This arrangement suggests that healing is not something that happens to patients, but rather, it is something that happens with them. Staff members are not only accessible, they are also there to collaborate and confer with each patient about health and healing.

Today's modern nursing units are designed either as clusters of four to six patient bedrooms, each with a small staff station, or private activity-adaptable rooms, each with a small staff workstation located directly outside the patient bedrooms. Both of those models serve to keep nursing staff close to patients in their bedrooms and will serve to make nurses more accessible to patients and their families. Feedback from early examples of these units, however, underscores the importance of also having a central workstation that is needed to support medical team

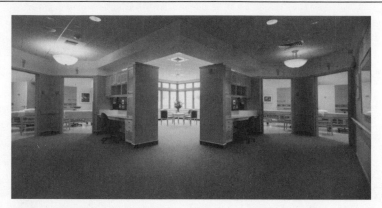

FIGURE 8.8. *Staff Workstation, Griffin Hospital.*

discussions and to provide work space for physicians and other ancillary staff. Also, private consultation and work areas are needed for confidential discussions or phone calls. See Figure 8.8.

EDUCATION SPACES

As discussed in Chapter Two, in the Planetree approach, patients are encouraged to become active participants in their own healing process. Open discussions with the staff are encouraged by the configuration of nursing stations, and health education is fostered by the presence of health resource centers or unit libraries. See Figure 8.9. At Sentara Williamsburg Regional Medical Center, a health resources library is located off the hospital lobby. Its convenient location and glass-walled entry create inviting space where visitors can access a range of health care information.

FOR EXAMPLE

"Greening" of Martha's Vineyard Hospital

Martha's Vineyard Hospital (MVH) is a critical access hospital located on an island off the coast of Cape Cod in Massachusetts. Planetree was introduced to the island hospital in 2004 and was greeted with enthusiasm by many inhabitants. The model's focus on a healing environment particularly resonated with this island community, whose residents, both year-round and seasonal, are concerned about the health of our global environment. It was therefore essential to keep these notions of both a healing and a healthy environment in mind when the time came to design a new hospital.

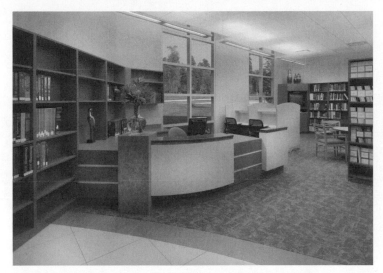

FIGURE 8.9. *Health Resource Center, Sentara Williamsburg Regional Medical Center.*

Source: Copyright © VanceFox.com.

It was obvious in the early stages of development that it would be imperative to plan a building that would be efficient and environmentally neutral while providing first-class medical care. Health care facilities have many regulatory requirements that compete with a "green" approach, and MVH faced many challenges in designing a building that not only met federal and state regulatory guidelines but also offered an opportunity to be environmentally friendly. Numerous meetings attended by community members, hospital leadership, architects, engineers, and contractors were held over several years in an attempt to define what was possible and what was probable.

Hospital leadership worked with community groups to develop the most efficient and "green" hospital possible, while staying true to many of the signature architectural features of the island buildings when feasible. The balance between fiscal responsibility to the community and civic responsibility to preserve the environment required many compromises, and community members varied widely in their expectations. One faction suggested that a wood-shingled construction was ideal, another wanted to limit power use to solar energy, and another individual challenged the concept of private rooms and water views for patients as being neither necessary nor advantageous to healing. Involving the community provided an opportunity not only to obtain their input but also to educate them about patient-centered design.

The Leadership in Energy and Environmental Design (LEED) program provided a point system by which the green initiative could be measured. Striving to attain a silver rating from LEED, MVH drew up building plans that included a variety of features that will both limit the impact on the environment and create a truly healing environment for patients. Some of the features that have been incorporated into the design of the new hospital include the following:

- Landscaped roof garden providing patients and visitors with access to fresh air and plantings
- Bike storage and showers to encourage employees to use non-emission-producing forms of transportation
- Special roof systems to reduce heat load
- Recycling plans that include the storage and collection of recyclables, utilization of recycled content in building materials, and the recycling of debris associated with demolition and construction
- The use of green products such as green seal carpet products and a green housekeeping program

Working with community members along with all components of the design team, MVH has planned a facility that will provide a compassionate and healing environment for many years to come.

CONTRIBUTED BY CAROL A. BARDWELL, MARTHA'S VINEYARD HOSPITAL

CONCLUSION

A Planetree environment is one that enables all inhabitants, no matter their role in the healing process, to care for the body, mind, and spirit of those seeking health care services from its facility. The Planetree experience appeals to all the senses, while incorporating aspects of privacy, control, access to nature, the nurturing and communal aspect of social interactions, and a sacred and honest approach to an environment that must be both high-tech and high-touch. When Angelica Thieriot envisioned a healing environment thirty years ago, she pictured a place where individuals were truly healed, not just a clinical setting for medical interventions. Her vision was to develop a treatment model that personalizes, humanizes, and demystifies the entire health care experience, encouraging design that would support these goals. At the center of that circle is the patient.

REFERENCES

Alcee, D. A. "The Experience of a Community Hospital in Quantifying and Reducing Patient Falls." *Journal of Nursing Care Quality*, 2000, *14*(3) 43–54.

Arneill, B., and Frasca-Beaulieu, K. "Healing Environments: Architecture and Design Conducive to Health." In S. B. Frampton, L. Gilpin, and P. A. Charmel (eds.), *Putting Patients First: Designing and Practicing Patient-Centered Care*. San Francisco: Jossey-Bass, 2003.

Berglund, B., Lindvall, T., and Schwela, D. H. "Guidelines for Community Noise." World Health Organization: Protection of the Human Environment, 1999.

Francis, C., and Cooper Marcus, C. "Places People Take Their Problems," Presented at the Twenty-Second Annual Conference of the Environmental Design Research Association, Oaxtepec, Mexico, 1991.

Francis, C., and Cooper Marcus, C. "Restorative Places: Environment and Emotional Well-Being." Unpublished paper, Berkeley, Calif., 1992.

Francis, C., and Cooper Marcus, C. "Gardens in Healthcare Facilities: Uses, Therapeutic Benefits, and Design Recommendations." Concord, Calif.: Center for Health Design, 1995.

Hagerman, I., and others. "Influence of Coronary Intensive Care Acoustics on the Quality of Care and Psychological States of Patients." *International Journal of Cardiology*, 2005, *98*, 267–270.

Hendrich, A., Fay, J., and Sorrells, A. "Courage to Heal: Comprehensive Cardiac Critical Care." Healthcare Design, Sep. 2002, pp. 11–13.

Kaplan, R., and Kaplan, S. *The Experience of Nature: A Psychological Perspective*. New York: Cambridge University Press, 1989.

Parsons, R., and Hartig, T. "Environmental Psychophysiology." In J. T. Cacioppo and L. G. Tassinary (eds.), *Handbook of Psychophysiology*. (2nd ed.) New York: Cambridge University Press, 2000.

Press Ganey Associates. "Patients, Physicians, and Employees: Satisfaction Trifecta Brings Bottom-Line Results." 2005. [www.pressganey.com/galleries/default-file/roiv2.pdf].

Ulrich, R. S. "Effects of Gardens on Health Outcomes: Theory and Research." In C. Cooper Marcus and M. Barnes (eds.), *Healing Gardens*. New York: Wiley, 1999.

Ulrich, R. S., and others. *The Role of the Physical Environment in the Hospital of the Twenty-First Century: A Once-in-a-Lifetime Opportunity*, Center for Health Design, Sept. 2004. [www.healthdesign.org/research/reports/pdfs/role_physical_env.pdf].

CHAPTER

9

HEALTHY COMMUNITIES: EXPANDING THE BOUNDARIES OF HEALTH CARE

RANDALL L. CARTER AND CATHERINE WHALEN

This chapter does the following:

- Examines how the Healthy Communities concept broadens the medical definition of health and expands the role that hospitals may play in providing health care for their communities

- Defines the five determinants of health and describes health care providers' efforts at collaboration and coalition building so as to address the biological, social, intellectual, environmental, and spiritual health care needs of their communities

- Encourages health care providers to look beyond demographics and geography in defining the communities they serve

Since its founding in 1978, the Planetree model has gone through continual enhancement and innovation as organizations uniquely apply the philosophy and its core components. Healthy Communities was added as a core component of the model in 2002 as a natural extension of principles already embraced and essential to patient-centered care: the importance of family, friends, and social support; architectural design conducive to health and healing; empowering patients through information and education; healing arts and spirituality. The Planetree mission and values have recognized the importance of community in assisting us with the healing process within hospital walls. Healthy Communities, as a component of patient-centered care, takes us outside those walls and helps us assist our communities to maximize the quality of their health.

Health—a condition of well-being

Healthy—conducive to health

Community—a group of people having common interests

THE HEALTHY COMMUNITIES MOVEMENT

The Healthy Communities concept has its roots in the Healthy Cities Movement, initiated by the World Health Organization (WHO). The movement was inspired by a speech given by Dr. Trevor Hancock at an international meeting in Canada in 1985. The theme was that health is the result of much more than medical care; people are healthy when they live in nurturing environments and are involved in the life of their community—in essence, when they live in Healthy Cities. The WHO began an initial pilot of a Healthy Cities program in 1986 with thirty-six European cities and slowly expanded to Australia and New Zealand. In December 1993, the first global conference on Healthy Cities and Communities was held in California. More than fourteen hundred participants from communities in over fifty countries came together to share Healthy Communities strategies and build upon one another's experiences, providing a catalyst for its implementation in the United States. Since then, the Healthy Cities and Healthy Communities movements have become interchangeable terms that reference the same basic tenets.

A BROADER DEFINITION OF HEALTH

In the late nineteenth century, hospitals played an active role in community health issues. Hospitals in large urban areas such as New York, Chicago, and Philadelphia forged partnerships with local public health agencies to combat high rates of injury and disease related to population density, poor housing, and sanitation; in rural areas, they often served as the public health clearinghouse for a broad array of public health services that could not afford infrastructure.

The twentieth century brought with it technological, pharmaceutical, and diagnostic advances at an unparalleled pace, leading to a major shift in focus that resulted in a *medical model* approach to health improvement, which today dominates our health delivery system. This medical model has also influenced the involvement of hospitals in community health. Patient education, health fairs, and screenings primarily focus on medical conditions, with little or no attention to community influences on health.

The healthy communities model broadens this medical definition of health: "a healthy city is one that is continually creating and improving those physical and social environments and strengthening those community resources which enable people to mutually support each other in performing all the functions of life and achieving their maximum potential" (Hancock, 1993, pp. 15–16). Defined in a variety of ways in today's literature and research, this model acknowledges the interdependence of the following five determinants of health.

Biological Health

The biological determinant of health refers to the physical state of health—that is, the presence or absence of chronic disease, genetic makeup, and history. It is the centerpiece of our medical model of care. The vast majority of hospital-sponsored community health initiatives have long been in this category, including initiatives such as pharmacy assistance programs, mobile health clinics, health fair screenings, and community vaccination clinics.

Social Health

Social determinants of health are factors in the social environment that contribute to or detract from the health of individuals and communities. These factors include but are not limited to socioeconomic status, transportation, housing, access to services, discrimination by social grouping (such as race or gender), and the social and environmental stressors that accompany each. Essentially, one can view it as the resources and support systems existing in an individual's life.

A number of patient-centered hospitals are addressing social determinants of health in a variety of ways. One such example is Mid-Columbia Medical Center's partnership with the Families First Program. Families First is a newborn to age three home-visiting program, which provides parenting mentorship for families identified as being at high risk for child abuse. Based in The Dalles, Oregon, it serves Wasco County, which has the highest rate of child abuse in the state. Faced with rising numbers of eligible families and decreased program funding from the state, Mid-Columbia Medical Center has committed to a multidimensional partnership with Families First, providing fiscal support and staff participation in the Welcome Baby community resource information program prior to discharge and volunteer and fundraising participation.

Intellectual Health

In its simplest definition, *intellectual health* is the ability to learn, reason, and understand. Does one know how to read, or how to speak the language common in one's community? Scientifically, research suggests that there are skills and social benefits that come with increasing educational levels. "Skills may include: (1) ability to process certain kinds of information or critical thinking and (2) ability to interact with bureaucracies, institutions, and health practitioners. Social benefits may include: (1) credentials and the economic access they provide, (2) social networks and extension of cultural capital, (3) socialization to adopt health-promoting behaviors; and (4) enhanced expectations for the future leading to helpfulness, planning, self-efficacy, and a sense of control" (Yen and Moss, 1999, pp. 350–351).

At Harborview Medical Center in Seattle, Washington, the Community House Calls Program was set up to decrease sociocultural barriers to care for non-English-speaking ethnic populations. The medical center serves a very diverse and changing ethnic population, which has required interpretation for over eighty languages and dialects. Bilingual and bicultural caseworkers facilitate an exchange of cultural information between Harborview's providers and King County's growing immigrant communities.

Environmental Health

In the first edition of *Putting Patients First,* Dr. Trevor Hancock, author of the chapter "Green Hospitals: The New Health Care Environmentalism," put forth the challenge for hospitals to be "the most environmentally friendly and healthiest building in the community" (Hancock, 2003, p. 262). In this edition, we look at environmental health from the perspective of the community. Many Healthy Communities initiatives include a visioning process, whereby participants are asked to envision their perfect community. Invariably, it includes green spaces, walkways, safe neighborhoods, clean water, and clean air.

In 1991, Via Christi Regional Medical Center (VCRMC) in Wichita began to explore possibilities to partner with local residents to improve their neighborhoods. The project chosen was the Healthy Hilltop Community Garden Project. VCRMC's role was to provide seed funding, facilitation, and volunteer coordination. After three years, the result was a garden that includes a greenhouse, pavilion, decks, and a gazebo, which has become a place of social gathering and community concerts, plays, and cultural activities for the community of Wichita.

Spiritual Health

Although a sacred or ecclesiastical interpretation of this component is most familiar, its essence is a sense of hope and a sense of meaning in one's life. *The Determinants of Health,* a report by the Canadian Institute for Advanced Research, found that on an individual level, a greater sense of belonging to a social group and control over one's circumstances and fate contributed more to health than medical care (Mustard and Frank, 1991).

COMMUNITY

Community, according to the *American Heritage Dictionary* (www.bartleby.com), refers to a group of people who live in the same locality, a group that has common interests, a group that has similar character or identity, or society as a whole.

Every hospital lives in a community. Its size and diversity can vary significantly. How does your hospital define the community it serves? For most hospitals, the description is one of location, its defined geographical or market-share boundaries. It can also be described as a community of experience (patients, families, and friends needing health care services). But the broader definition of health demands consideration of many other communities, including the following:

- *Communities of interest:* groups of people who enjoy the same thing, for instance, book clubs, bowling leagues, football fans, or Internet blogging

- *Communities of values:* people who share a sense of spirituality that is meaningful to them

- *Communities of age:* children, adolescents, adults, the elderly

- *Communities of a shared event:* WWII and Vietnam War veterans, participants in sports competitions, cancer survivors, graduates from the same college or high school

- *Communities of circumstance:* teen mothers, the homeless, the uninsured.

All of these community groups consist of members that have been shaped by their own and shared experiences, beliefs, and priorities. In her 1993 essay, "Concepts of Community," Emily Friedman writes, "Communities form and dissolve and develop into the places and people who will be the focus of future healthcare services" (p. 11). Regardless of the makeup of communities, it is imperative that we actively seek them out and discover their strengths, assets, and needs.

The Right Thing to Do

For many administrators and hospital board members, the work of Healthy Communities is often viewed through the lens of their community benefit strategy. With increasing pressure from local, state, and the federal government for nonprofit organizations to demonstrate and justify their tax exempt status, the focus on quantifying the positive impact hospitals have on the communities they serve has become a familiar exercise. Measures such as total dollar of charity care, educational offerings, health fairs, and screenings equate to community health initiatives.

For those organizations committed to a broader definition of health, the process is both more significant and rewarding. In these environments, visionary leaders and collaborators have covered the road traveled by their peer hospitals and continued on to higher ground. They have developed strategies and partnerships across the community with a focus to strike at the root causes of persistent health challenges before they respond to the need for significant medical interventions. Here you will find communities with a sense of common purpose, where health and caring come together in unique ways to meet the specific needs of the community's residents.

Historically, it is worth noting that when asked, an exceedingly high percentage of administrators, physicians, and board members state that a primary reason that they either went into or accepted their roles in health care originally was to make a significant difference in the lives of others. Today these altruistic motives are challenged by balancing reductions in reimbursement, increases in regulatory demands, new technology, and global competition. In this arena, the justification and prioritization to invest in healthy communities may boil down to the availability of resources and the effectiveness of how they are allocated. According to Tom Chapman, former CEO of Greater Southeast Health System, "People tend to say, 'This costs too much' or 'I'm not going to be reimbursed for it.' These are not only shallow reactions, they may not even be accurate. Many things can be done that cost little or no money. What they take is leadership, and energy" (Healthcare Forum Leadership Center, 1994, p. 8).

Over the years Healthier Communities and Cities pioneer Tyler Norris has observed which kinds of leaders have the most success in Healthy Communities efforts. His insights will sound familiar to anyone who has started or been actively engaged in the work of patient-centered care in an organizational setting. Tyler describes successful leaders as rooted in service and values, because it's the "right thing" to do for the communities they serve. He also notes the clarity of purpose and the spirit of collaboration needed to create partnerships that can reach a common, but difficult, destination. "These leaders have been selfless—not doing the work for the PR and marketing value—but rather as a path to realize the end-state objective of healthier people in healthier places. It requires . . . the long view: this is not a sprint, but a marathon" (e-mail communication between Tyler Norris and Randall Carter, 2008).

Today, and even more important in the days ahead, successful health care leaders will need to view the delivery of their services in a new and distinctively different way than the leaders who preceded them to their posts. Leaders will need to possess the patience needed to hold a vision that produces results over time. The good news for many communities is that the necessary character and individual qualities of leadership needed to make the transition to healthier communities may already be in place. Work in healthy communities can provide health care leaders, board members, and practitioners with some of the best opportunities available to express both their individual and their collective commitments to making a difference. Health care's mission is more significant than simply market share, the need for competitive advantage, tax status, or technology. Healthy Communities has proven to be a passionate rallying point for organizations committed to transcending the everyday pressures of health care, creating meaningful change in the communities they serve.

Getting Started

The Healthy Communities concept is universally applicable, but its implementation will vary community by community. Implementation will be specific, unique, and resource dependent. As illustrated in the previous examples and the case studies at the end of this chapter, the role of the hospital system may vary. It may be that of a facilitator, a catalyst, an advocate, a funder, or a leader. There are different methods advocated to engage the community and a myriad of successful examples shared in literature and on the Internet. But before you attempt to engage the community, your organization must make a commitment to the Healthy Communities concept.

Unlike the medical model, in the Healthy Communities model, there are few immediate results. It requires collaboration, flexibility, patience, and acceptance that not all results may be able to be measured. It requires a willingness to relinquish control, as partners bring their own perspectives, priorities, timelines, and resources to the table.

The broader definition of health must be part of your organizational culture, reflected in your mission statement and understood and promoted by everyone in the organization, from CEO to board to every staff member. Before walking out your doors, look at your own internal services and access points from the five determinants of health perspective. What could you do differently within your own walls?

Identify your natural access points. Are there community partners that could be engaged to add synergy to services you are already providing? Start with a partner with whom you have a shared mission. For example, in many communities the local public health department provides prenatal care for expectant mothers who are insured by Medicaid or uninsured and who deliver their babies at the local hospital. Are there synergies or improvements in continuity of care that could result from a dialogue?

Inventory your resources. What do you have to bring to the table in community partnerships? The economic pressures on our health care system are having an impact on hospitals' bottom lines and the ability to financially support community initiatives. But a hospital's resources go far beyond monetary donations. Staff has technical, administrative, problem-solving, and leadership skills to offer. Public relations can help with communications and media access. Information systems departments could assist with data analysis and extrapolation. Print shop assistance, food services, and meeting space are often in high demand.

Who Will You Ask? What Will You Do Then?

There are many ways to venture out and listen to your community. Group approaches may include town forums, community surveys, and focus groups. Another unique approach is the Community Plunge Initiative, developed by Memorial Health System in South Bend, Indiana (Newbold, n.d.). Facilitating a visioning process with the diverse communities you serve can identify common priorities and assist in coalition building. Attend your local community meal, have lunch at the senior center, go to a school meeting. The important thing is to ask the questions and listen closely as often as possible.

Many patient-centered hospitals have accomplished histories of working in their communities to make a positive impact on the quality of health. Once outside the confines of the organizational setting, they have found ways to collaborate, build on existing resources and assets, reduce duplication, and create sustainable improvements. Seek them out, learn from their experiences, and share your own. Some key resources and benchmark organizations are listed for you at the end of the chapter.

A successful journey begins with looking for new ways of seeing what we do through the eyes of those we serve. Open the door, begin your journey.

Dispensary of Hope

Following dramatic cuts made to Tennessee's Medicaid program in 2005, more than two hundred thousand newly uninsured individuals flooded the state's health care market, unable to afford their prescription drugs. Saint Thomas Hospital, a 541-bed hospital in Nashville, recognized the need to respond to this growing demand for medication assistance. Leaders turned to a model already being implemented by one of the hospital's

FOR EXAMPLE

physicians in his solo practice. Noting the number and monetary value of medication samples that went unused or expired in his practice, Bruce Wolf, MD, developed a program to help patients in need by collecting and distributing the unused sample medications. The program became known as the Dispensary of Hope and served as the model for Saint Thomas's hospital-based program.

A team of pharmacists and social workers met to adapt this concept, which had worked so effectively in solo practices, to a program that would be viable in a hospital setting. The Saint Thomas model had to fit into an existing retail outpatient pharmacy that already had a charity component. Unique challenges, such as keeping a separate stock of sample drug inventory, had to be taken into consideration.

Supplied with pharmaceuticals donated through physician practices or directly from pharmaceutical companies, this sample drug inventory and the additional prescription volume it created was initially staffed largely by existing staff within the retail pharmacy. A pharmacy technician was added to handle the inventory component of the program, and hospital volunteers were tapped to sort, break down packaging, inventory, and separate donated drug samples by expiration dates.

Because not all therapeutic drug classes have drugs that are routinely sampled, a safety net list of mostly generic drugs helped fill in the gap (for instance, diuretics and potassium). Sample drugs are dispensed at no charge, but safety net drugs are dispensed at a $3 dispensing fee. No controlled substances are provided under the program.

In June 2006, the program officially opened to any patient in need within the community, including patients from clinics, physician offices, and those discharged from the hospital. To qualify for the program, a patient must fill out an application and meet income criteria (200 percent of the Federal Poverty Guidelines).

Initially, pharmacists handled this application process, but this significantly affected the turn-around times of prescription order entry with all patients of the retail pharmacy. A state grant funded the hiring of a social worker who is now responsible for the initial application process, for the six-month renewal process, and for providing assistance with pharmaceutical companies' patient assistance programs.

To date, the Saint Thomas Hospital's Dispensary of Hope has gathered more than $3.4 million worth of samples and dispensed more than $1.25 million worth of sample drugs to patients in need (representing over 16,000 prescriptions). More than $89,000 worth of safety net drugs has been dispensed (representing over 14,500 prescriptions). More than $1.1 million worth of sample drugs has been given to other clinics or mission trips. This program allowed Saint Thomas to expand prescription assistance from an average of 45 patients per month to over 560 patients per month in a cost-effective manner.

CONTRIBUTED BY ROBIN CROWELL, SAINT THOMAS HOSPITAL

Block Buddies

Sentara Williamsburg Regional Medical Center established Block Buddies in 1998 as a Lay Health Promoter Program targeting at-risk neighborhoods. Residents in these areas were found to suffer from disproportionate rates of preventable chronic diseases because they do not access available health care in the community. The reasons go beyond a lack of health insurance and transportation. There is often a lack of trust. Many residents do not go to the doctor because they are afraid, or uncomfortable, or don't feel it is a priority. As one woman states, "It didn't matter how much my back hurt, the rent had to be paid."

Champions who would rise to the challenge of becoming their neighborhood health resource contact were recruited as Block Buddies. They encourage and coordinate neighborhood-based health education activities. Each week, they make contact with their neighbors, friends, and families to discuss health topics and community resources or check their blood pressure, making recommendations based on their findings. The Block Buddies are seen as community leaders and are frequently asked to help promote programs such as the free dental clinic, free cervical cancer and breast exam screening days, and church and school health fairs.

The Block Buddies Program provides fifteen weeks of intensive health education. Training is held at the hospital or other facilities to help the Block Buddies learn about local resources, and the instructors are local health experts who have volunteered their time to teach classes. Topics include safety, first aid, diabetes, cancer, nutrition, exercise, substance abuse, immunizations, and more. In exchange for this wealth of information, the Block Buddies agree to share what they have learned with their neighbors, friends, and family members. At graduation, they receive a *wellness kit*, which includes a blood pressure cuff and stethoscope, first-aid kit, and other items that will assist them in their promotion of health.

FOR EXAMPLE

The Block Buddies stay engaged through monthly alumni meetings, where they learn about topics that were not covered in the initial training.

Initial funding for the program was provided by the United Way and the Williamsburg Community Health Foundation. Ongoing funding is now provided by Sentara Williamsburg Regional Medical Center and corporate donations.

Since its inception, the Block Buddies Program has trained forty-five champions, representing seventeen different neighborhoods in the Greater Williamsburg Area. The neighbor-to-neighbor approach has been successful in countering many common reasons cited for not accessing health care. The Block Buddies have raised awareness of the importance of prevention and early detection as well as the importance of screenings available to many uninsured individuals who may otherwise neglect their health. In neighborhood-based health screenings, over 50 percent of the participants are found to have health risks that require a follow-up physician visit. The residents who return to the health screenings are proud to share their recent changes in health and lifestyle.

CONTRIBUTED BY HELEN CLENDENIN, CAROL WILSON, SENTARA HEALTHCARE; AND
MARGARET CULLIVAN, SENTARA WILLIAMSBURG REGIONAL MEDICAL CENTER

REFERENCES

Friedman, E. "Concepts of Community." *Healthcare Forum Journal*, May–June 1993, 36(3), 11–17.

Hancock, T. "The Evolution, Impact and Significance of the Healthy Cities/Communities Movement." *Journal of Public Health Policy*, Spring 1993, 14(1), 5–18.

Hancock, T. "Green Hospitals: The New Health Care Environmentalism." In S. B. Frampton, L. Gilpin, and P. A. Charmel (eds.), *Putting Patients First: Designing and Practicing Patient-Centered Care*. San Francisco: Jossey-Bass, 2003.

Healthcare Forum Leadership Center, National Civic League. *Healthier Communities Action Kit*. San Francisco: Healthcare Forum, 1994.

Mustard, J. F., and Frank, J. "The Determinants of Health." Population Health Publication Number 5. Toronto: Canadian Institute for Advanced Research, 1991.

Newbold, P. "Community Plunge: Learning History." n.d. [www.qualityoflife.org/ich/plunge/plunge.cfm].

Yen, I. H., and Moss, N. "Unbundling Education: A Critical Discussion of What Education Confers and How It Lowers Risk for Disease and Health." *Annals of the New York Academy of Sciences*, 1999, *896*(1), 350–351.

ADDITIONAL RESOURCES

Association for Community Health Improvement (ACHI). [www.communityhlth.org].

Association of Community Health Indicators. [www.achi.org].

Coalition for Healthier Cities and Communities. [www.healthycities.org/userTemplate.html].

Flower, J. "Healthier Communities: A Compendium of Best Practices Healthcare Forum Journal." *Healthcare Forum Journal*, 2003, *36*(3).

Guide to Community Preventive Services: Task Force Recommendations. Oct. 2003. [www.thecommunityguide.org].

Hancock, T. "Beyond Health Care: Creating a Healthy Future." *Futurist*, Aug. 1982, *16*(4), 4–13.

Hancock, T. "Creating a Healthy Community: The Preferred Role for Hospitals." *Dimension*. Sept. 1986, *63*(6), 22–23.

Hancock, T. "Seeing the Vision, Defining Your Role." *Healthcare Forum Journal*, May–June 1993, *36*(3), 30–36.

Healthy People in Healthy Communities: A Community Planning Guide Using Healthy People 2010. Washington, D.C.: Office of Disease Prevention and Health Promotion, Department of Health and Human Services, Feb. 2001.

National Civic League Healthy Communities Initiative. [www.ncl.org].

PART

2

CURRENT TRENDS IN PATIENT-CENTERED CARE

CHAPTER

10

BUILDING THE BUSINESS CASE FOR PATIENT-CENTERED CARE

PATRICK A. CHARMEL

This chapter does the following:

- Demonstrates how organizations that implement patient-centered care are positioned to reap a number of clinical and operational benefits

- Demonstrates how Planetree members are differentiating themselves by building a brand identity around a patient-centered approach to care that addresses patients' expectations for how their care will be delivered

191

- Asserts that patient-centered care is a viable strategy for improving employee recruitment and retention

Since Planetree's inception as a demonstration project serving as a model of patient-centered care delivery, its founders and their successors have been continually challenged to demonstrate its efficacy and value. Many of Planetree's early adopters found the model's underlying philosophy compelling. They were willing to adopt the model's programmatic elements based on an inherent belief that the delivery of personalized, compassionate care in a healing environment was "the right thing to do." However, many decision makers have subjected the Planetree approach to greater scrutiny. They have demanded documentation of the tangible benefits to be derived from adoption of the model. In particular, skeptics have asked for data substantiating a fair return on the investment of time, energy (both physical and emotional), and money necessary to implement Planetree and achieve its benefits. Until recently, the Planetree model's value proposition had not been clearly articulated, and failure to proffer a strong business case for the model had impeded its widespread adoption.

The first edition of *Putting Patients First* described data available at the time of publication that substantiated the business benefits of patient-centered care. In the intervening years, wider adoption of the Planetree model has contributed to the growth of this evidence base. The 2001 Institute of Medicine report that identified patient-centeredness among the six interrelated factors defining quality care further solidified patient-centered care as much more than a cosmetic strategy to create an outwardly more appealing patient experience, but rather as a practice fundamental to the provision of quality care. The national implementation of the CAHPS Hospital Survey (HCAHPS), a standardized patient experience of care survey, and the public release of HCAHPS survey results have also enhanced the visibility and operational importance of focusing on the patient experience. Considered together, these factors have resulted in a stronger business case for patient-centered care and the Planetree model to be examined in this second edition.

DEMONSTRATING PLANETREE'S EFFECTIVENESS

A review of the evolution of the Planetree model and a description of the rigor to which it was subjected as a condition of its development are helpful in establishing a foundation from which to build a credible business case. The Planetree Model Hospital Unit was established in 1985 at the then 272-bed Pacific Presbyterian Medical Center (PPMC) in San Francisco, with funding from The San Francisco Foundation and The Kaiser Family Foundation, to demonstrate the benefits of patient-centered care and to serve as a model for hospital and health care providers throughout the country. The founders of Planetree and the foundations that funded its development recognized that to gain acceptance in an industry dominated by the scientific method, patient-centered care would have to demonstrate its superiority to traditional care using a methodology that would withstand scientific scrutiny.

Researchers from the University of Washington School of Public Health were commissioned to conduct a randomized controlled trial to compare the patient outcomes on the Planetree Model Hospital Unit with those on PPMC's other medical-surgical units. The University of Washington study is believed to be the first comprehensive evaluation of patient outcomes on a patient-centered unit, compared with a traditional unit, ever conducted. Outcome indicators chosen by the researchers included patient satisfaction, patient education and involvement in the care process, patient health behavior and compliance, health status, hospital resource consumption (defined as length of stay), and hospital charges generated (Martin and others, 1998).

Patients were enrolled in the study for a period lasting more than three years, from late 1986 to early 1990. A total of 760 patients participated, 315 of whom were cared for on the Planetree unit, with 445 being cared for on other medical-surgical units. Study subjects underwent a thorough twenty-minute interview upon admission and completed a written questionnaire one week, three months, and six months after discharge. In addition, hospital bills were analyzed to quantify resource consumption during the initial hospital admission and subsequent hospital stays. Consumption of nonacute care services, such as home care, emergency room care, and ambulatory care in the year following enrollment in the study were also quantified.

The findings indicated that patients had significantly higher overall satisfaction on the Planetree Unit than on the other units studied, they had greater opportunity to see family and friends, they were more satisfied with their nursing care and the unit's architecture and environment, they learned more about their illness and self-care, and they were included more often in the care process. In addition, patients on the Planetree unit were more satisfied with the health education they received while hospitalized. These findings left no doubt that the model of care delivery was effective. However, for the remaining performance indicators studied, the Planetree unit failed to demonstrate an advantage.

Study participants cared for on the Planetree unit experienced essentially the same length of stay as patients on the other units. Charges generated, a proxy for hospital resources consumed, were also similar. Although study findings indicated that Planetree unit patients learned more about their illness and self-care requirements, that knowledge did not translate into improved health status or decreased use of inpatient hospital services and ambulatory services in the year following study enrollment. It is safe to say that given the hospital industry's relentless pursuit of operating cost reduction, had the University of Washington study found that engaging patients in the care process offered lasting benefits in terms of reduced use of health services or fewer resources when services were required, there would have been few obstacles to widespread adoption of the model.

In the years following the completion of the University of Washington study, the Planetree model has evolved considerably. Today, the model is much broader in scope, now incorporating the distinct components described in Part One of this book. It also exerts greater influence on the operation and performance of the hospitals that adopt it in that the model is now implemented hospital-wide as opposed to on a single unit. With these advances in the development of the Planetree model, the tangible and lasting operational benefits of providing patient-centered care are beginning to be revealed. A recent study examining data for two comparable hospital units over five years—one that had implemented the extensive patient-centered practices and processes of the Planetree model for the duration of five years and the other not—found significant differences in operating efficiency. In each of the five years studied, the Planetree unit consistently demonstrated

■ A shorter average length of stay than the control unit.

■ A statistically significant lower cost per case than the control unit.

■ The relative use of RN to ancillary staff—for example, clerks, aides, LVNs—shifted from higher-cost RN staff to lower-cost ancillary staff in the patient-centered unit.

■ Higher average overall patient satisfaction scores, as well as higher scores in seven of the nine specific dimensions of patient satisfaction measured (Stone, 2007).

FOR EXAMPLE

Improving Quality Outcomes

The link between patient-centered care and quality outcomes such as patient satisfaction, length of stay, readmission, cost per case, and productive nursing hours per patient day has been postulated; however, to date, little to no research has been conducted to examine this issue. A 2007 retrospective quasi-experimental study (Stone, 2007) has begun to fill this research gap. The study compared the performance of two units managed by the same organization, caring for the same types of patients, using the same skill mix, with standardized organizational pay rates, supply costs, policies, procedures, contracts, and regulatory compliance programs. The comparative study provided a unique opportunity to evaluate the impact of the Planetree patient-centered model of care practiced in the treatment unit on inpatient quality outcomes. The following research questions were posed: What is the impact of the Planetree patient-centered model of care on (1) patient satisfaction, (2) clinical outcomes (length of stay and readmission), and (3) the cost of providing care (cost per case and productive nursing hours per patient day)?

The sample size consisted of 869 hospitalized adults—67.5 percent (n = 587 patients) in the treatment unit and 32.5 percent (n = 282 patients) in the control unit—undergoing elective total knee or total hip joint replacement surgery, who completed and returned the English-speaking version of the inpatient Press Ganey satisfaction survey.

The patient satisfaction composite mean score evaluation, length of stay evaluation, and cost per case evaluation demonstrated that the treatment unit was different from the control group (p = <.05 with Eta squared = >.01). Which is to say, in this group of hospitalized adults undergoing elective total knee or total hip joint replacement surgery, the findings indicate that the Planetree patient-centered model of care positively influenced patient satisfaction, length of stay, and cost per case.

The study concluded that based on these findings, nursing and hospital administrators seeking to improve the inpatient hospital experience should consider implementation of the Planetree patient-centered model of care. See Figures 10.1, 10.2, and 10.3.

CONTRIBUTED BY SUSAN STONE, SHARP CORONADO HOSPITAL

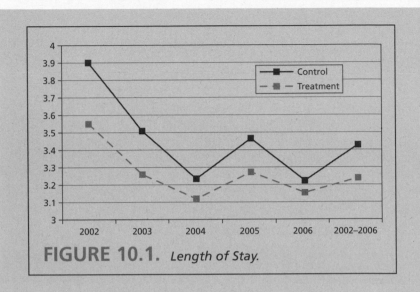

FIGURE 10.1. *Length of Stay.*

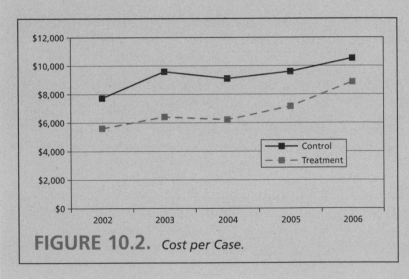

FIGURE 10.2. *Cost per Case.*

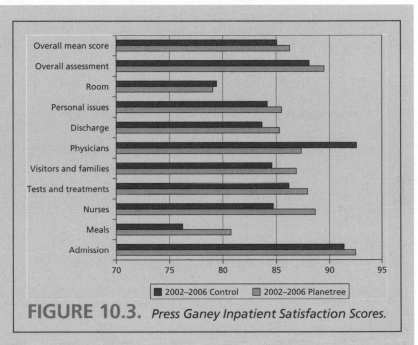

FIGURE 10.3. *Press Ganey Inpatient Satisfaction Scores.*

Note: Overall and composite scores.

THE INDUSTRY SHIFTS ITS FOCUS

Faced with growing federal budget deficits and the prospect that the demands of an aging baby boom generation might bankrupt the Medicare program, Congress passed the Balanced Budget Amendment (BBA) in 1997, in hopes of cutting the rate of Medicare expense growth in half. The BBA exceeded the expectation of Congress in that in the years immediately following its adoption, real Medicare expense growth declined for the first time since the program's inception. The dramatic reduction in Medicare spending was achieved primarily through reductions in payments to hospitals and physicians. The resulting loss of revenue reduced the profitability of all hospitals. More than a third of the nation's hospitals with thin operating margins saw their profitability disappear altogether. In reaction, hospitals aggressively cut their operating costs through efficiency enhancement and productivity improvement.

Efficiency of care delivery was enhanced primarily through length-of-stay reduction. Length-of-stay reduction was achieved by standardizing the care of patients with a similar diagnosis to eliminate, to the extent possible, variability among physicians. Practice guidelines, also called *care pathways,* were the principal tool used to standardize care.

Reduction in the average length of stay and the associated reduction in the average daily census of the typical U.S. hospital facilitated labor cost savings through staff reductions. The need to compensate for lost Medicare revenue drove many hospitals to eliminate staff members to a greater degree than was justified by reduction in workload resulting from shorter average length of stay. To the dismay of hospital executives, productivity improvement—that is, producing more work with less staff—was insufficient to restore profitability or enhance operating margins. It soon became apparent that economic viability could only be ensured by a strategy that combined cost reduction with revenue enhancement.

The hospital industry's shift in emphasis to revenue enhancement and business growth corresponded with the first appearances of the health care consumer movement. It has been said that health care consumerism will "alter how health care organizations operate, how they compete and, perhaps, why they exist" (Ernst & Young LLP, 1998). A growing appreciation that success through revenue enhancement and business growth cannot be achieved without responding to the forces of health care consumerism has motivated hospital leaders to become more customer focused. It may be that the Planetree model's greatest value is that it was designed from the perspective of the health care consumer, and therefore it is most effective in responding to the health care consumer movement.

PRODUCT DIFFERENTIATION

Health care consumerism is being driven by changes in society, improved access to information, and changes in the financing of health care. As levels of affluence have risen, consumers who are working more hours and have less free time have begun to demand improved service and convenience. The Internet has given consumers access to health care information and decision-making tools that enable them to play a more active role in their own health care. Finally, consumers have been given a choice of health insurance plans by government and private employers, but they are being asked to pay a larger share of the cost of their own health care. As illustrated in Figure 10.4, in 2005 (the latest year for which data are available), 63.9 percent of employees were enrolled in a health insurance plan that required a deductible, up from

47.6 percent in 2002 (Crimmel, 2007). Concurrently, deductibles themselves are increasing. In 2002, the average annual deductible for health insurance plan enrollees with single coverage was $446. Within three years, the average annual deductible increased to $652, a 46.2 percent increase (see Figure 10.5). In the same three-year time period, the average deductible for family coverage increased 28.6 percent, from $958 in 2002 to $1,232 in 2005 (Crimmel, 2007); see Figure 10.6.

Not only do consumers today have stronger incentives to differentiate among health care providers, but they also have more resources available to assist them in doing so. This intensified consumer scrutiny has presented a challenge for health care providers, many of whom have traditionally differentiated themselves on clinical excellence alone. Clinical excellence is essential, but consumers frequently will assume clinical competence and instead select providers based on other factors. To distinguish themselves in an era of health care consumerism, hospitals must view care through the eyes of their patients and improve the experience in ways that are meaningful to patients and their families.

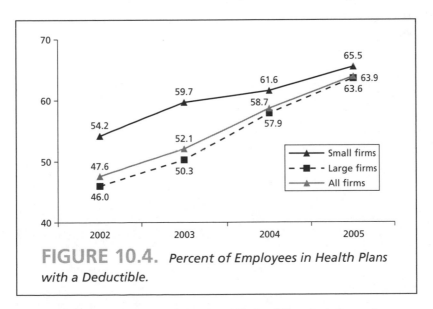

FIGURE 10.4. *Percent of Employees in Health Plans with a Deductible.*

Note: By firm size, private industry, 2002–2005. Small firms have fewer than fifty employees; large firms have fifty or more employees.
Source: Center for Financing, Access, and Cost Trends, AHRQ, 2005.

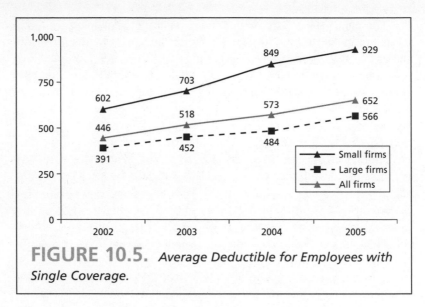

FIGURE 10.5. *Average Deductible for Employees with Single Coverage.*

Note: By firm size, private industry, 2002–2005. Small firms have fewer than fifty employees. Large firms have fifty or more employees.

Source: Center for Financing, Access, and Cost Trends, AHRQ, 2005.

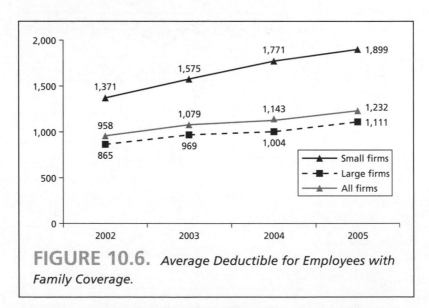

FIGURE 10.6. *Average Deductible for Employees with Family Coverage.*

Note: By firm size, private Industry, 2002–2005. Small firms have fewer than fifty employees; large firms have fifty or more employees.

Source: Center for Financing, Access, and Cost Trends, AHRQ, 2005.

The patient satisfaction ratings in Planetree member hospitals throughout the United States over the past several years document the success of the Planetree model in meeting patient demand for more responsive care and service. A 2002 study of patient satisfaction ratings of twelve Planetree hospitals (from one year before through twenty-four months after implementation) showed an average improvement across all hospitals studied of three or more percentage points in overall satisfaction, likeliness to recommend, and willingness to return (Iacono, 2002).

Among these twelve hospitals is Griffin Hospital, a 160-bed community hospital in Derby, Connecticut. Having adopted the model of care fifteen years ago as a strategy to combat eroding patient preference ratings and significant loss of market share, Griffin has since earned a reputation for innovation, service excellence, and superior clinical outcomes and has tracked a steady climb in patient satisfaction. At the same time, inpatient volume has increased by 31 percent (1998–2007, compared with a state average growth rate of 5.7 percent), and outpatient volume has increased 70 percent in the same time period.

Sharp Coronado Hospital, a 204-bed hospital outside San Diego, California, began implementing the Planetree model five years ago and approaches patient care by consistently returning to three core questions: Have we helped patients live their lives with dignity and in optimal health, heal to the highest degree of functioning possible, and grow in all ways that have meaning for them? Its effectiveness in meeting the needs of patients is measured using a community image survey tool that evaluates the hospital's image and consumer preference for the hospital's inpatient and outpatient services across all service lines. Between 2003 and 2006, the preference among those surveyed for Sharp Coronado Hospital increased 12 percentage points, with a 21 percentage point increase in "most responsive to the needs of the community." In addition, ratings for service line preference improved in every category, including a 17 percentage point increase for outpatient surgery (Charmel and Frampton, 2008).

FINANCIAL IMPERATIVE

Although several Planetree-affiliated hospitals have reported increases in their patient satisfaction scores following adoption of the model, the introduction of the HCAHPS survey—the first-ever nationally administered instrument to assess the patient experience—provides a powerful new tool to measure the impact of Planetree implementation in a standardized way. The survey focuses on critical aspects of the hospital experience from the patient's perspective, including communication with nurses and physicians, communication about medication, staff responsiveness, cleanliness and quietness of the physical environment, as well as overall satisfaction and willingness to recommend the hospital. Although participation in the HCAHPS survey was initially voluntary, the Medicare program provided a strong financial incentive for hospital participation beginning in July 2007. Use of the survey and participation in public reporting are now a requirement for acute care hospitals to receive the full Medicare Annual Payment Update (APU) for inpatient hospital services. Hospitals that do not participate will receive a 2.0 percent reduction in their defined APU payment.

The initial HCAHPS survey results publicly reported in March 2008 reinforce the link between HCAHPS performance and Planetree implementation. Six organizations that had fully implemented the Planetree model, as demonstrated by their participation in pilot-testing

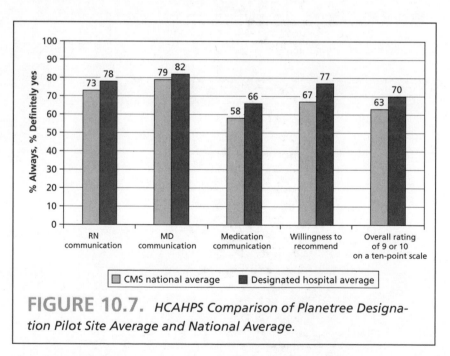

FIGURE 10.7. *HCAHPS Comparison of Planetree Designation Pilot Site Average and National Average.*

Note: Initial reporting period from October 2006 through June 2007.
Source: Brady, 2008.

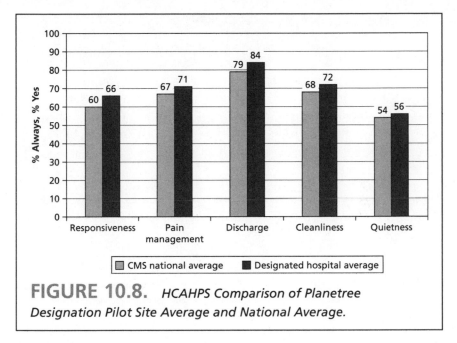

FIGURE 10.8. *HCAHPS Comparison of Planetree Designation Pilot Site Average and National Average.*

Note: Initial reporting period from October 2006 through June 2007.
Source: Brady, 2008.

Planetree's Patient-Centered Hospital Designation Program, as a group exceeded the HCAHPS national average as reported by the Centers for Medicare and Medicaid Services in all ten patient experience domains. See Figures 10.7 and 10.8.

As of October 2008, performance on the HCAHPS survey will take on even greater relevance when the Medicare program introduces *value-based purchasing* (VBP). With the launch of this program, no longer will hospitals merely be avoiding financial penalties for nonreporting; they will benefit from tangible financial incentives for superior performance on the HCAHPS survey and other patient care quality indicators. By publicly reporting HCAHPS survey results, the Medicare program has increased the visibility of hospitals successful in providing patient-centered care; through value-based purchasing, it has effectively made patient-centered care a financial imperative.

IMPROVED CLINICAL OUTCOMES

Patient-centered care is increasingly being recognized not only as a financial imperative but also as an essential foundation for safety. Following its 2001 report identifying patient-centered care as one of six essential aims to improve patient care quality, the Institute of Medicine has continued to emphasize the relationship between patient-centered care, quality, and safety, noting "patient-centered care that embodies both effective communication and technical skill is necessary to achieve safety and quality of care" (Institute of Medicine, 2007, p. 155). In addition, recent research reveals that "patient-reported service quality deficiencies are associated with adverse events and medical errors" (Taylor and others, 2008, p. 226). As described in more detail in Chapter Thirteen, a patient-centered approach to care supports quality and safety in many ways.

The topic of medical errors has received considerable consumer attention, and with increasing frequency patients with unanticipated outcomes are taking legal action against their caregivers. In the last decade, a combination of factors, including the number and size of medical malpractice payouts, has prompted insurers to dramatically increase their malpractice premiums or exit the malpractice insurance marketplace all together, giving the remaining insurers even greater pricing power. For many hospitals, this has equated to millions of dollars in increased operating cost.

Insurance underwriters base a hospital's malpractice insurance premium on a combination of industry experience and a hospital's individual claims history. Research shows that 1 percent of hospital patients nationwide are harmed in some way, but only 3 percent of those who are harmed file a lawsuit. Those who do sue do so because of one of four types of communication problems: deserting the patient, devaluing patient views, delivering information poorly, and failing to understand the patient's perspective (Kavalier and Spiegel, 1997). Communication issues also are a common root cause of adverse events, according to The Joint Commission's review of more than four thousand reports to its sentinel event database over the past twelve years (The Joint Commission, 2007).

Accordingly, the Planetree model's emphasis on improved caregiver-patient communication, patient and family involvement, and focus on the patient's perspective has the potential to reduce adverse events, malpractice claims, and associated operating cost increases. Although no study has been conducted to date on the impact of the model on these measures, one hospital has reported compelling results related to malpractice claims. Figure 10.9 displays a dramatic reduction in malpractice claims in the first nine years of Planetree implementation—despite an increase in patient care activity, which tends to increase claims.

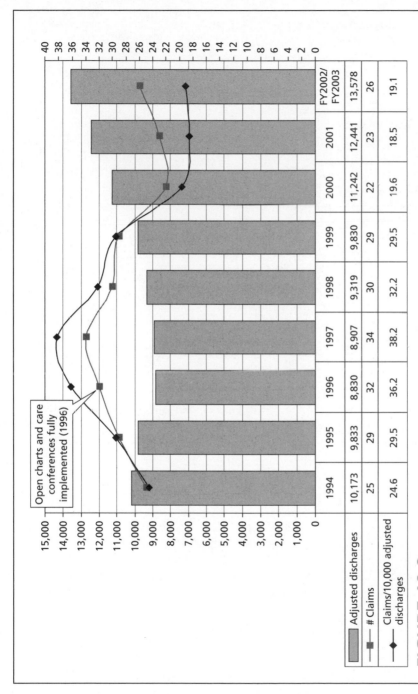

	1994	1995	1996	1997	1998	1999	2000	2001	FY2002/FY2003
Adjusted discharges	10,173	9,833	8,830	8,907	9,319	9,830	11,242	12,441	13,578
# Claims	25	29	32	34	30	29	22	23	26
Claims/10,000 adjusted discharges	24.6	29.5	36.2	38.2	32.2	29.5	19.6	18.5	19.1

Open charts and care conferences fully implemented (1996)

FIGURE 10.9. *Adjusted Discharges Versus Number of Claims and Claims per 10,000.*

Note: All departments, by policy years 1994–2002 (FY2003).

The importance of communication and attention to the patient's perspective is reiterated in Press Ganey's 2008 Hospital Pulse Report, which indicates that based on survey results from more than two million patients from approximately seventeen hundred hospitals nationwide, the top five issues identified by inpatients as priorities for hospitals all relate to communication and empathy. They are (1) staff responsiveness to patient concerns and complaints, (2) having one's emotional needs addressed while hospitalized, (3) being included in treatment decisions, (4) being kept informed by nurses, and (5) prompt responses to call buttons. Not surprisingly, each of these priorities is directly related to staff interactions with patients, underscoring the impact that frontline health care workers have on the overall experience of patients.

HEALTH CARE WORKFORCE SHORTAGE

Recruiting and retaining quality staff is key to a hospital's viability; however, these efforts are impeded by the nation's well-documented health care workforce shortage. The 2007 American Hospital Association Survey of Hospital Leaders found that hospitals had an estimated 116,000 RN vacancies as of December 2006—a national RN vacancy rate of 8.1 percent. This shortage is not limited to RNs—with the vacancy rate for speech, occupational, and physical therapists at 11.4 percent; pharmacists at 8.1 percent; nursing assistants at 8.0 percent; LPNs at 6.6 percent; laboratory technicians at 5.9 percent; and imaging technicians at 5.9 percent.

Financially, this translates into many hospitals being forced to use agency and travel staff and paying a premium of more than double their standard rate for the privilege. Alternatively, hospitals may be forced to turn away patients because of reduced capacity. Given the high fixed costs of operating a hospital, the resulting loss of revenue can be devastating. This is compounded by the high cost of nurse turnover, a subject that has been the focus of a number of studies conducted in the last several years, with estimates of the cost of replacing a single registered nurse ranging from approximately $22,000 to more than $60,000 (Advisory Board, 1999; Jones, 2005; O'Brien-Pallas and others, 2006; Stone and others, 2003; Waldman, Kelly, Sanjeev, and Smith, 2004—as cited in Jones and Gates, 2007).

Unfortunately, the shortage is going to be exacerbated by the imminent retirement and growing health care needs of the baby boomer generation. The Health Resources and Services Administration (HRSA) estimates that by 2020, the nation's nursing shortage will grow to more than one million nurses. The Bureau of Labor Statistics also projects severe shortages for a number of allied health professions.

The growing shortage obliges hospitals to create a workplace environment where current employees want to continue working and where prospective employees want to be hired. A 1999 Press Ganey study identified employee pride in their workplace as the highest predictor of overall employee satisfaction. The study further found that along with open communication and exceptional management practices, these qualities are more relevant to employee satisfaction than wages, benefits, and the work environment.

The fact that the Planetree philosophy resonates with so many caregivers by focusing on the needs of the patient contributes to a strong sense of employee pride and high employee satisfaction in Planetree affiliate hospitals. A recent evaluation of results from employee satisfaction surveys of Planetree hospitals conducted by Planetree found higher average scores for those hospitals having greater experience with implementing the Planetree model, with the most statistically significant improvements in the areas of orientation, fostering a healthy work environment, valuing the organization, leadership integrity, and employee engagement.

Eighteen months into implementing the Planetree model, Stamford Hospital, a 305-bed tertiary care center in Stamford, Connecticut, demonstrated an increase from the 33rd to the 60th percentile of its peer group in employee satisfaction. Hospital leadership credited in part a number of Planetree initiatives—including the attendance of all staff at a series of full-day, off-site retreats focused on gaining alignment around the principles of patient-centered care and community building—for the improvement in employee satisfaction scores (Charmel and Frampton, 2008).

The well-documented link between employee satisfaction and patient satisfaction is also reflected in the Planetree philosophy: a defining tenet is the importance of staff feeling cared for themselves so that they can best care for their patients. During the same eighteen-month period at Stamford Hospital, as employee satisfaction improved, satisfaction ratings by emergency room patients increased from the 44th to the 89th percentile, and ratings by hospital inpatients increased from the 18th to the 75th percentile (Charmel and Frampton, 2008).

An array of staff recognition and communication programs, employee wellness initiatives, and tremendous employee pride in the care and service they provide have contributed to Griffin Hospital being named by *Fortune* magazine as one of "The 100 Best Companies to Work For in America" for nine consecutive years (2000–2008), a designation based on workplace culture and satisfaction ratings by a random sample of employees. This recognition has meant that despite the health care workforce shortage, in 2007 Griffin received 6,691 applications for 180 job openings. Clearly, fostering a workplace environment where employees feel valued, recognized, and empowered can result in a meaningful impact on a hospital's bottom line.

IN CONCLUSION: A STRONG BUSINESS CASE

Nearly thirty years of experience with more than 140 diverse health care institutions practicing the Planetree model have demonstrated the concrete advantages of providing patient-centered care. These institutions have individually reported a host of clinical and operational-level benefits realized as a result of implementation of the model, among them increased patient satisfaction, increased staff retention, enhanced staff recruitment, decreased length of stay, decreased emergency room return visits, fewer medication errors, and improved liability claims experience. In the context of an increasingly competitive marketplace, growing health care consumerism, the trend toward greater transparency, and the impending launch of value-based purchasing, these benefits are more consequential than ever before. No longer will hospitals be able to dismiss patient-centered care as superficial or extraneous. On the contrary, in order to ensure quality care, patient satisfaction, and ultimately optimum reimbursement, savvy health care providers are recognizing the importance of heeding the voice of patients and finding ways to deliver care that responds to the feedback received. Institutions that endeavor to seek and respond to consumer expectations and preferences will be poised to withstand the rankings, measures, and exacting scrutiny of empowered consumers and increasingly discriminating payers, and will be distinctly poised to reap the benefits.

The investments of time, attention, and resources necessary to implement the Planetree model, though not insignificant, are clearly dwarfed by the potential returns. The value proposition has been demonstrated, and the strong business case should spur more widespread adoption of patient-centered care.

REFERENCES

Advisory Board Company. "A Misplaced Focus: Reexamining the Recruiting/Retention Trade-Off." *Nursing Watch,* 1999, *11,* 114.

American Hospital Association. *2007 AHA Survey of Hospital Leaders.* Washington, D.C.: American Hospital Association, July 2007.

Brady, C. "Making Patient-Centered Care More Visible." *The Patient: Patient-Centered Outcomes Research,* 2008, *1*(2), 77–84.

Center for Financing, Access, and Cost Trends, Agency for Healthcare Research and Quality. Insurance Component of the Medical Expenditure Panel Survey, 2005.

Charmel, P., and Frampton, S. B. "Building the Business Case for Patient-Centered Care." *HFM Magazine,* 2008, *62*(3), 80–85.

Crimmel, B. L. "Deductibles for Employer-Sponsored Health Insurance in the Private Sector, by Firm Size Classification, 2002–2005." *Agency for Healthcare Research and Quality.* Rockville, Md.: Nov. 2007. [www.meps.ahrq.gov/mepsweb/data_files/publications/st190/stat190.pdf].

Ernst & Young LLP. *Built to Last Means Built to Change: Medicare+Choice and the New Health Care Consumerism.* Score No. 0–00200. Cleveland, Ohio: Ernst & Young Publications for the Health Care Industry, June 1998.

Iacono, S. "Planetree Philosophy: A Study on the Relationship of Patient Satisfaction and Utilization of a Planetree Model in Care Delivery." *Plane Talk,* Sept.–Oct. 2002, pp. 1–4.

Institute of Medicine. *Crossing the Quality Chasm: A New Health System for the Twenty-First Century.* Washington, D.C.: National Academies Press, 2001.

Institute of Medicine. *Preventing Medication Errors.* Washington, D.C.: National Academies Press, 2007.

Joint Commission's Root Causes of Sentinel Events. Sept. 2007. [www.jointcommission.org/NR/rdonlyres/FA465646–5F5F-4543-AC8F-E8AF6571E372/0/root_cause_se.jpg].

Jones, C. "The Cost of Nurse Turnover, Part 2: Application of the Nursing Turnover Cost Calculation Methodology." *Journal of Nursing Administration,* 2005, *35*(1), 41–48.

Jones, C., and Gates, M. "The Costs and Benefits of Nurse Turnover: A Business Case for Nurse Retention." *Online Journal of Issues in Nursing,* 2007, *12*(3).

Kavalier, F., and Spiegel, A. D. *Risk Management in Health Care Institutions.* Sudberry, Mass.: Jones & Bartlett, 1997.

Martin, D., and others. "Randomized Trial of a Patient-Centered Hospital Unit." *Patient Education and Counseling,* 1998, *34*(2), 125–133.

O'Brien-Pallas, L., and others. "The Impact of Nurse Turnover on Patient, Nurse and System Outcomes: A Pilot Study and Focus for a Multicenter International Study." *Policy, Politics, and Nursing Practice,* 2006, *7*(3), 169–179.

Press Ganey Associates, Inc. "One Million Patients Have Spoken: Who Will Listen?" *Satisfaction Monitor,* 1999.

Press Ganey Associates, Inc. *Hospital Pulse Report: Patient Perspectives on American Health Care.* 2008. [www.pressganey.com/galleries/default-file/2008_Hospital_Pulse_Report.pdf].

Stone, P. W., and others. *An International Examination of the Cost of Turnover and Its Impact on Patient Safety and Nurse Outcomes.* Proceedings of the 37th Biennial Convention, Sigma Theta Tau International, Toronto, Ont., 2003.

Stone, S. "A Retrospective Evaluation of the Planetree Patient-Centered Model of Care Program's Impact on Inpatient Quality Outcomes." Doctoral dissertation, University of San Diego, 2007.

Taylor, B. B., and others. "Do Medical Inpatients Who Report Poor Service Quality Experience More Adverse Events and Medical Errors?" *Medical Care,* 2008, *46*(2), 224–228.

Waldman, J. D., Kelly, F., Sanjeev, A., and Smith, H. L. "The Shocking Cost of Turnover in Health Care." *Health Care Management Review,* 2004, *29*(1), 27.

CHAPTER

THE PHYSICIAN-PATIENT RELATIONSHIP IN THE PATIENT-CENTERED CARE MODEL

H. LEE KANTER AND STEVEN F. HOROWITZ

This chapter does the following:

- Places patient-centered care within the context of the current state of affairs in which physicians are practicing medicine
- Describes an optimal patient-physician relationship, in which the physician is a trusted adviser and the patient is empowered to be an active participant and decision maker in his or her care

■   Discusses the role that physicians play in promoting a culture of patient-centered care within their organizations

In the intervening years since the publication of the first edition of *Putting Patients First* in 2003, there has been a marked shift toward a greater level of physician involvement in the Planetree model of care. Physicians frequently ask, "What is Planetree and why should I get involved?" Planetree's vision statement is to serve "as a global catalyst and leader to promote the development and implementation of innovative models of health care that focus on healing and nurturing body, mind, and spirit." Planetree, then, is a vision or philosophy that promotes cultural change in health care. This cultural change has a positive effect on physician practice as well as on the sanctity of the physician-patient relationship.

Four of the first five model Planetree units located within hospitals consisted of individual floor conversions. After this experience, Planetree chose to convert entire hospitals rather than individual floors. It rapidly became clear that top administrative and physician leadership must buy into the concepts of patient-centered care to ensure the full success of cultural transformation. Thoughtful leaders who share the vision must be identified within the organization to help perform an honest organizational self-analysis and identify and prioritize suggestions for change. Originally the nearly exclusive domain of nursing and administration, Planetree has been joined by enthusiastic physician partners throughout its network, as a growing number of doctors acknowledge the need for profound cultural change within the health care system. At the Planetree Conference in 2007, thirty-six physician champions were honored for their work at sites around the country.

It is valuable to examine the current conditions of health care from multiple perspectives in order to better understand the need for the cultural change that accompanies Planetree hospital conversions and the role of the physician in this change.

THE CHANGING PHYSICIAN PERSPECTIVE

A recent survey of over eight hundred members of the Medical Society of Virginia revealed that doctors continue to care deeply about the needs of their patients and practice medicine because they are driven to help people in need (Medical Society of Virginia, 2007). What has changed dramatically, however, is the growing complexity of medicine and health care delivery and the inability of the physician to fully influence the care of the patient.

Outside influences, including insurers, regulators, government authorities, and attorneys, may create immense frustration among physicians and erode the public's trust in physicians to deliver the best care possible. For example, a physician may order a nuclear stress test to rule out coronary disease in a high-risk diabetic patient with exertional fatigue as the only symptom. The test request may then be rejected by the insurance company because the patient does not have chest pain. Should the test not be done and the patient later suffer a heart attack and sue, the lawyer would surely ask the doctor, "Isn't it true that atypical symptoms like fatigue may indicate the presence of coronary disease in a diabetic patient?" Physicians in emergency departments may feel the pressure to order medically unnecessary (but legally prudent) X-rays and other tests, and doctors working for HMOs may be under pressure to limit the number of specialty consultations they order. Whole communities may lose access to specialties like obstetrics because the high cost of malpractice insurance has driven obstetricians out of the region. These and many other influences have contributed to the decline in the public's trust of the medical profession.

"Trust is one of the central features of patient-physician relationships. Although evidence shows that the majority of patients continue to trust physicians to act in their best interest, concern is growing that the rapid and far-reaching changes in the healthcare system have placed great pressure on that trust and may be undermining it" (Pearson and Raeke, 2000, p. 509). When utilization review by insurers restricts choices or contradicts physicians' medical decisions, physicians lose control even though they still bear responsibility for outcomes. Although the patient's welfare is a physician's highest priority, the intrusion into medical decision making by third-party intermediaries may negatively affect the quality of the physician-patient relationship, and there is ample evidence that this relationship has therapeutic value in and of itself.

The findings of the Medical Society of Virginia Survey (2007) suggest that at no other time in history have physicians felt such an extreme loss of control and autonomy when it comes to practicing medicine. Physicians are especially frustrated because they often feel they are being dictated to by less-knowledgeable workers at insurance companies, rather than being able to practice medicine the way they believe it should be practiced. Tests that can be ordered, treatment options, and specific medications must frequently be tailored to meet the patient's insurance plans. A change in the patient's insurance plan sometimes even requires a change in physician. Many physicians feel that the public does not understand that they are working extremely hard to ensure that patient care will not suffer but are often powerless to control the situation.

In addition, the number of patients that physicians have to see just to meet overhead has gone up greatly; this too has tremendous impact on patient and physician satisfaction. Thus there is less time for the interpersonal dialogue that is both medically valuable and spiritually nurturing for both parties. The sum total of these intrusions can have damaging consequences, not only to the physician-patient relationship but also to patient outcomes.

In general, physicians are committed to the sanctity and trust of the physician-patient relationship and need a supportive health care environment to ensure that a strong relationship is cultivated. To accomplish these goals in our current environment, physicians need a restoration of trust in the system and increased patient confidence that the physician can truly be an advocate for the patient's health care needs within the system. The physician's desired outcome is acceptance that the physician and the patient together be the ultimate decision makers in health care matters within guidelines that allow freedom of choice, rather than a rigid one-size-fits-all approach that disregards an individual's needs.

A modern, well-run hospital that is both safe and financially solvent depends on hospital-based algorithms of care crafted from risk-benefit and cost-effective models and assessments. For instance, the use of national, evidence-based core measurements that reflect adherence to *best practice* protocols promote improved outcomes and standardized care for many common illnesses. For conditions like coronary artery disease, for instance, hospitals are graded by the frequency of use of key medications like statins for high cholesterol. Though there is evidence that this cookbook approach improves outcomes, it also reduces the focus on other therapeutic options that may in the long run be at least as valuable for the patient. These include weight loss, relaxation therapy, and proper nutrition, which, though difficult for many people, can markedly improve outcomes in highly motivated individuals. There is evidence that the best therapeutic approach to reducing the risk of coronary events in patients at risk is a combination of lifestyle change and medication, the former receiving too little attention and funding when compared with the latter.

THE PATIENT PERSPECTIVE

First and foremost, patients need confidence and trust that their providers and the health care system will be there for them when they are in need and will provide safe and high-quality health care to achieve the best possible outcomes. Patients expect to be treated with dignity and respect, to be communicated with and listened to, and to be empowered to make their own decisions about their body and their health. Patients expect that their health care providers effectively share information resulting in coordination and integration of care. Furthermore, patients expect caring attention and respect for emotional and spiritual needs. In other words, patients expect to be treated as a whole person and not as a broken body part. This is also frequently accompanied by an expectation of communication with and involvement of the family in order to promote support for the patients at home. Increasingly, as patients pay more of the bill, they will expect more economic value and choices of treatment received. Finally, patients expect an enhanced quality and length of life, which puts constant pressure on technological, pharmaceutical, and scientific innovation, which, of course, increases costs. Ultimately, we are all patients and can agree that these needs are reasonable and shared universally. These concepts represent what we as physicians would expect for ourselves and our loved ones.

A review of how well our current model of health care fulfills patient expectations is valuable to understand potential opportunities for improvement served by innovative patient-centered care initiatives.

The first patient expectation is access to health care. In a poll of twelve hundred Americans ("Six Prescriptions for Change," 2008) more than 80 percent expressed concerns about coverage and continuity of care. Increasingly, even well-insured patients, as well as the uninsured and Medicare patients, find it difficult to find and establish a permanent relationship with a primary care physician. Many patients in our highly mobile society move or change jobs (and insurers) and are left without a long-term relationship with a primary health care provider. The lack of a trusted provider results in frustration for a patient trying to navigate a complex system of medical specialists. Emergency departments and hospitals frequently become the providers of last resort for patients who can find no other access to the health care system. Even for patients with a regular primary provider, access to specialty care in a timely manner is frequently difficult. Inadequate health care access and fragmented care in emergency departments reinforce the patient perspective of poor service in a service industry. Beyond poor service, delays in diagnosis and appropriate care may result in adverse clinical outcomes. In addition, for those patients who require hospitalization, the trend is toward care by hospitalists rather than primary care physicians. This loss of continuity of providers may result in less integration between inpatient and outpatient care and may result in a perception by the patient of less personal care.

A second and fundamental patient expectation is safe and high-quality health care. Increasing media attention about hospital-acquired infections, medication errors, and other safety lapses has appropriately heightened patient concerns. Current and future public reporting of outcomes, from surgical results to adherence with evidenced-based practices, will increasingly influence patient health care decisions. Public reporting of quality indicators are being demanded by employers, such as Leap Frog, and payers, including Centers for Medicare and Medicaid Services (CMS). Increasingly, data will be collected, analyzed, and publicly reported as a "scorecard" for all levels of providers, including hospitals and individual physicians. These trends are designed to force quality and safety improvements in order to meet the very reasonable patient expectations of safe and high-quality care.

The third patient expectation is that a patient be treated with dignity and respect and be communicated with and listened to effectively. These expectations reflect the innate desires and rights of human beings and should be especially honored in issues of personal decisions regarding one's own body. The medical profession needs to understand and respect the increasing importance to the patient of these essential expectations. Medical knowledge is a specialized area of understanding that requires intensive study to comprehend. It uses specialized language or jargon that is unfamiliar to most patients. Therefore, it falls to the physician to translate for the patient, a skill that requires not only knowledge but also sensitivity. This *knowledge deficit* on the part of a patient results in the necessity to grant decision making about his or her own medical condition to another person, usually a physician, in a blind and dependent manner. This paternalistic approach was a constant in medicine until relatively recently, even though the word *physician* means teacher. Giving up control of decisions over one's own body requires great trust, which runs counter to most people's desire for self-determination in the current era.

The availability of medical information through the Internet and other sources has empowered patients to self-educate and to expect and demand improved communication and information sharing with providers. At the same time, patients need physicians more than ever to answer more informed questions and sort out often conflicting Web-based information. Patients are demanding a shared decision-making model, where they are communicated with, educated, and empowered to make their own decisions regarding their personal health care. Physician communication skills and respectful treatment of patients are being assessed for the first time as publicly reported quality indicators as part of a movement to standardize the survey tools and thus the data collected by them. Examples of these include the HCAHPS survey now being used in the United States and the CQI survey in the Netherlands. Participation in use of such surveys— and ultimately reimbursement for care based on performance—will increasingly influence hospital reimbursement.

Beyond being treated with dignity and respect and being communicated with effectively, patients expect caring attention, compassion, and understanding of their emotional needs under the stressful conditions of illness. In the focused drive toward efficient diagnosis and treatment of physical ailments, it is easy to underestimate and overlook the powerful emotions of fear, anxiety, loneliness, depression, and hopelessness that can influence perceived health and ultimately affect outcomes. Besides health care, few other avocations provide the privilege and honor to serve other people in moments of need and vulnerability. It is these special moments of caring and connecting with others that provide the fulfillment for both patient and caregiver. With medical advances, we must never forget our equal responsibility to listen compassionately, communicate clearly, and meet the emotional and spiritual needs of the patient.

THE PAYER PERSPECTIVE

Despite the fact that the United States leads the world in health care expenditures, life expectancy in the United States lags behind that of many other countries. Clearly, current and future economic realities of health care costs will serve as catalysts to evaluate new models of health care. According to the Director of the Congressional Budget Office, Peter Orszag, in the *New England Journal of Medicine,* "The long-term fiscal balance of the United States will be determined primarily by the future rate of growth of health care costs" (Orszag and Ellis, 2007, p. 1885). If the same rate of growth continues, in 2050 federal spending on Medicare and Medicaid will equal 20 percent of the gross domestic product, which equals the share accounted for now by the entire federal budget. Dr. Orszag suggests that opportunities be created to constrain health care costs without incurring adverse health consequences. He suggests providing more information about relative effectiveness of medical treatments and enhancing incentives for providers to supply, and consumers to demand, effective care. Dr. Orszag's observation that "treatment choices often depend on the experience and judgment of the physicians involved, as well as on anecdotal evidence and local practice norms" (p. 1885) does not appropriately acknowledge the tremendous effort expended by physicians to define and pursue evidence-based medicine. He further argues that substantial changes would probably require public and private insurers to modify their coverage or payment policies and alter the incentives offered to doctors and patients. This *value-based insurance* design will likely require enrollees to pay higher deductibles and the additional costs of more expensive treatments that are shown to be less effective or less cost-effective.

These comments from the Director of the Congressional Budget Office are consistent with the current movement toward *consumer-driven health care.* In order to slow the rate of increase of health care costs, consumers would pay a larger part of the real cost and therefore would be more discerning in how their money is spent. In order to empower the consumer, there will be mandatory public reporting of accurate outcomes, data, and costs. This cost-and-quality transparency is designed to promote value-driven decision making, where consumers seek the best quality for cost. In addition, the electronic medical record will be highly portable and likely *individually owned,* which will allow consumers to shop and cost-compare. The problem with the free market approach to health care delivery is an assumption of "perfect information" and unlimited access to and supply of health care providers, neither of which is likely to occur.

In addition to consumer-driven health care, another current trend is *pay-for-performance.* Payers such as Centers for Medicare and Medicaid Services (CMS) provide financial incentives to hospitals and physicians in order to promote improved outcomes or patient satisfaction. The HCAHPS survey results of recently discharged patients will be performed every quarter, publicly reported, and used to determine if a hospital receives a bonus payment from CMS. The HCAHPS survey demonstrates that payers will use financial incentives to encourage physician behavioral changes as well as to reward certain prespecified outcome measures. The HCAHPS survey asks patients three questions regarding care from their doctors:

- During this hospital stay, how often did doctors treat you with courtesy and respect?

- During this hospital stay, how often did doctors listen carefully to you?

- During this hospital stay, how often did doctors explain things in a way you could understand?

It is obvious that CMS places real value on communication and respect and will use financial incentives to try to improve these measures of quality.

Who defines performance and how it is defined will be increasingly important to physicians and patients. Measures of performance must be valid, important, useful to patients, and useful to organizations to guide quality and safety improvements. In addition, we must ask where physician performance ends and patient performance begins. Ultimately, there is a shared responsibility for outcomes, which requires increased personal responsibility for health maintenance on the part of patients.

THE ROLE OF PLANETREE

The HCAHPS survey and financial incentives for improved physician courtesy and communication represent important steps in the right direction. However, given the current, fragmented status of patient care, a new model of health care is needed, one that addresses and improves conditions from the combined perspectives of patients, physicians, and payers. Such a model would do well to preserve physician autonomy and the physician-patient relationship. The model should promote safety, quality, and access and should empower patients' decision making through communication and education. The model should guarantee a compassionate atmosphere of caring for the emotional and spiritual needs of patients, should encourage supportive involvement of family and a seamless connection between hospital and outpatient care, and should improve integration between providers and continuity of care throughout the entire health care system. Encouraging patients to be personally responsible for their health should be advocated and rewarded. Ultimately, the result should be high-quality and cost-effective health care.

Planetree promotes an evolving framework of shared decision making, which is frequently referred to as *patient-centered care.* Over time, there has been a shift in the locus of control in terms of health care decision making. In the traditional paternalistic model, the decision making was vested in the physician alone, as the keeper of specialized medical knowledge. Over time, the informed-consent model or informed-choice model has shifted decision making toward the patients. Logically, people prefer to be involved in decisions affecting their own body and life. The locus of control over these personal decisions rightfully belongs to the individual, even though some patients and doctors still cling to the old paternalistic approach.

Patient-centered care promotes respect for patient values, preferences, and expressed needs. Other important components are information, communication, and education to empower patient decision making. The role of the staff is to meet the needs of each patient individually. Involvement of family and friends is encouraged, and they are welcomed as partners in both care and caring. The healing environment is designed to support patient dignity, decrease barriers, feel homelike, and encourage family participation in care. Emphasis on the transition to home and the continuity of care is designed to make sure patients continue to receive the support they need. The Planetree model also espouses that to effectively care for patients, we must also care for our staff members, so the system must support the health care worker as well.

Patient-centered care appropriately places the focus on serving the patient. However, the Planetree model also acknowledges the importance of enabling staff in their roles as caregivers so that they feel appreciated and supported. In patient-centered care, there is an emphasis on the *therapeutic relationship,* which requires both serving the patient and supporting caregivers. *Patient relationship centered care* is designed to empower providers (physicians, nurses, and others) and patients to work together through the provider-patient relationship to promote health, to prevent illness, and to treat diseases in order to achieve the best possible outcomes.

In this new and idealized model of health care, a key role and responsibility for the physician is to communicate effectively and educate the patient in order to empower the patient to make appropriate health care choices. The system itself is designed to support this educational component and encourage the patient to participate in the process as an informed health care consumer. The patient's role and responsibility is to understand his or her medical condition, to assume personal responsibility for adherence to a treatment regimen, and ultimately to achieve a better outcome by being an active participant on the health care team. For instance, a patient may have successful shoulder surgery, but recovery of function depends heavily on the commitment of the patient to do the work required in physical rehabilitation. Ultimately, the physician is a trusted adviser who is valued and needed for medical advice, therapeutic recommendations, and caring attention. Just as physicians' communication skills may vary, it is also the case that not all patients are equally capable of absorbing the information or taking on the same degree of personal responsibility in matters of health care. More research is needed to understand the characteristics of successful patients, specifically regarding the effects of medical literacy, personal motivation, social support, and physician communication.

According to the World Health Organization (2003), "Poor adherence increases with the duration and complexity of treatment regimens . . . duration and complex treatment are inherent to chronic illnesses. Across diseases, adherence is the single most important modifiable factor that compromises treatment outcome" (p. 148). Although it may seem a matter of semantics, the distinction between the terms *compliance* and *adherence* reflects the differences between a paternalistic care model and a patient-centered care model. The *American Heritage Dictionary* defines *compliance* as "yielding to a wish, or demand; acquiescence."*Adherence* is defined as "the act or quality of sticking to something; faithful attachment." Adherence means that a patient understands the reasons, buys into the treatment, and accepts personal responsibility for staying with the plan. Therefore, it is anticipated that empowered, adherent patients should have improved outcomes. A number of Planetree affiliates are in the process of devising and conducting studies to further validate the hypothesis that patient-centered care improves outcomes and not just patient satisfaction (Stone, 2007).

PHYSICIAN INVOLVEMENT IN PLANETREE

There are various opportunities for direct physician involvement in the implementation of the Planetree model of patient-centered care. Many of the model's core components, including education and human interaction, represent natural opportunities for physician involvement.

These key components often surface in patient surveys as opportunities for improvement, as many physicians focus on medically essential tasks at the expense of spending the time necessary for full discussions about treatment options and patient and family dynamics. Interested Planetree physicians may address this opportunity by giving prescheduled, advertised public lectures or offering to engage in informal discussions with patients and family members in a lounge area on the floor. Physicians can contribute by simply becoming better listeners or arriving earlier than usual to a clinic to afford patients more time for dialogue.

Dr. Louis Teichholz, a Harvard-trained physician who is chief of cardiology at Hackensack University Medical Center in New Jersey, relies on Dr. Francis Weld Peabody's statement as a guide to physicians: "The secret of the care of the patient is in caring for the patient" (Peabody, 1927, p. 882). Dr. Peabody, also a Harvard physician, wrote these words at the age of thirty-five while dying of cancer.

A common role for Dr. Teichholz and other Planetree physician champions is to lend voice to the Planetree philosophy during administrative meetings. This is especially valuable for decision-making meetings where the physician leader may be the only person in the room with clinical experience. The impact of the physician breaking loose from the expected role of providing a medical opinion to offer instead the patient's perspective is often dramatic, reframing the hospital experience in human terms for the rest of the administrative team.

Many physicians express support for the principles of patient-centered care, but few feel they can afford the time to become more actively involved. Dr. Lisa Sombrotto, a psychiatrist who is the clinical director of rehabilitation medicine at New York–Presbyterian Medical Center's New York site, says, "If you meet people's needs on many levels, it will save you time" (personal interview, December 2007). To help meet those needs, a family and patient bulletin board has been set up, and additional, readily available educational tools are provided. The result is that there are more-informed questions directed to the physicians. Each of the members of the Planetree executive committee at the medical center is responsible for spearheading a Planetree initiative. Dr. Sombrotto's project is spirituality, a sometimes controversial concept in nonsectarian hospitals because of its relationship (and confusion) with religiosity. A solution to the controversy was the creation of a *meditation room* for quiet reflection, which has become popular with patients and staff members.

A common thread among physicians who have become more active at Planetree sites is the shared recognition that the patient-centered care model fostered by the Planetree philosophy is not a new or alien concept, but a practical, hospital-wide implementation of a type of health care that many physicians have been practicing for years. Some physicians are drawn to become Planetree activists because of an intrinsic affinity for the Planetree philosophy and the recognition of an opportunity to join a community of like-minded health care professionals, even though most are not physicians.

This concept is summarized well by Dr. Paul Summerside of Aurora Baycare Medical Center in Wisconsin, who states simply, "It's the right thing to do." In fact, he considers his involvement a bit selfish because "it makes practice more fun. I can't understand physicians who do this job for the money. If you do not get anything back emotionally, it is too hard a job" (personal interview, December 2007). This is echoed in the words of Dr. Rachel Naomi Remen, a pediatric oncologist and best-selling author, who says that *fixing* a patient's problem is the work of the ego and eventually leads to burnout. In contrast, *serving* a patient's needs is the work of the soul and is a nurturing experience for both patient and physician.

Physician resistance is a common challenge for local physician advocates at many Planetree sites. Resistance may come from concern that precious hospital resources are being diverted to so-called soft, nonmedical modalities, such as the emotional support of patients and families, rather than going toward the purchase of much-needed "hard" medical resources, like imaging equipment.

Unfortunately, physician resistance may also originate from the wounded healer with a limited ability to empathize with patients and family members. It is always fascinating to look at the history of medical education and hospital practice to more fully realize that an industry with a mediocre track record for compassionate care of its own personnel expects its workers to be models of compassionate patient care. Depression has traditionally been rampant in medical schools, and physicians themselves have a high incidence of divorce, drug abuse, and suicide (Center and others, 2003; Schernhammer and Colditz, 2004). In the 1950s, at least one hospital in New York would not hire house officers if they were married because they would not be able to devote their full energies to their medical responsibilities. Residencies commonly demanded fifty-six hours of continuous weekend on-call well into the 1990s. These practices, long since prohibited in airline and transportation industries, ultimately required governmental regulation to create more tolerable work shifts in the health care industry. Codes of behavior had to be drafted to limit exploitation of house staff and medical students. It is not surprising that some physicians emerge from the brutality of training programs unable to give what they do not have or have lost along the way.

Physician leaders who model the patient-centered care philosophy of Planetree often serve as catalysts for change among the other health care workers in the hospital setting. Working committees with broad representation (including physicians) are important to encourage creativity and participation. If there are too few staff members involved, there will not be sustained cultural change. Staff retreats are invaluable to promote understanding of purpose, show value, and achieve buy-in. Workers must see a positive impact of a Planetree conversion and improvement in both their own and the patients' satisfaction to overcome cynicism. It is critical that staff members see physician leaders participate in these retreats and that adequate numbers of workers become directly involved. Mini-retreats or dinners for physicians may allow for more intimate discussions and open dialogue, presenting opportunities for physician-inspired changes in patient-centered care.

Each Planetree hospital and affiliate has wonderful examples of successful implementation. As an organization, Planetree should function as a repository of *best practices* in order to help participating affiliates learn from one another and facilitate rapid spread of successes. Affiliates have led the way in creating an open culture of patient-centered care through promoting expanded visitation times, open medical records, and many other creative innovations.

An important example of patient-centered care is the creation of a palliative care consultation service. Utilizing a multidisciplinary approach, including physicians, nurses, social workers, and hospice experts, this consult service offers substantial value to patients, families, and referring physicians in dealing with end-of-life issues. This service of trained and committed professionals provides understanding, compassion, and frank discussion of options and is truly an important example of the value of patient-centered care.

Another example that has led to cultural change is the patient assistance liaison (PAL) program at Sentara Virginia Beach General Hospital. This program and others like it at other Planetree affiliates is designed to encourage family and friend participation in hospital patient care so as to provide emotional and social support for the patient and create a smoother transition to care at home. The Patient Advisory Council is a hospital-based Planetree committee that involves interested patients in the cultural change of the hospital. This committee encourages organizational transparency and responsiveness to real patient needs and encourages creative input from the community the hospital serves. Active encouragement and involvement of community volunteers further contribute to cultural transformation to openness and provide opportunities for volunteers, who offer caring and attention to patients. These and many other innovations serve to supplement and support the counsel provided by physicians.

The introduction of in-house complementary therapies that patients commonly use outside the hospital is growing in popularity but remains controversial. At Hackensack University Medical Center, Dr. Teichholz offers evidence-based complementary therapies to inpatients. At Stamford Hospital in Connecticut, Chief of Cardiothoracic Surgery, Dr. Li Poa, offers acupuncture for nausea control and Reiki therapy to enhance general well-being for all heart surgery patients. Massage therapy, healing touch, and reflexology are examples of modalities implemented at various hospitals throughout the Planetree Network as traditional techniques that offer comfort to many patients with little downside.

A new program using the Getwell Network, implemented at Sentara Virginia Beach General Hospital, is designed to enhance patient education through the creative use of different educational resources to try to improve patient outcomes. This four-day patient education pathway is directed at patients with congestive heart failure (CHF) and uses the television in the patient's room to deliver information and solicit patient responses to assess understanding. The pathway is designed to educate patients about the diagnosis of congestive heart failure and explain where they are in the disease process. In addition, the pathway educates patients about their individual test results and the importance and potential side effects of their medications. The pathway teaches patients self-assessment skills in order to manage their chronic disease process. The goal of the CHF pathway is to empower patients to understand their disease; manage their medications, diet, and exercise; and perform self-assessment to help them be in control of the treatment of this chronic disease process. Outcomes data will be collected regarding length of stay, thirty-day readmission rates, and patient satisfaction. The objective is to provide evidence that patient-specific education services improve outcomes and patient satisfaction. Many physicians say that what is needed now is more research, especially in assessing efficacy, cost, and risk benefit of the many new approaches emerging throughout the Planetree network. This need is currently being addressed within the organization. It is hoped that it will result in Planetree not only providing leadership in implementing patient-centered care but also in providing additional evidence to assess its full value as the model of care for the future.

REFERENCES

Center, C., and others. "Confronting Depression and Suicide in Physicians: A Consensus Statement."*Journal of the American Medical Association,* 2003, *289,* 3161–3166.

"Medical Society of Virginia Physician Survey." Unpublished. 2007.

Orszag, P. R., and Ellis, P."Addressing Rising Health Care Costs: A View from the Congressional Budget Office."*New England Journal of Medicine,* 2007, *357,* 1885–1887.

Peabody, F. W."The Care of the Patient."*Journal of the American Medical Association,* 1927, *88,* 877–882.

Pearson, S. D., and Raeke, L. H."Patients' Trust in Physicians: Many Theories, Few Measures, and Little Data."*Journal of General Internal Medicine,* 2000, *15,* 509–513.

Schernhammer, E. S., and Colditz, G. A. "Suicide Rates Among Physicians: A Quantitative and Gender Assessment Meta-Analysis." *American Journal of Psychiatry,* 2004, *161,* 2295–2302.

"Six Prescriptions for Change." *Consumer Reports,* Mar. 2008, pp. 14–17.

Stone, S. *"A Retrospective Evaluation of the Planetree Patient-Centered Model of Care Program's Impact on Inpatient Quality Outcomes."* Doctoral dissertation, University of San Diego, 2007.

World Health Organization. *Adherence to Long-Term Therapies: Evidence for Action.* Geneva: World Health Organization, 2003.

CHAPTER

12

ADAPTING PATIENT-CENTERED CARE TO DIVERSE HEALTH CARE SETTINGS

HEIDI GIL, WENDY W. PECHE, AND PHILIP J. WILNER

This chapter does the following:

- Describes effective ways that patient-centered care has been adapted from an acute care model to behavioral health, continuing care, and integrated health care system settings, both in the United States and abroad.

Planetree's beginnings were largely limited to health resource centers and acute care hospitals, but the fundamentals of providing patient-centered care resonate across the health care continuum. With its intent to provide personalized care, the flexibility and adaptability of the model are in fact defining characteristics of patient-centered care. In a series of in-depth case studies, this chapter recounts the culture change journeys of three pioneering organizations, one in a behavioral health setting, one in a continuing care environment, and one throughout an expansive integrated health care system. Each organization faced a unique set of challenges and considerations that required innovative adaptations to the model, to its core components, and to the infrastructure necessary to initiate and sustain organizational culture transformation.

BEHAVIORAL HEALTH: NEW YORK–PRESBYTERIAN HOSPITAL

Behavioral health is arguably the most difficult service to adapt to a patient-centered approach. The essential element of partnering with the patient is limited in a subtle way by our tendency toward paternalism and in a very obvious way by the very illnesses that the patients experience and the consequent impairments of judgment, insight, and in many cases cognitive organization. Empowerment and education are noble and needed but often difficult to effect with the mentally ill. Manifestations of these challenges include difficulty with maintaining an open record, efforts to educate and share decision making, and the feasibility and advisability of extensive involvement of families in treatment. Environmental issues also pose major challenges: being homelike, being private, and encouraging individual expression versus an overregulated climate of patient safety concerns.

That said, patient-centered care completely resonates with the Moral Treatment antecedents of quality psychiatric care and its emphasis on respecting the healthy human core of even the sickest patients, the value placed on meaningful engagement with the world through work and activities, and the importance of sustaining leisure endeavors such as appreciation for and engagement in the arts.

The introduction of *Moral Treatment* at the end of the eighteenth century in England marked a turning point in the history of psychiatry and the approach to caring for patients with mental illness. Prior to this period, impairments of reason, judgment, and behavior—currently understood as mental illness—were treated as disordered behaviors requiring control and punishment. Concepts of mental illness emerged that demanded that the insane be treated as ill human beings, with compassion and caring.

The New York Hospital was at the forefront of the Moral Treatment movement during the nineteenth century, with the establishment of the Bloomingdale Asylum and the move to White Plains, New York. The design of the new Westchester facility and its extensive property offered expanded opportunities for the use of psychosocial, occupational, and recreational therapies—important elements of Moral Treatment and patient-centered care. The Moral Treatment model had much in common with the concept of *putting patients first*. Unfortunately, over the ensuing century, with the advent of sophisticated psychological and biological treatments, the humane aspects of caring were marginalized in favor of productivity, efficiency, and protocol. The Planetree model, embraced in 2003 by the Weill Cornell Psychiatric Services of what is now New York–Presbyterian Hospital, represents a return to our roots.

New York-Presbyterian Hospital is a large academic medical center, established in 1997 with the full asset merger of The New York Hospital and The Presbyterian Hospital. New York–Presbyterian maintains academic affiliation with both Weill Cornell Medical College and Columbia University's College of Physicians and Surgeons. The hospital operates 2,250 beds on five campuses, generates about 1.2 million ambulatory visits, and employs over seventeen thousand employees. The Westchester Division is home to one of the largest freestanding psychiatric facilities in the country. The program is composed of 269 psychiatric and addiction inpatient beds and a broad array of ambulatory services. The chief operating officer responsible for the campus, interested in fulfilling the hospital's goal to improve the patient experience at New York–Presbyterian, had knowledge of the Planetree model from a previous position he had held. He was eager to bring it to the Westchester Division as a pilot, with the long-term goal of bringing Planetree to the rest of New York–Presbyterian. It was his determination that Planetree would be an easy fit for the psychiatric program and that there were advantages to piloting Planetree first in a homogeneous program before subjecting it to the challenges and complexities of the large, complex, urban academic medical center.

The Journey

The hospital's Planetree journey began in autumn 2003, with site visits by the leadership team to Griffin Hospital, the Planetree flagship in the northeast. Planetree Retreats were held during 2004 to inspire and orient all staff, physicians, and administrators, with an achieved goal of 100 percent participation. In December 2004, the Westchester Division became the first freestanding behavioral health facility in the nation to implement the Planetree model. A committee structure was established to support unit-based initiatives and to continue evaluating the program along the components of the Planetree model. The components were reviewed, adopted, and of necessity adapted to meet the needs of the behavioral health clinical program and setting. For example, to maintain patient and staff safety, psychiatric inpatient units must maintain a rigorous structure and schedule, limiting in certain instances flexibility to facilitate specific patient and family requests. Group and community benefit often trump individual accommodation. Governmental regulations mandate environmental safety measures and features that at times conflict with comfort and aesthetics. Nonetheless, staff felt excited and empowered to assess their assumptions, practices, and attitudes and to embark on a journey of creativity and change.

Human Interactions. Not surprisingly, the Planetree approach fit easily into the culture of the psychiatric hospital and resonated well with staff. The interdisciplinary nature of behavioral health care allowed for the early establishment of annual staff retreats, comingling staff of all roles and disciplines, including physicians. A quick focus was building teamwork through individual and unit recognition, social and sports events for staff, and an internal newsletter. The position of front door receptionist was created to support and guide visitors through a facility where their loved ones will stay days or weeks, compared with an earlier era when patients stayed one to two years.

Family, Friends, and Social Supports. Small changes to established practices yielded huge early gains for patients, for their family members and friends, and for staff. The implementation of more flexible visiting hours and unit programming during those hours for visitors was easily achieved, despite the fact that many practices had not changed for many years because of concretized rules and protocols. More private visiting space was created on the units, and family members, no longer seen as intrusive enemies of care, were better integrated in treatment planning and implementation. Staff face the challenge of managing the confidentiality of patient information, where often patients do not choose to disclose to family and friends personal aspects of their clinical history or treatment program. Similarly, a balance must be struck between open visitation and the need for patients to engage in the clinical program on the unit and participate in the milieu and its activities.

Access to Information. Complex rules and regulations often govern patient access to behavioral health information. There was little interest on the part of administrators and clinicians to develop an open medical record program. Greater emphasis was placed on providing health information to patients. The Patient Resource Center was created adjacent to the entrance to the main building, and health information resource carts were developed to bring materials to patients who could not leave their unit. Patient-dedicated hours were established at the Medical Library, and medication education programs were instituted on all the units.

Architectural Design. A number of important projects were completed in the public areas of the facility, including redesigning the main lobby entrance. A reception desk was created, a comfortable waiting area with a fish tank was installed, an electronic information kiosk was put in, and a café area was opened. A nondenominational chapel was designed and built adjacent to the reception area. Improvements were made to the grounds, with upgrades to and beautification projects in the courtyards and playgrounds and the installation of gazebo sitting areas.

Patient safety concerns on psychiatric inpatient units have resulted in a national campaign toward eliminating all looping hazards on the units. Traditional door hinges and knobs, and bathroom faucets and fixtures, all pose potential chances for self-destructive behavior, resulting in many hospitals installing prison-type hardware to guard against potential risks. It continues to be a struggle to provide the homelike environment that is conducive to healing in the face of these regulatory and safety challenges.

Nutritional and Nurturing Aspects of Food. Simple steps, such as allotting more time for meals and changing meal times, have gone a long way to creating a more nurturing environment. Psychiatric patients eat their meals family style, offering an easy opportunity to use the dining experience as a chance to build community. Soft music is often played during meals, and menus and food selections have been reevaluated. Unit tea times, once a standard amenity on all units, have been reintroduced. For staff, a twenty-four-hour vending lounge was established to provide easy access to food for staff.

Healing Arts. Many events now fill the day, bringing the therapeutic arts to patients and their visitors. Many volunteers donate time to provide movie afternoons, jazz ensembles, storytelling, dance performances, choral singing, and special holiday events. New artwork has been displayed in patient and public areas.

Spirituality. Behavioral health specialists have always been at the forefront of medicine, in their efforts to integrate mind, body, and spirit. The biopsychosocial model is at its core the implementation of these principles. With the introduction of Planetree to the campus, creative new ways were explored to support patients' efforts to nurture their spiritual needs. Mindfulness meditation is offered to patients, spirituality groups meet regularly, and spaces and places of quiet contemplation have been created. A patient-designed labyrinth is now available as well.

Human Touch. In a behavioral health setting, given the impaired reality testing that some patients may experience, restrictions are placed on physical contact between patients and staff. The Pet Therapy Program has been introduced, which provides a wonderful way to provide tactile pleasure to patients and visitors. Hand massage is used with geriatric patients, and staff have been trained to provide hand massage for one another. At the annual Employee Appreciation Event, free massage is made available for all employees.

Complementary Therapies. Aromatherapy has been introduced on the units, often as an alternative support to induce sleep. Movement classes are provided for patients on the units, and yoga is available for staff.

Healthy Communities. The resources of the hospital have been opened to the community. Community education classes are offered on campus and the Resource Center is open to the public. The hospital sponsors health fairs and related events, a speakers' bureau, screening days, and school outreach. The number of volunteers supporting the program has increased significantly, as a result of the partnership established with the community.

Lessons Learned and Future Challenges

The Planetree model has proved ideally suited for the behavioral health setting. In fact, in our experience, the easy adaptability of behavioral health to the Planetree approach has at times made it more difficult to convince other services within the academic medical center to adopt the Planetree methodology, as the synergy with behavioral health seems so tight.

No program is capable of surviving the rigors of the health care system today without metrics to support its efficacy. New York–Presbyterian uses a validated mailed survey to measure its patient satisfaction results and to identify areas for improvement. An important early lesson was that despite their mental disturbances, psychiatric patients are capable of carefully discriminating good from bad service and indicating it on the survey forms. Staff were able to see that when areas were targeted for improvement and changes were made, the patient satisfaction scores quickly reflected the improvements. When the focus was taken off a priority area, scores often declined.

Overall, patient satisfaction scores improved significantly. Since the introduction of Planetree, scores have increased 10 percent on the inpatient service and 5 percent in the outpatient service, both now approaching the 75th percentile for behavioral health facilities. The program is well on its way to achieving the stated goal of reaching the 90th percentile. At the same time and just as important for the success of the initiative and as a stimulant for change, employee engagement survey scores are rising as well. The Westchester Division staff report the highest levels of employee satisfaction across all New York–Presbyterian Hospital services. The Planetree approach has been credited by hospital leadership for the remarkable improvement in scores.

A continuing challenge for our program is to provide measurable outcomes to support the institution's investment in Planetree. It has been critical to teach staff to understand and speak the language of measurement while conveying the attitudes of high-quality, patient-centered care. Staff are asked to report their initiatives, with their supporting data, to groups large and small, underscoring the partnership that has been promoted of evidence-based and data-driven practice with humanism, compassion, and healing.

CONTINUING CARE: WESLEY VILLAGE

The long-term care industry is in the midst of exciting and dramatic changes. In continuing care environments, including independent and assisted living and skilled nursing communities, the culture change movement has emerged as a response to the growing disenchantment voiced by residents and caregivers alike. Addressing their dissatisfaction has involved a heightened sensitivity to both quality of care and quality of life for residents; it has also involved understanding why employees chose to enter health care professions in the first place. Even the best organizations are reshaping and redefining the meaning of service excellence. While long-term care undergoes this critical renaissance, it remains vulnerable to regulatory, clinical, operational, and financial challenges.

For Wesley Village, a community in Shelton, Connecticut, grappling with these complex challenges ironically led to a simple solution: that caring relationships are fundamental to a meaningful life. From this notion arose Planetree Continuing Care, a philosophy of systemic change that embraces resident-directed care while responding to the importance of the relationships between residents and employees, as well as among residents, family members, staff, supervisors, volunteers, physicians, and friends. Creating a relationship-centered environment is the first step toward becoming sensitized and committed to the possibilities that exist for growth, change, and improvement as individuals, and ultimately as a health care community.

The Journey

Owned by the nonprofit United Methodist Homes, Wesley Village consists of three communities that provide independent living, assisted living, and skilled nursing care to more than four hundred residents. When they first embarked on their culture change journey in 2001, the three communities at Wesley Village all had high satisfaction scores, strong reputations, and longevity in staffing. At the same time, leadership was top-down, and individual departments as well as the three communities were working in isolation. The caring staff worked diligently at perfecting their tasks and institutional routines. When the notion of culture change was introduced, many leaders had trouble accepting the concept and asked instead, "If it's not broken, why fix it?"

Despite the hesitation, the leaders of Wesley Village knew that moving from institution-directed to resident-directed care was essential for its health care communities. Wesley Village had examined and applauded the significant improvement made at nearby Griffin Hospital and believed that Planetree concepts made even more sense when applied to long-term care. Furthermore, they saw the potential for improving the patient transition experience by connecting the Planetree philosophy across the continuum of care. A national advisory council, including Planetree founder Angelica Thieriot, reviewed data collected from initial focus groups held with residents, family members, and staff from all levels. The information gathered from these multiple perspectives helped shape the Planetree components and their appropriate expression in long-term care.

Wesley Village began testing and refining these continuing care components and subsequently developed a set of guidelines for effective implementation in longer-term environments. Most of the components remained essentially the same as the acute care components, whereas others were modified to meet the needs of individuals served in continuing care environments.

Planetree Continuing Care Components

It is important to note that individualizing and personalizing care is not about developing programs; rather, it is about deep-rooted systems change. Listed under each component is a sampling of the innovations that emerged at Wesley Village as the larger vision of relationship-centered care took shape.

Recognizing the Primary Importance of Human Interactions. The Wesley Village employee retreats explore the meaning of caring relationships and emphasize putting the person before the task. Staff participate in two days of experiential exercises on the aging process, teamwork, and relationship building. The retreat experience offers a significant departure from the didactic, task-oriented approach typical of many employee training sessions. In an interactive and supportive environment, the staff reawaken their inner passion and remember what brought them to health care in the first place. The retreats serve as a springboard to building a common sense of purpose across the campus and acknowledging the role each individual plays, regardless of department, in creating a community of strong, trusting relationships.

Enhancing Each Individual's Life Journey. Long-term care facilities have long been seen as places of last resort. The concept of *enhancing life's journey* emerged to change this stereotype. This component supports the notion of *creating destinations,* places where people want to live and can continue to learn and grow, regardless of limitations or life expectancy. The resident journey begins at Wesley Village in a community that honors each individual's history while at the same time supporting the continued need for meaning and purpose and fulfillment of dreams. The Journey of Dreams program, for example, invites residents to share their dreams; and staff, family, and volunteers come together with care and creativity to make the dream come true. Emphasis is placed on affirming that the move into continuing care environments is not the *last* chapter in an individual's life, but in fact the *next* chapter.

Supporting Independence, Dignity, and Choice. Expanding resident choice is at the core of transforming long-term care. At Wesley Village, a consistent team of staff is assigned to each individual. This helps ensure that individual routines and preferences are honored, and care and services are well coordinated. The consistent team includes representatives from all clinical and nonclinical departments. To ensure that residents have autonomy and control, each team member is also given autonomy and management support to personalize the care experience in a way that is consistent with individual resident preferences.

Incorporating Family, Friends, and Social Support Networks into the Community. Families, friends, and social support networks are vital resources that can also significantly influence quality of care and quality of life for residents. The Care Partner Program has formalized ways that family members can support and respond to the resident's needs. To encourage more frequent and meaningful visits, the staff created a resource guide of 101 ways that family members, friends, and others can enhance their visits with loved ones.

Supporting Spirituality as a Source of Inner Strength. Being in touch with the spiritual life of the community has fueled an individual and a collective sense of purpose at Wesley Village. There is a time to reflect, a time to grieve, a time to celebrate, and a time to pull together as a community. Shortly after a resident dies, a reflection program brings family, residents, and staff together to honor that resident, allowing an opportunity for closure and a celebration of the uniqueness of each individual. An emphasis is placed on the role that faith plays in the workplace for staff.

Promoting Paths to Well-Being. Complementary therapies and other wellness programs have been extremely well received by residents, family, and staff. The wellness center offers comprehensive classes, including yoga, tai chi, and specialized fitness equipment for elders. A naturopathic clinic integrates acupuncture, aromatherapy, massage, dietary consultation, and herbal supplements. These programs have supported the management of chronic diseases, including pain, depression, and incontinence. A heightened sensitivity to the impact that the five senses have on quality of life has inspired a variety of on-site clinics, including those for vision, hearing, dental, and pharmacological services.

Empowering Individuals Through Information and Education. Promoting resident access to open medical records and providing a health resource library were important new developments for continuing care. It was also recognized that intellectual and personal growth are not limited to a classroom or a particular time in life. A Planetree community provides the information necessary to maximize the physical, mental, emotional, and financial well-being of all of its members. A focus on the importance of lifelong learning has increased educational programs, provided access to computers with Internet capability, and provided the impetus for library expansions. Quality improvement indicators are posted to raise awareness and promote transparency in an environment that strives to exceed quality standards. A career ladder program for line staff has resulted in a leadership culture that is no longer top-down, but where decisions are made by the residents and the staff closest to the residents.

Recognizing the Nutritional and Nurturing Aspects of Food. In continuing care settings, food is often the focal point of the day. When a more flexible meal service was implemented, there was a domino effect that took place on the rhythms and routines of all departments. The changes started with providing a breakfast buffet for short-term rehabilitation residents to enhance their choice of waking and rehabilitation times and to create a separate dining experience. Because staff and residents responded so positively to the changes (including the aroma of fresh cooked food, hot toast, expanded menu choices, fewer calls to the kitchen for adjustments to the food provided, bonding of residents with one another and with dietary staff, increased resident consumption of food, and an atmosphere of normality), within nine months, a tray-less buffet system had been implemented for the benefit of every resident during all meals. The main dining room is also open for several seatings at each meal, which provides flexibility of mealtimes and alternate choices in dining atmosphere.

Offering Meaningful Arts, Activities, and Entertainment. Responding to individual interests and supporting spontaneity have been fundamental to making changes at Wesley Village. Activity staff had previously been evaluated by how many residents attend a program, rather than by how many residents are actively engaged. The focus has now shifted from the quantity of programs and number of residents served to the level of engagement of each resident in meaningful, individualized programs. Resident-directed programs that support teaching, mentoring, sharing, and the building of skills and talents are also emphasized. For example, a drama club of residents and staff evolved when a resident with a background in and love for theater moved into the community. When nurtured, one individual's passion can benefit the entire community.

Providing an Environment Conducive to Quality Living. On the Wesley Village campus, each resident now has a room with a view. Beautiful landscaping, waterfalls, and walking paths connect the campus. Inside, overhead paging has been eliminated, along with the institutional equipment and clutter from hallways. The Environmental Services Department has implemented an Earth-friendly cleaning program using all nontoxic cleaning supplies. The Alzheimer's unit has been unlocked so residents are free to safely integrate into the general community, and all residents can independently enjoy outside areas with the use of a wireless pendant system that ensures their safety by allowing staff to determine a resident's location remotely.

Lessons Learned and Future Challenges

Ultimately, the implementation of Planetree Continuing Care far exceeded expectations and enhanced clinical, financial, and operational outcomes as well as resident and staff satisfaction. Since 2003, in the nursing home on campus

- Restraints were reduced by 91 percent while the national rate declined by 35 percent.

- High-risk pressure ulcers were reduced by 59 percent while the national rate declined by 14 percent.

- For residents with moderate to severe pain, their pain was reduced by 40 percent while the national rate declined by 30 percent.

In addition, just two years after the model had been implemented, the nursing home reported that no certified nursing aides had left due to dissatisfaction with their jobs. In fact, all turnover was involuntary at a rate of 18 percent, compared to a national average of 70 percent.

An important lesson to be gained from Wesley Village's experiences is that transformation is not about a project, a building renovation, or a plethora of mandatory staff in-services or meetings. Rather, it is about awakening passion, creating a strong sense of purpose, and engaging everyone in the process of improvement.

The Planetree process is key to implementing and sustaining changes. On an annual basis, Planetree engages residents, families, staff, and volunteers in evaluating progress and identifying improvements in each of the ten component areas. Weighing these perspectives with other clinical, financial, and operational data ensures that Planetree serves as a comprehensive vehicle for all performance improvement initiatives. By evaluating both qualitative and quantitative data, resident-centered goals are prioritized by a committee composed of managers, staff from all departments, residents, and family members, and they are posted visibly throughout the community. Subsequently, there are regular community updates on the progress toward annual goals and celebrations to acknowledge accomplishments.

In continuing care, it is all about *putting relationships first*. A Planetree community brings everyone together not only in believing in the same vision but also in creating and owning it. As one Wesley Village resident shared, "Planetree means we have to get together because we are all on the same side. What we are building here is something that will make your life worth living, a community. When you are building something, it takes awhile, but this will be beyond you and me, it's bigger than all of us." Staff, residents, and families already know what is important for culture change to occur. The challenge is to assist them in discovering the value of their own unique contributions.

Planetree in the Netherlands, Case One

Woonzorggroep Samen is a continuing care and rehabilitation organization located in the Netherlands. A Planetree member since 2006, the woonzorggroep Samen has been implementing the core Planetree components adapted to reflect the Dutch culture and its health care practices. Planetree Nederland organized the components into three clusters that reinforce one another: Better Care, a Healing Environment, and Healthy Organization. The overriding premise remains the same: to create a patient-centered organizational culture. Through the staff retreat process, staff at the organization was familiarized with the Planetree concept of delivering care the way patients want it delivered. Staff from eight locations attended comingled retreats, created as such to promote sharing of ideas and best practices. The curriculum included exercises in improvisation, communication, creativity, hospitality, and open, friendly behavior. It inspired the creation of a new verb in the Dutch language, which translates into "de-groove your thoughts." An organizational culture once defined by a "that-is-not-allowed" mentality was challenged and changed step-by-step, as staff participated in the retreats and became increasingly engaged in the transformation of the organizational culture.

FOR EXAMPLE

Turning to patient feedback to direct its Planetree efforts, woonzorggroep Samen's first component team was charged with developing meaningful arts and entertainment activities for its residents, an area identified by residents themselves during focus groups as needing improvement. In devising this arts and entertainment program, team members were reminded that putting patients first means listening to what patients have to say. Staff was convinced that residents would enjoy dogs, cats, and rabbits in their homes, but resident input made it clear that staff's expectations did not necessarily mirror resident preferences. In fact, 80 percent of clients asked indicated that being in contact with animals every now and then was more than enough! As a result, a modified pet therapy program was introduced, which includes dog-training center visits and scheduled days with pets. A traveling circus was set up for a week in the parking lot, amusing residents with free performances and loving interactions with animals.

Outcomes measures in the following months have been encouraging. One of the nursing homes, Magnushof, was among a hundred comparable organizations that participated in a client satisfaction measurement pilot. The facility's Alzheimer's unit scored at the highest level and the somatic care scored above the average. A follow-up Planetree assessment conducted one year after the site began implementing the model corroborated these results, showing a 10 percent increase in client satisfaction and a 22 percent increase in staff satisfaction. In addition, 97 percent of those interviewed indicated that they would refer a loved one to woonzorggroep Samen. The follow-up assessment also identified those areas where client's needs are not being satisfied, helping to guide the future direction of the organization's Planetree journey.

CONTRIBUTED BY THEO WINDER, WOONZORGGROEP SAMEN, AND
MARCEL SNIJDERS, STICHTING PLANETREE NEDERLAND

FOR EXAMPLE

Planetree in the Netherlands, Case Two

The Judith Leysterhof in Hardinxveld-Giessendam in the Netherlands was established with the vision that it must feel like home for its psychogeriatric residents. It is designed to offer a warm, safe, and familiar environment in which the employees, residents, and their loved ones form a household. By running this household together, everyone makes a meaningful contribution to daily activities, which helps enhance residents' feelings of self-worth, dignity, and respect.

To reinforce this familial atmosphere, residents live in groups of six, each with his or her own room. Bathrooms are shared by two people and there is a communal living room with an open kitchen. The environment is light, clean, tidy, and tastefully decorated and furnished. Residents' own possessions fill their rooms. Personal ornaments, paintings, and objects from the past serve as anchors, helping to provide a feeling of calm and a sense of familiarity. A garden, which offers an array of sensory experiences, is a safe and pleasant place to sit and widens residents' radius of operations and environment. Each day finds residents engaged in recognizable activities, oftentimes as part of a fixed routine. Common daily activities include polishing shoes, doing the dishes, folding the laundry, weeding, and peeling potatoes. Daily deliveries are made by the grocer and butcher, and residents participate in preparing fresh meals. Even if residents are no longer able to take an active part in these daily activities, they still experience them by being present and observing, smelling, feeling, or hearing what is going on around them.

A permanent team of caregivers staffs each living unit to encourage the cultivation of long-term relationships with residents and their families. Actively involved in residents' care, relatives participate in multidisciplinary meetings about the care and living plan of their loved one and work with staff to identify tasks that they as relatives will be responsible for. What develops is a partnership between staff and loved ones, as they mutually care for the resident.

Staff receive special training to work in this small-scale residential facility. All have been trained in caring skills and have completed various courses on well-being and welfare. This type of focused training and coaching has enabled all caregivers to develop their own competencies so that they can function confidently in a broad range of situations. Staff look after residents, prepare meals, do the shopping, dress wounds, and maintain contact with loved ones. Nursing tasks are sometimes necessary and are carried out by trained clinical staff. The work of staff is complemented by the presence of students, who are present at mealtimes and in the evenings to provide extra supervision, a friendly atmosphere, and assistance with simple care tasks. Staff at the Judith Leysterhof report high job satisfaction, solidarity, and loyalty, and this is reflected in minimal staff turnover.

Only one year after opening, the Judith Leysterhof has earned a reputation as a facility where the experience of the residents and their relatives are prioritized. This is evidenced by the growing waiting list of psychogeriatric individuals and their loved ones who have selected the Judith Leysterhof as the place they would like to live.

CONTRIBUTED BY HEIDI RUIS AND C. M. HEIJBLOM, RIVAS ZORGGROEP

INTEGRATED HEALTH CARE: AURORA HEALTH CARE

Integrated health care providers are unique in that they include in- and outpatient settings to care for patients across a broad continuum of services. Aurora Health Care, a not-for-profit Wisconsin integrated health care provider, was created around a single idea: there is a better way to provide health care. Established in 1984, Aurora has patient access points in more than 90 communities throughout Eastern Wisconsin, including 12 hospitals, a psychiatric hospital, more than 120 clinics, over 130 community pharmacies, home care and hospice services, and a social service agency. Two additional community hospitals will be opening in 2009 and 2010.

Aurora employs more than a thousand physicians. In addition, over thirty-four hundred physicians are affiliated with Aurora. With more than twenty-seven thousand employees or caregivers, Aurora is the largest private employer in Wisconsin.

Although this integrated approach benefits patients in many ways, this scope of service, expansive service areas, and sizeable team of caregivers introduces added complexity when transforming organizational culture.

The Journey

In 2001, Aurora Health Care joined the Planetree membership network and opened its first Planetree hospital, Aurora BayCare Medical Center in Green Bay. Aurora BayCare Medical Center was conceived and built to reflect the Planetree patient-centered model. This new hospital provided a wonderful and unique healing environment to its patients; however, Aurora realized that limiting its Planetree vision to just the inpatient hospital experience was shortsighted. Patient interaction most frequently occurs in the outpatient or clinic setting where patients develop long-term relationships with their physicians and the staff. Today only a third of Aurora's care is delivered in inpatient settings. Being an integrated health care provider meant it would not be fulfilling Aurora's vision of Planetree if it was only being implemented in its hospitals.

In 2003, the formal integration of the Planetree model into Aurora's outpatient settings began. With the guiding vision that a consistent, patient-centered experience across hospitals and clinics is paramount, the five clinics closest to Aurora BayCare Medical Center began transforming their cultures. The Planetree philosophy and components fit well into the outpatient setting and enabled Aurora to provide health care consistency for its patients. The adaptation of the Planetree inpatient model to the outpatient setting was enthusiastically embraced by staff and physicians, who had seen the positive impact on their patients in the hospital and could see the rationale for integrating a patient-centered approach in their clinics. Between 2003 and 2005, three more hospitals and ten clinics transitioned to the Planetree model of care.

Later in 2006, Planetree was identified as the patient-centered model of care to be integrated into Aurora's ten-year, long-term strategy. This commitment meant taking the Planetree model of patient-centered care to every entity and service area within Aurora. Patient care needed to be integrated across the continuum. Limiting its patient-centered vision to its hospitals and clinics would jeopardize Aurora's outcomes. Every employee, every department, every service line, would need to identify how they support patient-centered care and how they can better personalize, humanize, and demystify the work they do for the people they serve. The foundation of the Planetree message that everyone is a caregiver and that each individual directly affects the environment they work in resonates throughout Aurora. It is its pharmacies creating a single medication list for patients and the business office simplifying the patient bill. It is the human resources staff redesigning the interview process to ensure that staff are hired who believe they are caregivers and the corporate communications department personalizing messages from Aurora's CEO and having his picture on key messages to the twenty-seven thousand employees. It is the Care Management team reviewing patient education materials to meet the plain language guidelines and the system logistics (purchasing) department simplifying the ordering process for supplies. It is the information services staff designing a Web site that demystifies the medical resources.

Three critical steps were taken early on that set the foundation for this ambitious journey. First, Aurora's chief financial officer, later to become the chief operating officer and executive vice president, took the leadership role of Planetree System Champion. This culturally unusual step ensured leadership alignment and support throughout the entire Aurora system. Second, the regional director of medical operations took the leadership role of Planetree System Physician Champion to ensure medical staff leadership and support. Finally, the Department of Employee and Organizational Development defined the Planetree journey as a cultural transformation, which required a defined, consistent strategy and implementation process. Organizational Development's role was to support and guide the process, whereas site leadership owned its defined outcomes. Organizational Development staff were assigned to each entity/site within Aurora.

Believing that patient-centered care is a necessary cultural shift for the entire health care industry (beyond just hospitals) made the discussion and need for Planetree relevant to all Aurora's sites and services. The infrastructure of the model defined by Planetree—which recommends steering committees, work teams, and staff action committees—proved to be flexible and adaptable to fit additional components and the continuum of care in the health care system (including home care, pharmacies, clinics, business office, human resources, and so forth). The fact that each area or department would charter its own course and not follow a "cookie-cutter approach" gave leadership the ownership they required to *buy in* to the model.

Learning from its first Planetree hospitals, Aurora developed four phases that clearly defined the cultural transformation. The Management Committee of Aurora, which includes the chief executive officer, the chief operating officer, the senior clinical vice president, and several other senior vice presidents, approved the Planetree Phases of Implementation, which made the commitment and expectations clear to everyone. These four phases set clear parameters and allowed flexibility to ensure success. The Phases of Implementation are as follows:

Phase I: Leadership Readiness. This is for the senior leadership of each entity or service line only. This is their opportunity to learn, over approximately eight to twelve weeks, about Planetree and define their vision for their staff. Leaders are asked to participate in several of the following learning opportunities:

- Attend a Planetree Steering Committee at another site.

- Read *Putting Patients First* by Planetree.

- Interview two to three leaders of other Aurora sites about their personal leadership transformation, adapted behaviors, and lessons learned.

- Watch the Planetree video *Creating Patient-Centered Care in Healing Environments.*

- Attend a Planetree Initial Retreat.

- Visit the Planetree Web site and Aurora's Planetree Web site to become familiar with the Planetree member network and details around Aurora's Planetree journey.

- Read recommended articles on patient-centered care and research found on the Aurora Web site.

The flexibility of the model, the core components—personalize, humanize, and demystify (PHD)—are then discussed for relevancy and applicability to their area. This phase culminates in a formal leadership meeting, in which a *leadership commitment* document is created. It defines the dream/vision of patient-centered care for their area, why it is critical for success, and what leadership behaviors must be role-modeled.

Phase II: Organizational Assessment. This assessment is done by Planetree and can be site-based (a single hospital) or can be for a community of services (hospital, clinic, home care, pharmacy) that all serve the same geography or community. This latter approach makes sense in smaller communities and promotes how all of these entities serve the same patient and family. The assessment process includes a series of meetings and focus groups with key constituencies, such as patients and families, staff, leadership, and physicians. It also encompasses an evaluation of the physical environment and current outcomes data. The organizational assessment guides the leadership in the decision-making process by identifying the priorities and suggesting areas for quick, visible "wins" and greatest impact. All leaders also attend a Planetree leadership retreat. This retreat focuses on the role of leadership in the cultural transformation and helps leaders identify Planetree possibilities. It answers the question, "How does Planetree apply in my area?"

Phase III: Implementation. This is where the most visible outward activities take place over the first few years. The eight-hour initial retreats, the steering committee, the work teams, and the staff action committees begin as appropriate, following the guidance provided in the organizational assessment. Training is provided to all committees regarding their roles and responsibilities. Annual review of outcomes assessment and of initiatives is done at the steering committee. The ultimate measure of Planetree success is improved scores in patient loyalty and the employee engagement index. This accountability creates focus and purpose across Aurora.

Phase IV: Sustaining/Ongoing. The greatest challenge is sustaining the gains and continuing innovation. The Planetree organization's commitment to the progress assessment is the foundation of this ongoing work. The progress assessment is a biannual checkup, including many of the elements in the initial organizational assessment, but it focuses on progress made and refinement of goals and objectives.

As part of Aurora's continuing effort to break down silos or invisible walls between sites within its system, which spans several hundred miles, Aurora identified a number of ways to foster a sense of collaboration and shared purpose organization-wide. Having one consistent Planetree staff retreat ensures consistency of Aurora's message (no matter what the person's role is), and having employees from multiple sites attend the same retreats affords employees the opportunity to get to meet other colleagues who also "serve the patient." Aurora also created a number of internal sharing networks, including monthly Planetree co-champion conference calls (Aurora uses the term *co-champion* instead of *coordinator*—each site leader is the champion and they choose a co-champion); biannual workshops for all Aurora Planetree co-champions; quarterly Aurora Physician Advisory Councils; and an Aurora Planetree Web site for sharing stories, innovative ideas, and research articles. The creation of an Aurora Planetree Advisory Council chaired by the system champion helps provide system leadership and problem-solve system challenges.

Lessons Learned and Future Challenges

Certainly, as Aurora's journey of cultural transformation has continued, many lessons have been learned, each of which has helped to refine the structure and processes that have been put in place to ensure continuity, consistency, and sustainability. Among them are the following:

- Visible senior leadership is key to organization commitment.

- Clarifying how Planetree integrates with all past and current initiatives around service, patient safety, and other key organizational initiatives reduces confusion and promotes a greater buy-in. Aurora strives to "connect the dots," to prevent Planetree from being perceived as "one more thing I have to do."

- One of the greatest single messages of Planetree is that everyone is a caregiver, which itself is a cultural transformation. The health care team is much larger this way. Everyone can make a difference no matter how closely each person works with patients and families. For example, the hospital transporter is one more person who can make sure every patient has an identification band on.

- Storytelling is the single most powerful tool in cultural transformation.

- Leaders will not let go of control easily, so the success of the staff action committees requires focused training and communication.

- Peer-to-peer education about Planetree is the most credible, so using panels or taped presentations is very helpful; for example, doctor-to-doctor, manager-to-manager, staff-to-staff.

■ Understanding the change process and having a visual model can help create patience with the cultural transformation journey. We tend to want change to occur quickly. Aurora uses the Managing Complex Change Model from Howick Associates (Madison, Wisconsin). It resonated with leadership.

■ Clarifying roles and expectations of Planetree champions, co-champions, organizational development liaisons, and senior leadership is critical.

Taking care to address these key lessons has helped to ensure that a patient-centered culture is established and maintained within this highly diverse organization, from acute care hospitals to physician office practices, home care services, and community-based clinics.

CONCLUSION

Disparate regulatory requirements, patient and resident populations, physical environments, organizational structures, and service lines are not in themselves barriers to culture change. Whether we focus on behavioral health, continuing care, or large integrated health systems, these organizations have much more in common than what makes them different. Modifications have been made in the various settings and new innovations have emerged, but the Planetree process of engaging all stakeholders has remained constant. This process, which begins with listening to internal and external customers, not only provides health care leaders with a multitude of perspectives but also helps overcome one of the greatest challenges: *creating buy-in to change.* As touched on in each case study, collective awareness and commitment to transparency drives accountability and a collective vision to implementing and sustaining changes. The Planetree hallmark of becoming *sensitized* and responding to the uniqueness of each individual builds an unwavering ethos that enables an organization to accomplish what it once thought impossible.

The opportunity for Planetree to support transformational change of an entire health care system is vast. While the work to adapt the model in a variety of settings continues, there must also be recognition of the challenges that exist as patients and residents become more deeply engaged in their own care. Progress is accelerated when we can break down the silos between constituencies and work together to transform the transitions between these environments. Undoubtedly, the Planetree philosophy fosters a powerful collective vision across the entire continuum of care.

CHAPTER

13

INTEGRATING QUALITY AND SAFETY WITH PATIENT-CENTERED CARE

CARRIE BRADY AND JAMES B. CONWAY

This chapter does the following:

- Explores the connection between patient-centered care, quality, and patient safety
- Provides concrete examples of effective patient-centered quality and safety strategies used by health care organizations

The engagement of consumers (the public, patients, and families) in a true partnership is essential to achieve transformational improvement aims in quality and safety (American Hospital Association and Institute for Family-Centered Care, 2005; Conway and others, 2006; National Patient Safety Foundation, 2003; Robert Wood Johnson Foundation, 2007; World Health Organization, 2006). Over the last ten years, the patient safety movement has been driven by the face, experience, and voice of patients and those who have cared for them (Conway, 2007; see Gibson and Singh, 2003). The 1998 Salzburg Seminar (Delbanco and others, 2001) suggested that efforts to improve care might take strikingly different shape if patients worked as full partners with health professionals to design and implement change, and that resulted in adoption of the principle of "Nothing about me, without me." Education and activation Web sites are being developed, educational materials are ubiquitous, coalitions (see, for example, [www.partnershipforhealth.org]) and regional alliances (Robert Wood Johnson Foundation, 2006) are forming, patient-centered patient safety goals are being set (Pillow, 2007), and public reporting is being implemented to guide accountability, education, advocacy, and decision making (National Patient Safety Foundation, 2008).

Despite this broad array of activities, true partnerships between patients, families, and providers remain rare. Quality improvement and patient safety efforts in the hospital and community largely continue without involving patients and those who care for them, even in areas where they have a lot to add and a lot at stake, including medication management, communication and disclosure, team training, and care at the bedside/clinic. Well-intentioned organizations still frequently take action *for* their consumers, not *with* them (Entwistle, Mello, and Brennan, 2005).

A comprehensive approach to patient-centered care can help bridge this gap. Patient- and family-centered care has been the focus of extensive experimentation, application, and research for more than thirty years (Gerteis, Edgman-Levitan, Daley, and Delbanco, 1993) and has been the subject of emphasis, expectations, and endorsement from the Institute of Medicine, the White House and presidential campaigns, foundation reports, state and national health reform, medical specialty groups, communities, and improvement and accreditation/standards–setting organizations, such as The Joint Commission and National Quality Forum. National policy leaders and the public alike are saying this partnership is just the ethical practice of *patient* care; it is the right thing to do. We have moved past the question of whether providers should partner with patients and families on quality and safety: the question now is *how*? (Johnson and others, 2008).

This chapter highlights several strategies that are successfully being used not only to engage patients as partners in their care and safety but to make providers better partners as well. Seven areas of focus are explored:

1. Human interactions and communication

2. Patient education and access to information

3. Involvement of family and friends

4. Nutrition

5. Community partnerships

6. Structures and processes that support patient involvement

7. Patient-centered care when things go wrong

Taken together, these areas form a foundation on which to build effective partnerships between consumers and providers to improve quality and patient safety.

HUMAN INTERACTIONS AND COMMUNICATION

Patient-centered health care organizations focus on human interactions as the core of their service. It is not enough to provide the right clinical treatment; treatment must be provided in the right way—in partnership with patients, respecting their diversity, and meeting their clinical and nonclinical needs. Patient-centered care has a significant effect on both patient and staff satisfaction, and it also can significantly affect safety, in part by affecting patients' communication with providers.

As The Joint Commission (2007) and other organizations have documented, communication failures are the most frequent root cause of adverse events. A common method to involve patients in their safety is to encourage them to speak up, ask questions, and engage in a dialogue with providers (see, for example, Agency for Healthcare Research and Quality, Questions Are the Answer Web site [www.ahrq.gov/questionsaretheanswer]; Ask Me 3 Web site [www.askme3.org]; and The Joint Commission's Speak Up Initiatives Web site [www.jointcommission.org/PatientSafety/SpeakUp]). But if patients feel like they are "imposing" when speaking with staff, they may not ask questions (Entwistle, Mello, and Brennan, 2005) and may not even ask for help when they need it (Gibson, 2007). Patient-centered care improves communication by promoting an open, effective, and ongoing dialogue between and among patients, families, and staff, not just about safety issues, but about all aspects of care.

In order to refocus staff on the experience of being a patient and to reinspire staff to connect with and truly *care* for patients instead of merely treating them, Planetree affiliate hospitals conduct patient-centered orientation and retreats with their staff members. The retreats enhance staff sensitivity and understanding of the patient perspective, and they encourage staff to use this perspective to find additional ways to deliver service in a kind, caring, and respectful manner. This philosophy of caring is recognized by patients, who frequently express in focus groups that they are more comfortable interacting with staff because the staff seem to really care about them as individuals.

FOR EXAMPLE

Aurora Sinai's Patient Safety Refresher Retreats

Fundamentally, patient-centered care must be safe care. Recognizing this, Aurora Sinai Medical Center (ASMC), a 233-bed hospital in the heart of downtown Milwaukee, Wisconsin, has developed a "refresher" staff retreat, which goes above and beyond reviewing the Planetree model and reenergizing staff around providing patient-centered care. The sessions also enhance the hospital's culture of safety by reinforcing that as caregivers, *all* employees are responsible for patient safety and must therefore be actively involved in the vigorous pursuit of a safer hospital.

Like the hospital's eight-hour, new-employee Planetree retreats, these four-hour refresher retreats are designed to promote sharing and interaction. They are run by staff who have been trained to facilitate the curriculum, which includes interactive exercises, opportunities for dialogue, and real-life stories of patients and caregivers within ASMC.

The curriculum is structured around five core areas critical to ensuring patient safety: patient identification/patient handovers, plain language, Banish the Bugs, Silence Kills, and making safe choices. Within each topic, participants are urged to share their own experiences and identify ways that they personally may contribute to creating a safer environment. As with the new-employee retreat, a number of exercises aim to sensitize staff to the patient experience. One activity illustrates the value of plain language versus confusing, unfamiliar medical jargon. A hand-washing exercise demonstrates the importance of vigilant hand hygiene. And small group discussions help identify effective strategies for crucial conversations addressing behaviors that may jeopardize patient safety.

At the conclusion of the retreat, participants complete an evaluation that is used for continual improvement of the format and curriculum. In addition, they are asked to name one thing that they will commit to doing differently to make ASMC a safer hospital. The two most common responses are more conscientious hand hygiene and speaking up when something is being done that may put a patient at risk.

Participation in the Patient Safety Planetree Retreat is only one step along the journey to becoming a safer, patient-centered hospital. ASMC encourages employees to continue learning while earning credits toward a Safety PHD (personalize, humanize, and demystify). Participation in the retreat earns 250 credits toward the 1,000 needed for the PhD. Participants then have two years to earn the additional 750 credits. Examples of other ways to earn credits include reporting great catches, getting a flu shot, and completing the annual safety review.

Some of the outcomes observed within the first nine months of the program have been the following:

- 900 (out of 1500) caregivers had participated in the retreats.
- There was an 11 percent increase in the annual employee survey Patient Safety Index.
- There was a 10.2 percent increase from 2005 to 2007 in "Nonpunitive Response to Error" on the Agency for Healthcare Research and Quality Patient Safety Culture Survey.
- They had the highest-ever percentage of observed use of hand sanitizer and lowest-ever percentage of caregivers who were observed doing nothing to sanitize their hands.
- Over 250 had enrolled in ASMC's Patient Safety University PhD Program.

CONTRIBUTED BY THE AURORA SINAI MEDICAL
CENTER PLANETREE SAFETY WORK TEAM

Patient-centered hospitals seek to anticipate and respond to the full range of patients' needs, clinical and nonclinical, which also may promote communication. Responsiveness of hospital staff is one of the areas in which hospitals nationwide perform the least well on the HCAHPS survey (Agency for Healthcare Research and Quality, 2007). Responsiveness of hospital staff is based on two questions, one of which is speed in getting patients to the bathroom when they need assistance. Beyond the immediate consequences related to potential falls, skin deterioration, or infection from patients soiling themselves or getting up unassisted while waiting for staff to respond, the lack of response to a request for toileting sends a powerful message to patients that may have broader patient safety consequences. Toilet training occurs at a young age, and the majority of patients are confident that they know their bodies well enough to tell providers when they need to go to the bathroom. If providers do not respond to patients when the patients *know* they need help, will patients ask questions or raise concerns if they aren't certain? Partnership is a two-way street; providers shouldn't ask patients to take on more responsibility to communicate unless the providers are prepared to be responsive.

Patient-centered hospitals perceive every person as a caregiver who has the ability to affect the experience of patients and their families. Consequently, such hospitals foster an organizational culture in which all staff members recognize that their role is to meet patient needs. This focus on the patient translates into all activities at the organization. At Wellmont Health System hospitals in Tennessee and Virginia, for example, each employee's tasks are reframed to focus on patient outcomes. Instead of telling the housekeeping staff that their responsibility is to complete the tasks of cleaning the rooms, Wellmont Health System hospitals tell the housekeepers that their role is to make sure that patients in the rooms they clean do not get an infection in the hospital. This reframing from a task-oriented role to a patient-focused role may inspire staff in their work and promote enhanced teamwork, in addition to empowering all staff members to communicate with patients and act on safety concerns. Hospitals have reported that nonclinical staff members are frequently involved in identifying patient concerns, in part because some patients feel more comfortable raising issues with nonclinical staff. Nonclinical staff also may be involved in anticipating falls and seeking appropriate assistance if they are attentive to the fall risk and the activities of the patient. If all staff members, clinical and nonclinical, are focused on listening to the patient, there is more opportunity for issues to be addressed.

In addition to empowering all staff to respond to individual patient needs, recognizing all staff as caregivers reinforces the role nonclinical staff can play in developing safer systems. At Aurora Sinai Medical Center, the Patient Escort Team was instrumental in developing a plan to reduce the incidence of nosocomial skin wounds. The team developed a system to move patients in their beds in order to reduce the exposure a patient might have if transferred from bed to stretcher when being transported for tests. The result was a sharp decrease in nosocomial wounds from 8.5 percent to 1.5 percent in one year. Following this successful initiative, Aurora Sinai also engaged the Patient Escort Team to help eliminate identification band incidents by implementing a *hard stop* approach, in which the team would not transport a patient for a treatment or procedure without an identification band in place. This change in practice has virtually eliminated the chance of a patient being transported without an identification band.

PATIENT EDUCATION AND ACCESS TO INFORMATION

Research demonstrates that patients who are more actively involved in their care tend to have better results (Institute of Medicine, 2007). As described in more detail in Chapter Two, patient-centered hospitals engage patients in their care by providing access to understandable health information in a variety of ways, including consumer libraries, community education, customized information packets, patient pathways, and easy access to medical records.

Planetree began as a consumer health library that was designed to provide the community with a comprehensive collection of health resources written for nonclinicians, as well as access to clinical information. Although a librarian was available to assist users in locating information, Planetree also developed a library indexing system still in use today, which organizes materials by body system and common diagnostic terms so that lay persons can easily find the information they are looking for without asking a librarian. This ability to conduct self-directed research is important because it allows individuals to keep the subjects of their research private if desired.

Today, the Planetree network includes five full community health resource centers, as well as many smaller hospital libraries that make health care resources available to patients and the public. To supplement the resources available in the libraries, Planetree affiliates engage in a variety of short-term and long-term community education activities related to empowering patients, such as a ten-week Mini-Med School, offered one evening per week by Griffin Hospital in Derby, Connecticut (described in detail in Chapter Two).

In addition to making information broadly available to the community, many Planetree affiliates use each inpatient hospitalization as an opportunity to provide patients with detailed information about their condition and treatment plan in an information packet that includes a form for the patient to request more information from the health librarian. Containing information about the patient's diagnosis and previous medical history, treatment plan, medication information, nutritional information and needs, exercise plan or physical limitations, and community resources, Sentara Virginia Beach General Hospital's customized Personal Health Book for patients (described in Chapter Two) has proven to be a useful resource for both patients and providers. Patients have reported that the book makes them feel more in control of their illness because they are organized and informed. And with the hospital asking patients to bring the book to each inpatient or outpatient visit for use as a reference and for updating, local physicians have reported that the book is a valuable tool for them as well. Some hospitals begin the education process even earlier for patients whose hospitalization is planned. At Mid-Columbia Medical Center in The Dalles, Oregon, for example, patients who are undergoing a total joint replacement receive extensive education before the procedure, including a half-day education session and a comprehensive resource binder, containing a variety of checklists, specific expectations for each day of the hospital stay, physical and occupational therapy, and community resources.

Another way to empower patients to take an active role in their care is to encourage patients to review their medical record. In a random survey of forty-five hundred adults, 79 percent expressed interest in reading their medical record (Fowles and others, 2004), but patients are frequently not aware that they can review their chart or do not know how to access it. Patient-centered hospitals actively encourage patients to read their medical chart, such as by posting signs in patient rooms or informing patients upon admission about the opportunity to review their records. Staff members go through the chart with the patients to help interpret medical terminology and other information, which can help proactively address any areas of concern or confusion. Based on a survey of ten Planetree affiliate hospitals with active open chart programs, 95 percent of patients who reviewed their chart reported that it was helpful to them. Planetree affiliate hospitals also have reported that in some cases the patients' review of the chart has directly improved patient safety because the patients have identified missing or incorrect information, such as the omission of an allergy.

INVOLVEMENT OF FAMILY AND FRIENDS

The social support of family and friends has been shown to have a direct effect on the health of patients, and patient-centered hospitals encourage participation of family and friends. Twenty-four-hour patient-directed visitation policies and family presence protocols (each described in Chapter Three) foster an environment in which family members remaining with the patient whenever the patient desires is the standard, not the exception to the rule. Two specific activities that may affect safety are programs to involve a partner in the patient's care and programs that enable family members to initiate a rapid response team.

Many Planetree affiliate hospitals enable patients to identify a person who will assist in taking care of the patient in the hospital. This *care partner* is frequently the same person who will care for the person after discharge. During the hospitalization, the care partner is trained by hospital staff to perform tasks that are appropriate given the condition of the patient and the interest and skills of the care partner. The program is voluntary, and the care partner or patient may choose to discontinue participating at any time. The involvement of the care partner may reduce complications following discharge because the care partner receives more training and experience in caring for the patient while the patient is still hospitalized. Northern Westchester Hospital in Mount Kisco, New York, takes the program a step further by allowing parents who are taking a child home from the NICU to spend a couple of nights before the anticipated discharge with their child in a hotel-like room with a crib and bathroom directly across from the NICU in order to become more comfortable in caring for their child at home.

In addition to empowering family members or friends as care partners, some patient-centered hospitals allow family members to directly initiate rapid response teams if they become concerned about a change in the patient's condition. North Carolina (NC) Children's Hospital in Chapel Hill implemented a pediatric rapid response team in 2005, and family-member concern was a basis for staff to activate the team. When NC Children's Hospital reviewed the data from the first year of the system, they determined that in the cases where the rapid response team was initiated based on family concern, more than half of the time the patient's condition warranted transfer to the ICU. As a result, NC Children's Hospital created the *family alert system* as an addition to its pediatric rapid response system, which allows family members to directly initiate the rapid response team by calling a phone number within the hospital. NC Children's Hospital involved family members in designing and rolling out the system and also designed a study to evaluate the system. The research is in process, and NC Children's Hospital hopes to demonstrate that the system maintains call numbers at a level that does not require a change in team structure or staffing, improves family confidence and comfort with emergency responses, and provides an additional reliable method of identifying patients with clinical instability. NC Children's Hospital received the National Patient Safety Foundation's Socius Award in 2007 for its work on this initiative to partner with patients on safety.

NUTRITION

Patient-centered hospitals recognize the importance of nutrition in health, and many provide unusual flexibility for patients in accessing food. This flexibility relates not only to the type of food available but also to the times of day during which it is offered. Some Planetree affiliates allow patients to select preferred times for food to arrive, and others allow patients to order food on demand similar to hotel room service. During the hours when a full-service menu may not be available, Planetree hospitals provide patients and family members with access to healthy food options, in some cases through unit kitchens with stocked refrigerators and pantries. Family members also may use these kitchen facilities to prepare meals for patients if desired. For diabetic patients in particular, the availability of food can become a safety issue. In focus groups, diabetic patients have commented on the need to ensure that they have access to food at all times and on the anxiety that they experience when food is not readily available. Even for nondiabetic patients, the recent studies indicating that glycemic control affects outcomes in critically ill patients (see, for example, Krinsley, 2006) may prompt additional interest in the connection between food and safety in hospitalized patients.

COMMUNITY PARTNERSHIPS

In addition to engaging the patient and family during their visits to the hospital, patient-centered hospitals engage the community in innovative partnerships to improve health and enhance patient safety. Aurora Health Care in Wisconsin, for example, created an innovative community-based advisory council that developed medication safety tools.

Similarly, Fauquier Hospital in Warrenton, Virginia, has partnered with an electronic prescriptions vendor to pilot-test a system that allows the hospital to access a patient's pharmacy records in order to assist in medication reconciliation. This effort is designed to provide the hospital with more information to reduce medication errors, particularly in situations where a patient may know he is taking the "blue pill" at lunch time, but he does not know what the blue pill is or the purpose of the pill.

The Albany Stratton VA Medical Center in New York also has partnered with an outside organization to implement a system that helps locate wandering patients. The Medical Center recommends this system to appropriate patients and family members identified through their interactions with the medical center. If the patient agrees, a locator device is placed on the patient. The locator device allows the police to quickly locate the patient if the patient is wandering. The service promotes quick recovery of wandering patients, whether they elope from the hospital or in the community, and therefore reduces the span of time during which adverse events could occur before the patient is located.

Broader partnerships also are developing to engage consumers as active participants in their care. Examples include MN Community Measurement [www.mnhealthcare.org/~wwd.cfm], the RWJ Aligning Forces for Quality Efforts with the National Partnership for Women and Families (www.forces4quality.org), and the Partnership for Healthcare Excellence [www.partnershipforhealthcare.org] in Massachusetts. Composed of more than forty organizations—including the Massachusetts Health Care Quality and Cost Council, consumer associations, disease and advocacy organizations, doctors, nurses, hospitals, community health centers, insurers, business groups, labor, public health advocates, and other health care leaders—the Partnership for Healthcare Excellence (2008) was formed to attain three goals:

- Educate people about variations in the quality of health care

- Encourage patients to become more informed and involved in their own care

- Mobilize consumers to become advocates for the kind of overall change necessary to improve the quality of health care

The Massachusetts Partnership is encouraging patients to speak up and speak out because one of the strongest barriers against medical errors—and among the most powerful resources for improving the quality of health care—is an informed, empowered, and engaged patient.

SUPPORTING PATIENT INVOLVEMENT

Consideration of the patient perspective is essential to providing patient-centered care, so patient-centered hospitals engage in a variety of strategies to obtain perspectives from patients on an ongoing basis. Patient and family advisory councils are common, as are efforts to add patients to existing hospital committees. National initiatives such as the IHI 5 Million Lives Campaign Boards on Board Intervention are instructing governing boards and executive leaders that there is no lever more powerful to drive quality and safety than their personal engagement and the inclusion of the patients and those who care for them (Institute for Healthcare Improvement, 2007a). Evidence from the Institute for Healthcare Improvement (IHI) suggests that an industry affirmative response is growing (Conway, 2008).

At Wellmont Health System hospitals, actual patients are used as "mystery shoppers," who report on their experiences as inpatients and outpatients. The inpatient mystery shoppers are recruited by the infection control coordinator and are asked to track hand-washing practices of staff members. The patient makes a check mark every time a staff member enters the room and indicates whether the staff member washed hands in the presence of the patient. The staff members are aware of the program, but they do not know which patients are participating. This program engages patients and staff and also provides an opportunity to educate patients about infection control practices. Because the patient is not asked to confront the staff member about hand washing, some patients may be more comfortable participating in this manner (see Hibbard and others, 2005). This initiative complements the more common practice of encouraging patients to ask staff if they have washed their hands and to speak up if they have any questions or concerns about their care. In patient-centered hospitals, these conversations should be more comfortable for patients because of the ongoing focus on patient-provider partnerships.

Several hospitals use patient surveys to obtain specific feedback on patient safety issues, including West Park Hospital in Cody, Wyoming, and Aurora Health Care in Wisconsin. In addition to asking specific questions about whether the patient observed staff performing specific safety practices, such as hand washing and verifying the patient's identity, some surveys provide patients with the opportunity to comment on any issues that could affect their safety. At Aurora Health Care, the patient safety officer complements the surveys with personal rounds with patients to obtain their direct feedback on safety issues. Dana-Farber Cancer Institute in Boston has also developed a program to engage patients and families in rounds (Dana-Farber Cancer Institute, 2007).

Delnor Community Hospital in Geneva, Illinois, has created a dedicated patient safety hotline for patients and staff to use in reporting any concerns about safety. The hotline is promoted to patients in their guest services book, as well as in stickers, prominently displayed in each patient room. The hotline is accessible from inside and outside the hospital and is also a speed-dial number on inpatient phones, which is intended to reinforce to patients that the hospital wants patient feedback. The hotline is a reflection of the hospital's deep-rooted commitment to partnering with patients; patients also regularly attend board meetings, each of which starts with a patient story.

The patient perspective on safety is invaluable. At Northern Westchester Hospital in New York, for example, a patient pointed out that she was not readily able to wash her hands before a meal in the hospital. As a result, the hospital now provides a disposable moist towelette to patients to clean their hands, along with a notice wrapped around the napkin explaining why patients should cleanse their hands before eating to reduce the chance of infection.

WHEN THINGS GO WRONG

It is essential for organizations to maintain their patient-centered approach even when things go wrong. The effect of poor communication with patients and families after a medical error is well-documented, and there are many efforts under way nationwide to promote full and open disclosure to patients of adverse events (Institute of Medicine, 2007; Leape, 2006). It is much more than disclosure. A patient-centered approach to adverse events also involves ongoing communication (not just when there is a problem), disclosure when there is, apology, support, resolution, and learning (Institute for Healthcare Improvement, 2007b). The referenced support must be inclusive of the patients, families, and staff members who are involved in the event (see, for example, Kenney and van Pelt, 2005). Some pioneering patient-centered hospitals not only provide disclosure and support but also engage the affected patient or family member in educating staff when appropriate. At Wellmont Health System hospitals, some patients and family members who have been dissatisfied with their experience at the hospital are invited after discharge for a face-to-face family focus conference with the staff that cared for them. The hospital has reported that the family focus conferences have a powerful effect on staff members, who are often surprised by how their actions were interpreted. Sentara Williamsburg Regional Medical Center in Virginia has engaged family and health care providers in sharing their experiences with adverse events in order to reinforce specific safety behaviors, expectations, and personal responsibility for error prevention techniques for all employees. In order to spread the messages of the patients and their families even more broadly, some hospitals, including Calgary Health Region, have videotaped patients discussing their experiences. Members of Calgary Health Region's Patient/Family Safety Council also regularly make presentations about their experiences and the importance of safety in patient care.

FOR EXAMPLE

Calgary Health Region Patient/Family Safety Council

The Calgary Health Region has been working to integrate patient and family feedback into organizational processes for many years now. Providing patients and families with opportunities to share their experiences continues to provide the Region with invaluable feedback that is informing the development of many new services and helping to make improvements to existing ones. Incorporating this input into patient safety began in earnest in 2004, following a triggering safety event. The Region deliberately sought out the input and advice of patients and families as it began to develop a new framework for quality and patient safety. In beginning this dialogue, many common themes and concerns emerged, and leaders quickly acknowledged the need for more opportunities for listening to patients and families. Their stories and experiences were very powerful motivators for change.

In March 2006, the Region established a forum aimed at engaging patients and families as patient safety advisers. Beginning as a pilot, the program consisted of a group of patients and family members who came together, each having a safety-related experience and an interest in collaborating with health care providers and the Region to make improvements. Today, the council is composed of fourteen patients and families, health care providers, and Region staff. The work of the council is not about assigning blame, but rather about partnering with health care providers and the Region to identify hazards and areas where improvements can be made. In this spirit of collaboration, the council is co-chaired by a patient/family member and a region staff member.

Enabling patients and families to have discussions with health care providers and to provide advice and make recommendations on operational patient safety issues has taken the Calgary Health Region to a new level of openness, transparency, and collaboration. Monthly council meetings are supplemented with small group meetings to discuss, plan, and help advance specific initiatives. As opportunities for improvements are identified and discussed, the council then makes recommendations to the Region's president and chief operating officer.

In its first two years of operation, the council has taken its mandate very seriously. Examples of its work include providing input into the development of new patient safety policies and procedures and working with operational leaders to help roll the policies and practices out to the Region's twenty-four thousand employees. Members participate in monthly clinical patient safety meetings with Region leaders and have attended provider disclosure training sessions. In fact, one member has been trained and now helps teach the Region's disclosure course. The council has participated in the development of a multimedia patient safety information campaign, Safer Together, and has recommended that the Region conduct a feasibility study to pilot patient and family activation of its rapid response services.

Initially as one of only two patient/family safety councils in Canada, Calgary's council has been a strong advocate and supporter of the voice of patients and families at the provincial and national levels, working with the Health Quality Council of Alberta and Patients for Patient Safety—Canada.

CONTRIBUTED BY THE CALGARY HEALTH REGION
PATIENT/FAMILY SAFETY COUNCIL

CONCLUSIONS

Patient-centered care and patient safety are interrelated goals. To succeed, efforts to engage patients as partners in their safety should be grounded in a comprehensive patient-centered approach that recognizes patients as partners, listens to and respects their input, anticipates and addresses patient needs, and simultaneously cares for staff so that they can more effectively care for patients. Safety from unintended harm is a basic need for any patient; it is not possible to be truly patient-centered without being safe. It is also not possible to be safe without being patient-centered. As the Institute of Medicine (2007) noted, "patient-centered care that embodies both effective communication and technical skill is necessary to achieve safety and quality of care" (p. 155). To make significant improvements in quality and safety, hospitals must effectively partner with patients and families. This chapter provides a framework and stepping stones for building that partnership. Transformation of the health care system in partnership with consumers is a right that requires urgent and immediate attention. Do not wait. Decide today what you will do and by when.

REFERENCES

Agency for Healthcare Research and Quality. *2007 CAHPS® Hospital Survey Chartbook.* Pub. No. 07-0064-EF. Rockville, Md.: Agency for Healthcare Research and Quality, May 2007.

American Hospital Association and Institute for Family-Centered Care. "Strategies for Leadership: Patient and Family-Centered Care." 2005. [www.aha.org/aha/key_issues/patient_safety/resources/patientcenteredcare.html].

Conway, J. "The Contributions of Patient Advocacy to Patient Safety." In J. L. Earp, E. A. French, and M. B. Gilkey (eds.), *Patient Advocacy for Health Care.* Boston: Jones & Bartlett, 2007.

Conway, J. "Patients and Families: Powerful New Partners for Healthcare and for Caregivers." *Healthcare Executive,* Jan.–Feb. 2008. [www.ihi.org/IHI/Topics/PatientSafety/Safety General/Literature/PatientsandFamiliesPowerfulNewPartners.htm].

Conway, J., and others. *Partnering with Patients and Families to Design a Patient- and Family-Centered Health Care System: A Roadmap for the Future.* Institute for Family-Centered Care and Institute for Healthcare Improvement, 2006. [www.Ihi.Org/Ihi/Topics/Patientcenteredcare/Patientcenteredcaregeneral/Literature/Partneringwithpatientsandfamilies.Htm].

Dana-Farber Cancer Institute. *Patient Safety Rounds Toolkit.* 2007. [www.dana-farber.org/pat/patient-safety/patient-safety-resources/patient-rounding-toolkit.html].

Delbanco, T., and others. "Healthcare in a Land Called Peoplepower: Nothing About Me Without Me." *Health Expectations,* 2001, *4,*144–150.

Entwistle, V. A., Mello, M. M., and Brennan, T. A. "Advising Patients About Patient Safety: Current Initiatives Risk Shifting Responsibility."*Joint Commission Journal on Quality and Patient Safety,* 2005, *31*(9), 483–494.

Fowles, J. B., and others. "Patients' Interest in Reading Their Medical Record."*Archives of Internal Medicine,* Apr. 2004, *164,* 793–800.

Gerteis, M., Edgman-Levitan, S., Daley, J., and Delbanco, T. L. (eds.). *Through the Patient's Eyes: Understanding and Promoting Patient-Centered Care.* San Francisco: Jossey-Bass, 1993.

Gibson, R."The Role of the Patient in Improving Patient Safety." *AHRQ Web M&M (Morbidity and Mortality Rounds on the Web): Perspectives on Safety.* Mar. 2007. [www.webmm.ahrq.gov/perspective.aspx?perspectiveID=38].

Gibson, R., and Singh, J. P. *Wall of Silence: The Untold Story of the Medical Mistakes That Kill and Injure Millions of Americans.* Washington, D.C.: LifeLine Press, 2003.

Hibbard, J., and others. "Can Patients Be Part of the Solution? Views on Their Role in Preventing Medical Errors."*Medical Care Research and Review,* 2005, *62*(5), 601–616.

Institute for Healthcare Improvement. *"Boards on Board."* 2007a. [www.ihi.org/IHI/Programs/Campaign/BoardsonBoard.htm].

Institute for Healthcare Improvement. "Communicating After an Adverse Event: Selected Bibliography and Resources." 2007. [www.ihi.org/IHI/Topics/PatientCenteredCare/PatientCenteredCareGeneral/Tools/CommunicatingAfteranAdverseEventBiblioIHITool.htm].

Institute of Medicine. *Preventing Medication Errors.* Washington, D.C.: National Academies Press, 2007.

Johnson, B., and others. *Partnering with Patients and Families to Design a Patient- and Family-Centered Health Care System: Recommendations and Promising Practices.* 2008. [http://familycenteredcare.org/pdf/PartneringwithPatients.pdf].

Joint Commission, The. "Root Causes of Sentinel Events." Sept. 2007. [www.jointcommission.org/SentinelEvents].

Kenney, L. K., and van Pelt, R. A."To Err Is Human; The Need for Trauma Support Is, Too: A Story of the Power of Patient/Physician Partnership After a Sentinel Event." *Patient Safety and Quality Healthcare,* 2005, *2*(6), 8–9.

Krinsley, J. S. "Glycemic Control, Diabetic Status, and Mortality in a Heterogeneous Population of Critically Ill Patients Before and During the Era of Intensive Glycemic Management: Six and One-Half Years Experience at a University-Affiliated Community Hospital." *Seminars in Thoracic Cardiovascular Surgery,* 2006, *18*(4), 317–325.

Leape, L., *When Things Go Wrong.* Burlington: Massachusetts Coalition for the Prevention of Medical Errors, 2006. [www.macoalition.org/documents/respondingToAdverseEvents.pdf].

National Patient Safety Foundation. *National Agenda for Action: Patients and Families in Patient Safety—Nothing About Me, Without Me.* 2003. [www.npsf.org/download//AgendaFamilies.pdf].

National Patient Safety Foundation, Lucian Leape Institute. Discussion Documents. Feb. 4, 2008.

Partnership for Healthcare Excellence. Home page. 2008. [www.partnershipforhealthcare.org].

Pillow, M. (ed.). *Patients as Partners: Toolkit for Implementing National Patient Safety Goal 13.* Oakbrook Terrace, Ill.: Joint Commission Resources, 2007.

Robert Wood Johnson Foundation. "Aligning Forces for Quality." 2006. [www.rwjf.org/programareas/resources/product.jsp?id=21884&pid=1142&gsa=1].

Robert Wood Johnson Foundation. "Improving Quality Health Care: The Role of Consumer Engagement." 2007. [www.rwjf.org/pr/product.jsp?id=23071].

Vincent, C. A., and Coulter, A."Patient Safety: What About the Patient?"*Quality and Safety in Health Care,* 2002, *11*, 76–80.

World Health Organization. *London Declaration: A Patient Manifesto.* 2006. [www.who.int/patientsafety/patients_for_patient/London_Declaration_EN.pdf].

CHAPTER

14

PATIENT-CENTERED CARE AS PUBLIC POLICY: THE ROLE OF GOVERNMENT, PAYERS, AND THE GENERAL PUBLIC

CAROLYN M. CLANCY, JANET M. CORRIGAN, AND
DWIGHT N. MCNEILL

This chapter does the following:

- Examines the role of public policy in amplifying patients' voices in decisions about health care priority setting, performance measurement, payment policies, research agendas, and delivery system design

- Encourages a *journey-based* approach to redesigning the health care system, which focuses on the impact of care on outcomes
- Explores how pay-for-performance initiatives and performance measurement of the patient's perception of care, care transition, and patient safety may influence provider behavior and foster a more integrated, patient-centered health care system

Patient-centered care has become a central goal for the nation's health care system in response to the wishes of patients and families to be more involved in their health care as well as a growing number of studies demonstrating that active engagement of patients is associated with superior care outcomes. Yet the Institute of Medicine's seminal report, *Crossing the Quality Chasm* (2001), noted that at least part of the yawning gap between best-possible and actual care can be attributed to the reality that too often patients and their families must adapt to the usual customs and procedures of health professionals and organizations, rather than receiving services designed to focus on individual needs and preferences. This chapter explores the role of public policy in improving patient-centered care, an intrinsic part of quality care.

The role of government in improving health care quality and safety, including patient-centered care, is best understood in the unique historical context of U.S. health care delivery. The U.S. health care system includes a mix of public and private sector financing and is governed by both federal and state laws and regulations. For example, federal laws passed by the Congress and administered by the Department of Health and Human Services govern Medicare payment policies and conditions of participation for hospitals and other facilities. States, conversely, regulate which professionals can provide care under specific circumstances. Last, the public-private mix of services, coupled with the fact that the vast majority of publicly financed services are provided by private sector organizations and professionals, has resulted in substantial delegation of authority for oversight of care quality to private entities. For example, medical societies provide oversight for the education, training, and board certification of health care providers; The Joint Commission is responsible for inspecting hospitals; and the National Quality Forum (NQF) provides oversight for care quality measurement for public reporting. In short, policy development and implementation are rarely straightforward and include legislation, regulation, and market forces such as financial incentives to deliver high-quality, patient-centered care.

The creation of the 1997 Presidential Advisory Commission on consumer protection in the health care industry underscored the need for the federal government to clearly articulate its role in improving health care quality and safety. Tang, Eisenberg, and Meyer (2004) identified ten specific roles for the federal government:

1. Purchase health care: the federal government is the largest single purchaser of health care

2. Provide health care; for example, to active duty military, veterans, and Native Americans

3. Ensure access for vulnerable populations; for example, through community health centers

4. Regulate health care markets

5. Support acquisition of new knowledge

6. Develop and evaluate health technologies and practices

7. Monitor health care quality

8. Inform health care decision makers

9. Develop the health care workforce

10. Convene stakeholders from across the health care system

How these functions are translated into action varies. For domains where the federal role is predominant (for example, research, direct care delivery for specified populations), the government plays a more direct role. For areas that require close collaboration with multiple stakeholders (for example, monitoring health care quality), the evolution of policy is far more deliberate and may occur in very small increments. A clear consequence of the current system is that there is no single entity with sole authority over and accountability for overall quality of care.

This conclusion offers both challenges and opportunities. Multiple levers promote patient-centered care as a key part of overall care quality. Thus, consumers, patients, and their advocates should work to influence these levers. For example, they can take opportunities to comment on legislation, regulation, and policies, such as priorities for care quality measurement and reporting. They can also explore more local opportunities, such as participation in state activities and hospital boards. The good news is that although oversight for care quality mirrors the fragmented nature of health care delivery itself, there are numerous ways for consumers to build on the history of activism to inform policy both directly and indirectly. Today, the development of measures, research agendas, leadership groups, and informal alliances that affect the final pathway for quality strategies are all informed by the patient voice. The patient voice can be heard via consumer representatives on boards of The Joint Commission, the National Quality Forum, advisory councils, foundation boards, medical boards, and other multi-stakeholder efforts. Indeed, the absence of consumer engagement would now be seen as a serious deficit in efforts to improve care quality. Moreover, public reporting of patients' experience of care is clearly part of mainstream efforts to improve care quality. In this chapter, we describe a few promising initiatives to promote patient-centered care that require direct involvement of consumers. These initiatives range from selection of care quality measures for public reporting to the redesign of health care at a very local level.

USING PUBLIC POLICY LEVERS

Public policy levers to promote patient-centered care include setting priorities, performance measurement, transparency and public reporting, redesigning the delivery system, payment and reimbursement policies, and research to determine evidence-based practices and diffusion of best practices.

Setting Priorities

An important function of public policy is to allocate resources for society's needs. This involves understanding these needs; achieving political consensus; setting goals, priorities, and targets; and supporting strategies with resources. However, setting national priorities is difficult, because the U.S. health care delivery system is a mixture of public and private programs, many settings and providers, multiple stakeholders and interest groups, and a variety of funding and insurance approaches. And although spending on U.S. health care has soared to over $2 trillion annually, it is often ineffective, inefficient, unsafe, inequitable, and working at cross-purposes.

Because health care delivery and its oversight are so fragmented and difficult to navigate, notable advances in patient-centered care have addressed very specific areas, such as the right of patients to formulate advance directives, as provided by the Patient Self-Determination Act, and state laws requiring women to provide informed consent about whether to have (possible) breast cancer surgery in one or two surgeries. However, promoting policies that support a systemwide focus on patients' needs and preferences has been far more difficult. There is a growing appreciation that efforts to assess and improve health care quality and safety can only succeed with multi-stakeholder agreement on priorities.

There needs to be a national agenda-setting process that results in a clear strategy to focus attention and scarce resources on high-leverage areas that will yield the greatest gains in terms of better health and health care—such as improving management of chronic illness, on which America spends 8 of every 10 health care dollars.

Such a process began in early 2008. The National Priorities Partners (NPP), a collaborative of twenty-seven influential health care organizations convened by the National Quality Forum (NQF), established a list of national priorities, identified goals for improvement over the coming three to five years, and developed action plans for implementing the priorities with their constituencies.

NPP is committed to putting patient-centered care at the forefront of its agenda, as evidenced by its choice of criteria to determine care improvement goals, priorities, and performance measures (see www. qualityforum.org/about/NPP).

NPP Criteria for Selecting Priorities, Goals, and Performance Measures for Health Care Quality Improvement

- Emphasize desired patient outcomes more commonly than desired care processes.
- Include direct measures of patients' voices regarding the experience of care.
- Include priorities involving the continuum of care, not just entity-based performance.
- Be important to every provider of care, no matter what the current level of achievement.
- Incorporate measures of efficiency, as well as of outcomes and experiences of care (for example, outcomes of effective care, safety of care, waste, and patient-reported experiences of care).
- Be useful (and used) for local improvement as well as external assessment.

FOR EXAMPLE

NPP Priorities

Priority Areas as of 2008

- Patient and family engagement
- Population health
- Safety
- Palliative care
- Care coordination
- Overuse
- Patient-focused care

These leaders recognize that if the health care system wants to know how it is doing, it should ask and listen to the people it is trying to help. It is not enough to focus on improving the quality of medical procedures or even practice settings, such as hospitals and ambulatory practices. A *journey-based approach* to understanding the value of care is needed. The journey-based approach addresses the outcomes of a spell of illness and relates this to the processes of care and to the multiple caregivers who contributed to the care of the patient. Although it is difficult to hold providers accountable in a precise way in a journey-based approach, it is important to develop goals and measures and learn more about attribution along the way.

Health care quality measurement has been mostly provider-centric and usually tracks the application of evidenced-based clinical practices. For example, there are a variety of widely used process measures of good heart care, including the provision of beta-blockers and measurement of left ventricular ejection fraction, for example. But there are few agreed-upon measures of good heart care that patients can relate to, such as death rates, quality of life, and experiences of care.

Concentrating on outcomes is important in order to engage patients in the care process by using a language that is meaningful to them. Economists stress the importance of concentrating on outcomes as part of *value determination* in driving health care toward higher quality at lower cost. They assert that quality ought to refer to patient outcomes and that value is created through the total care of a patient's condition, rather than by a single specialist or a discrete treatment, and that care needs to be measured over an extended time period (Porter and Teisberg, 2006). Capturing patient outcomes alongside care process measures also provides ongoing feedback to practitioners on the results associated with alternative practice styles. This approach also helps identify important areas for future clinical and health services research.

There are a variety of reasons why the journey-based approach has been slow to catch on, including challenges and concerns about the measures, who to hold accountable for outcomes that span multiple caregivers, payment policies that actually do not provide incentives for high quality and efficient care, and traditional concepts of professional autonomy that sometimes work against the reorganization of care processes to achieve best outcomes. Also, patients and providers view the world of health care quality differently. For example, from a patient's point of view, being seen in a timely manner for an appointment is a good barometer of efficiency, considering their opportunity costs of running late (for example, lost time from work). Yet, a provider may find it more "efficient" to overbook patients to ensure that all appointments are filled in order to sustain the practice. Committees that set care priorities and measures are increasingly concluding that the primary criteria should be the patient's perspective.

This convergence of the need to measure value, as seen from the patient's eyes with a concentration on outcomes over an extended period of illness, suggests a paradigm shift in the design of health care delivery systems.

Redesigning the Delivery System

The Institute of Medicine's groundbreaking report *Crossing the Quality Chasm* stated that fundamental redesign is needed and that "the current care systems cannot do the job. Trying harder will not work. Changing systems of care will" (Institute of Medicine [IOM], 2001, p. 4). Delivery systems organized to meet the IOM's "systemness" challenges include organized, integrated delivery systems, such as Kaiser Permanente, Geisinger Health System, and Health Partners. Many, but not all, of these models have as a foundation a multispecialty physician group practice. There are about 250 such practices in the United States, most with a hundred or more physicians (Council of Accountable Physician Practices, 2007).

Yet the vast majority of care is not delivered through these types of systems. In fact, most doctors practice in one- to two-person offices (Casalino and others, 2003). Therefore, there need to be plug-and-play system design features that can be adopted by the majority of players in the decentralized care delivery enterprise.

One key aspect of this redesign is the coordination of care among caregivers, patients, and families, across settings and time. Patients with chronic diseases and associated comorbidities often see different specialists for each condition, who often do not communicate with one another. This often results in medication errors, duplicate tests, and inefficient care. Care coordination is defined as a function that helps ensure that the patient's needs and preferences for health services and information sharing across people, functions, and sites are met over time. Coordination maximizes the value of services delivered to patients by facilitating beneficial, efficient, safe, and high-quality patient experiences and improved health care outcomes (National Quality Forum, 2006). Care coordination encompasses a number of areas. It includes the medical home, which is a usual source of care and enduring relationships; communications across team members, including patient and family; care transitions between settings of care; a proactive plan of care that includes goals, progress, and follow-up; and information systems that use standardized, integrated electronic information systems.

Very promising and innovative work in these areas includes the chronic care model (Wagner, 1998), coaches who educate and train patients and family members to be engaged in their care (Coleman, Parry, Chalmers, and Min, 2006), and the advanced practice nurse transitions model (Naylor and others, 2004), among others. A great deal of attention is also being placed on the concept of a designated medical home. The *medical home,* as defined by the American Academy of Pediatrics, the American Academy of Family Physicians, and the American College of Physicians, is viewed as the place responsible for ensuring coordination of care through the primary care provider team in partnership with patients and families. The Centers for Medicare and Medicaid Services (CMS) will start a demonstration of the medical home concept in 2009. It will include design elements of a monthly fee for a personal physician, who coordinates all patient care, ensures patient access to care and health information, and encourages patient involvement in his or her own care.

Another redesign element is data. "Data is the mother's milk of systems improvement," according to the CEO of Kaiser Permanente (Halvorson, 2007, p. 23), and there is very little of it to guide system change in health care. Data are needed to understand what works or not, to manage goals, and to innovate. Performance data are widely used to improve processes in other industries, but health care lags far behind. There are plenty of data about health care in hundreds of journals, but there is little relevant performance data.

Health information technologies must be adopted to improve the collection of appropriate performance data and to provide decision support at the point of clinical service. Today, the collection of performance data is cumbersome and burdensome. It often is based on abstracting data from paper records, which places a great burden on providers. This approach limits the type of information that can be used and often misses the mark on collecting the right information. Electronic medical records offer the promise to seamlessly collect, track, and report on a whole array of care performance measures, which allow for real-time reporting of care performance as well as decision support to improve the clinical process.

A redesigned health system focuses on outcomes rather than on individual units of care. It takes the journey-based view, encourages multidisciplinary collaborative relationships, and aims for high quality at the lowest cost. One example of this approach is the Geisinger Health System warranty program for its heart program. It ensures that all the necessary evidence-based care is provided at a fixed cost and that "rework" due to medical errors or omissions of care is not charged to the patient or payer.

Finally, a redesigned system needs the patient's voice. Quite simply, patients need to decide what treatments are best for them relative to their preferences, because the scientific evidence, more likely than not, does not prescribe one universal solution for all patients. For example, men need to decide whether surgery or watchful waiting for benign prostatic hyperplasia is appropriate relative to tradeoff decisions about sexual functioning vis-à-vis reduction of symptoms. Patients need to have the opportunity to share in the decision making, and appropriate tools need to be made available to patients to do so (Hibbard, 2004; Sepucha, Fowler, and Mulley, 2004).

Measurement and Public Reporting

There has been great progress in measuring and improving care quality. For example, today, nearly every hospital in the United States publicly reports data from at least a few performance measures on heart attack, heart failure, and pneumonia, and there is widespread commitment to develop and standardize a growing number of measures for a variety of conditions and settings. Performance measurement is widely accepted as essential to improvement in all sectors. For example, it facilitates consumer choice of products and services and thereby drives market share and revenues to the best performers. Also, it motivates health care providers to improve through public reporting. Major purchasers of care, including CMS, state governments, and large employers, require reporting on nationally endorsed measures and provide incentives for reporting and for good performance. For example, CMS publishes performance data online by specific hospitals [www.medicare.gov/Hospital], nursing homes [www.medicare.gov/NHCompare], and home health agencies [www.medicare.gov/HHCompare].

Although performance measurement has picked up momentum over the last ten years, wide gaps remain, as reported by the Institute of Medicine's Performance Measurement Accelerating Improvement report. Examples of these gaps are the few measures of patient-centered care, the narrow time frame over which care performance is measured, the provider-centric focus of care, and the limited focus of accountability with emphasis placed on individual provider's actions (Institute of Medicine, 2006).

There are three general areas of patient-centered performance measures that have received broad national consensus: the patient's experience of care, care transitions, and patient safety.

The leading survey instrument for assessing the experience of care is the Consumer Assessment of Healthcare Providers and Systems (CAHPS®), developed by the Agency for Healthcare Research and Quality (2008). It is a national effort to measure, report on, and improve the quality of health care from the perspective of consumers and patients. CAHPS surveys address settings of care that include health plans, hospitals, nursing homes, dialysis centers, and ambulatory care centers. Results of these surveys are used for public reporting, accreditation, quality monitoring at federal and state levels, and quality improvement at the health plan level.

One example is the CAHPS Hospital Survey (HCAHPS®), which measures the hospital patient's experience of hospital care. Certain measures address the patient's communication experiences with doctors and nurses, as well as the adequacy of care-related information they receive. As reported in the National Healthcare Quality Report (Agency for Healthcare Research and Quality, 2008):

- 6.1 percent of hospital patients reported sometimes or never having had good communication with their doctors during their stay.

- 8.0 percent of hospital patients reported sometimes or never having had good communication with their nurses during their stay.

- 27.1 percent of hospital patients reported sometimes or never having had good communication about new medications during their stay.

- 22.9 percent of hospital patients reported not receiving good discharge information.

Care transitions from the hospital or other care sites to new care sites, including home, are often fraught with anxiety and uncertainty for patients. They are also times when patients are vulnerable to medical errors and oversight. Care coordination is critical to ensure continuity of care and patient safety during care transitions. There are three NQF-endorsed measures on care transitions specific to hospital discharge care coordination, which focus on the patient's understanding of their care plan (National Quality Forum, 2006):

- The hospital staff took my preferences and those of my family or caregiver into account in deciding what my health care needs would be when I left the hospital.

- When I left the hospital, I had a good understanding of the things I was responsible for in managing my health.

- When I left the hospital, I clearly understood the purpose of taking each of my medications.

Clearly, there is a need to develop—and for NQF to endorse—more measures for care coordination. The NQF will convene a consensus development panel to consider appropriate measures in 2008. The important work of implementing the endorsed measures is accomplished by many organizations, including CMS, the Hospital Quality Alliance, the Ambulatory Quality Alliance, the nationwide value exchanges, and many community collectives, including the Robert Wood Johnson Aligning Market Forces communities.

Patient safety has become an overriding concern to patients, who are more aware than ever before of the potential for medical errors and care-related complications, such as hospital-acquired infections. Patient safety measures are not oriented to the patient's perspective or experiences. Instead, they focus on procedures likely to threaten patient safety. Examples of patient safety measures include central line–associated bloodstream infections and surgical site infection rates. There is growing interest in reporting on hospital-specific rates of infection. To date, twenty-two states have enacted legislation requiring public reporting of hospital-acquired infections, and four (Florida, Missouri, Pennsylvania, and Vermont) have begun posting data on their Web sites (National Quality Forum, 2008).

Does provider behavior change as a result of measurement and public reporting? The number of public reporting and pay-for-performance programs is expanding (Epstein, 2007), and early published results demonstrate promising improvements in quality. For example,

■ Deaths from cardiac surgery fell 41 percent over the first four years of New York's public reporting program of hospitals and surgeons (Chassin, 2002).

■ Hospitals reporting publicly on obstetrics performance were almost three times more likely to show significant improvement in quality over a two-year period as compared with hospitals with no public reporting (Hibbard, Stockard, and Tusler, 2005).

■ The Premier Hospital Quality Incentive Demonstration Program showed that pay-for-performance incentives and public reporting almost doubled the overall gains for heart and pneumonia care in hospitals relative to no reporting (Lindenauer and others, 2007).

Payment

There are nearly ten thousand billing codes for individual health care procedures, services, and separate units of care, but there is not one for patient improvement or cure. The bottom line is that providers are given incentives to produce more and more medical services. However, there are no codes for good handoffs between doctors; nor are there payments for coaches to help patients navigate the health care maze, to support a medical home, for fewer unnecessary services resulting from health information technology, or for decision tools for patients. One of the biggest barriers to improving coordinated care is payment policies that simply provide the wrong incentives (National Quality Forum, 2008).

There is an emerging movement to pay for performance, and it has met with demonstrated success and support by key care purchasers and provider groups. Yet, for the most part, it is still oriented toward performance on procedures—for example, whether or not a diabetes exam was performed or a series of medication treatments was given for the care of a specific condition in a specific setting. As mentioned earlier, in order to improve patient-centered care, there needs to be a shift to payments for outcomes, over an episode of care, which will foster collaborative, efficient, and better care among a variety of providers and will thereby facilitate a more integrated delivery system. It is the impact of care on patient health that matters, not the volume of services delivered. Specific models that have been proposed include these:

■ A shift to bundled reimbursement models for medical conditions, in which all physician fees, services, facilities, and drugs are included in a single price

■ Episode-based payments that include bundled reimbursements over a longer period of time

Examples of other payment innovations being considered to improve care coordination include these:

■ Risk-adjusted payments for the medical home to provide better support for the primary care team, support for information technology (IT) infrastructure, and inclusion of patient coaches

■ Referral sources on billing forms as a condition for payment

■ Classification of mismanaged transitions as nonreimbursable "never events"

Comprehensive, vertically integrated delivery systems may demonstrate a greater capacity to respond to these payment challenges, but only time will tell. Organizational supports are clearly needed to effectively manage care for the chronically ill, across settings and over time, to achieve the best patient outcomes.

Research and Education

Research is an essential component of efforts to transform health care from a disease-centered model to a patient-centered model, one that matches treatment intensity with a patient's needs, values, and preferences. This premise is central to all of health care, but it is particularly important for individuals with chronic illnesses. The chronic care model of care, developed by Ed Wagner, has inspired multiple demonstrations that informed, activated patients can achieve better outcomes than those who are passive recipients of care.

In fact, a major theme of health care research within the past fifteen years is evaluation of treatments from the patient's perspective—for instance, improved visual function after cataract surgery and relief of pain after surgery. Studies have shown that individuals may value alternative outcomes differently and that the ultimate decision maker for which treatment is best should be the individual. As the availability of health care information from online and other sources has exploded, a growing number of individuals expect to have their treatment preferences considered by clinicians. A very active focus for current research takes advantage of advances in health information technology, such as electronic health records, to provide evidence-based information to clinicians and patients and to support shared decision making.

Within recent years, a broader focus on patient-centered interventions that transcends specific conditions has emerged within health care organizations. This broader focus emerged from concerns about patient safety and clear evidence that ineffective communication between health care professionals and patients is a common root cause of subsequent adverse care outcomes. For example, poor communication at hospital discharge results in 15 percent of patients returning to the emergency department of the hospital within the next two weeks. A synthesis of published literature on the impact of low health literacy found that patients' inability to understand common instructions is very common and associated with adverse outcomes (Berkman and others, 2004). These findings motivated investments by the public and private sectors in evaluating strategies to address this critical problem. Similarly, both the Institute for Healthcare Improvement's 100,000 Lives Campaign and patient safety practices encouraged by The Joint Commission have focused attention on effective communication during transitions in care, including discharge, to prevent avoidable errors with medications and other treatments. Public reports of patient experience in hospitals (HCAHPS) are likely to continue the focus on organization-wide efforts to enhance patient-centered care.

Health care delivery in the United States covers a broad spectrum of effort, which ranges from individual hospitals struggling mightily to reconcile admission and discharge medications for all patients to leading-edge hospitals and systems that are engaging patients and families in redesigning care. Cincinnati Children's Hospital launched their efforts with patients and families with cystic fibrosis, and the Dana-Farber Cancer Institute has used a similar approach for cancer patients. Not surprisingly, patients in these settings brought important and previously overlooked insights to this work. These efforts substantially improved both patient care and the satisfaction of health care professionals in these organizations.

Educational efforts to promote patient-centered care have emerged as well, albeit slowly. There is an increased emphasis on patient communication within undergraduate training, and many practicing physicians have pursued continued education in this arena as well. In addition, anecdotal reports regarding current medical students suggest that the new generation is far more team oriented than their predecessors, and there are numerous efforts to help trainees understand the patient experience in new ways. For example, one residency program has all interns spend the night in a hospital before starting work. However, it is unusual that health care professionals share any common training experience—and there is not yet a clear requirement for education in patient-centered care or quality that extends to all institutions.

These examples should inspire both optimism and humility for patient-centered care advocates. Demonstrating that patient-centered care is not only achievable but also has widespread benefits is needed to drive the requisite changes in health care delivery. However, the path from promising—even exciting—possibilities to systemwide change has traditionally been incremental and evolutionary rather than dramatic. The need and opportunity for individual patients and patient/consumer organizations to continue to push the envelope is clear. In particular, an important frontier is translating the expressed concerns of individual patients and families into systematic action and organization-wide improvements.

CHALLENGES, PROSPECTS, AND OPPORTUNITIES

People have different roles when it comes to public policy, including that of citizen, consumer, advocate, and participant. As citizens, people elect officials who represent them on public policy issues. Beyond voting, the hard work of crafting policies is mostly delegated to representatives. People act as consumers in making economic choices, which are important drivers in a market-driven society. Choices about what to buy at what price can affect the global economy, as lower-priced goods command consumer loyalty and shift capital to innovative producers worldwide. People act as advocates in public policy as a special-interest group vying for public resources and recognition for their cause. Individuals also act as participants in public policy, for example, as voters demanding higher budgets for special programs or as a parent advocating for curriculum changes.

However, we would argue that the patient's role as participant in health care is different. The patient's role in health care does involve *election* and *delegation* to medical representatives, who by and large make decisions or frame the decision options on a patient's behalf. Some patients also take on the role of advocate, oftentimes due to some injustice that had befallen them or a family member. Patients are also expected to be consumers in making wise financial decisions about their health care choices. Yet, the big difference between decisions in health care and those in other arenas is the large personal stakes involved in health care decisions, including life and death, and health, prosperity, and disability.

The needs and preferences of patients are all too often overlooked in the very decisions that affect them, because of the nature of the seven-minute office visit, the presumption that medicine is a wholly technical formulaic task "once the lab tests are in," as well as the lack of communication and information among providers. Patients can be a drag on efficiency. They may be viewed as disoriented and unable to attend to complex issues. And all too often, the practice of medicine is centered on the needs of the provider and not the patient.

Public policy can change that by ensuring that the patient voice is the most important voice to listen to in decisions about priorities, performance measurement, payment policies, research agenda, and delivery system design. It can accomplish this through legislative action, professional standard setting and education, public and private partnerships, leadership that takes a stand, and board governance. The design elements of such a patient-centered public policy agenda include the following:

- Consideration of all decisions through the filter of the patient's voice

- Focus on outcomes of episodes of care and related bundled payment approaches

- Use of tools that engage patients and families in care decisions

- Performance metrics that drive system performance on behalf of patients

- Systematic use of patient incident reports on quality concerns to make system changes

There has been good but slow progress in all of these areas over the last decade, largely due to the persistent drumbeat of a growing cadre of dedicated health care professionals and consumer and patient representatives. Also, there is the emerging realization that health care is much more about chronic care and less so about acute care. Chronic care requires ongoing patient involvement for making behavior changes and self-monitoring of their condition, rather than a time-limited medical fix. Employers have had a strong influence on advancing patient-centered care, mostly through the motivation to reduce costs and the realization that patients can play an important part in improving provider performance by selecting providers based on cost and quality information. This has had a spillover effect to support patient-centered care. Patient-centric performance metrics are beginning to show up on governance dashboards as organizational critical success factors, thus reinforcing the organizational imperative to be customer-driven. Government purchasers and regulators are including patient-centered metrics in public reporting of hospitals, nursing homes, home health care, and ambulatory care. And government is providing leadership in developing clear policies and procedures to set the expectations for better patient-centered care.

Going forward, the pace of change needs to be accelerated. A piecemeal approach to one improvement at a time will not be sufficient. There must be a full-court press on all the policy levers. We are hopeful that we are approaching a tipping point in transforming the American health care delivery system toward one that is patient-centered.

REFERENCES

Agency for Healthcare Research and Quality. *2007 National Healthcare Quality Report.* AHRQ Pub. No. 08-0040. Rockville, Md.: U.S. Department of Health and Human Services, Feb. 2008.

Agency for Healthcare Research and Quality. *CAHPS®: Assessing Health Care Quality from the Patient's Perspective.* 2007. [www.cahps.ahrq.gov/content/cahpsOverview/07-P016.pdf].

Berkman, N. D., and others. *"Literacy and Health Outcomes."* Evidence Report/Technology Assessment No. 87. AHRQ Pub. No. 04-E007-02. Rockville, Md.: Agency for Healthcare Research and Quality, Jan. 2004.

Casalino, L., and others. "Benefits of and Barriers to Large Medical Group Practice in the United States."*Archives of Internal Medicine,* 2003, *163*(13), 1958–1964.

Chassin, M."Achieving and Sustaining Improved Quality: Lessons from New York State and Cardiac Surgery." *Health Affairs,* 2002, *21*(4), 40–51.

Coleman, E. A., Parry, C., Chalmers, S., and Min, S."The Care Transitions Intervention."*Archives of Internal Medicine,* 2006, *166*(17), 1822–1828.

Council of Accountable Physician Practices. *"Frequently Asked Questions."* July 5, 2007. [www.amga-capp.org/faq.html].

Epstein, A. "Pay for Performance at the Tipping Point." *New England Journal of Medicine,* 2007, *356*(5), 515–516.

Halvorson, G. *Health Care Reform Now! A Prescription for Change.* San Francisco: Jossey-Bass, 2007.

Hibbard, J. H. "Moving Toward a More Patient-Centered Health Care Delivery System." *Health Affairs,* 2004, VAR-133-135.

Hibbard, J. H., Stockard, J., and Tusler, M. "Hospital Performance Reports: Impact on Quality, Market Share, and Reputation." *Health Affairs,* 2005, *24*(4), 1150–1160.

Institute of Medicine. *Crossing the Quality Chasm: A New Health System for the Twenty-First Century.* Washington, D.C.: National Academies Press, 2001.

Institute of Medicine. *Performance Measurement: Accelerating Improvement.* Washington, D.C.: National Academies Press, 2006.

Lindenauer, P., and others. "Public Reporting and Pay for Performance in Hospital Quality Improvement." *New England Journal of Medicine,* 2007, *356*(5), 486–496.

National Quality Forum. *NQF-Endorsed Definition and Framework for Measuring Care Co-ordination.* 2006. [http://216.122.138.39/pdf/reports/ambulatory_endorsed_definition.pdf].

National Quality Forum. *Care Coordination: Membership Survey Results.* 2008. [www.qualityforum.org].

National Quality Forum. *Issue Brief: Battling Health Care-Associated Infections Through Public Accountability,* 2008.

Naylor, M. D., and others. "Transitional Care of Older Adults Hospitalized with Heart Failure: A Randomized Clinical Trial." *Journal of the American Geriatrics Society,* 2004, *52*(5), 675–684.

Porter, M. E., and Teisberg, E. O. *Redefining Health Care: Creating Value-Based Competition on Results.* Boston: Harvard Business School Press, 2006.

Sepucha, K. R., Fowler, F. J., Jr., and Mulley, A. G., Jr. "Policy Support for Patient-Centered Care: The Need for Measurable Improvements in Decision Quality." *Health Affairs,* 2004, VAR-54-62.

Tang, N., Eisenberg, J., and Meyer, G. "The Roles of Government in Improving Health Care Quality and Safety." *Joint Commission Journal on Quality and Safety,* 2004, *30*(1), 47–55.

Wagner, E. H. "Chronic Disease Management: What Will It Take to Improve Care for Chronic Illness?" *Effective Clinical Practice,* 1998, *1*(1), 2–4.

CHAPTER

15

BREAKING DOWN THE BARRIERS TO PATIENT-CENTERED CARE

CARRIE BRADY AND SUSAN B. FRAMPTON

This chapter does the following:

- Identifies barriers to the widespread implementation of patient-centered care and presents strategies to overcome them

- Suggests tangible ways that individuals—organization leaders, staff members, or patients themselves—can contribute to the effort to redesign the health care delivery system into one that is patient-centered

The previous chapters have presented a compelling case for embracing patient-centered care practices. The evidence supporting the impact of such practices on everything from patient and staff satisfaction, patient safety, quality of care, and financial outcomes is growing ever stronger. Why, then, is a comprehensive model of patient-centered care not practiced in more hospitals and health care environments in the United States and abroad? What are the continuing barriers to widespread adoption of a model like Planetree, and how can we begin to overcome these barriers?

EXPLORING THE BARRIERS

In numerous interviews with health care leaders about perceived barriers to widespread adoption of patient-centered practices, the consensus seems to fall into several categories that can be best defined as (1) a general resistance to change, (2) the perception that it will cost too much in both time and resources, and (3) a lack of clarity on how to initiate and maintain a culture change of this magnitude.

Health care has often been referred to as an entrenched, change-averse industry, with average lag times between emergence of effective, innovative practices and widespread dissemination of fifteen to twenty years (Balas and Boren, 2000). The focus in health care over the past several decades on quantitative versus qualitative outcomes has hampered an appreciation of the importance of the patient experience until very recently. In a culture in which financial incentives have been tied to lowering lengths of stay and medical errors over improving the patient experience, conservative approaches and accomplishments have been rewarded and thus encouraged. It was not until the Institute of Medicine's report (2001) identified patient-centeredness as one of the key elements of quality patient care that innovations affecting the qualitative aspect of the health care experience have begun to be taken seriously. Even with the recent emergence of publicly reported standardized survey data on patient ratings of these qualitative aspects of care, many health care leaders have yet to fully understand and embrace the importance of the patient perspective. The ongoing efforts of agencies like the Centers for Medicare and Medicaid Services (CMS) to link ratings of patient satisfaction to financial incentives will likely change this situation in time.

The patient's experience of care is of course a very personal and thus subjective measure of quality. With the advent of scientific medicine in the nineteenth and twentieth centuries and the amazing progress brought about through biomedical research, a bias toward objective, "hard" data has prevailed in health care up until the present time. Focusing on the "softer," human need for caring, comforting, and respectful delivery of medical care has been marginalized and devalued. Medical culture is itself characterized by an extremely demanding, Olympian ethos of inhumanely long work hours during training, which often extends into practice as well. This culture is entrenched and resistant to change and likely impairs the adoption of patient-centered practices as well.

Inasmuch as human nature prefers the known to the unknown and relies on habit formation to function, the ability to change behavior becomes more challenging as we age. The malleability and adaptability of the actively developing young professional solidifies over time into the experienced, mature practitioner. This has many advantages, particularly in medicine and nursing, but disadvantages as well. The average age of our nursing workforce, for example, is approximately forty-seven (Health Resources and Services Administration, 2006). These seasoned professionals are extremely competent at performing nursing duties as defined during their training and at incorporating additional discrete skills as necessary during their professional careers. Never before, however, have there been so many changes in so short a time, as have faced nurses in particular over the past decade. The move to electronic medical records has challenged many professionals with little prior experience using computers. The amount of required documentation itself by both government and private third-party payers has increased exponentially. Collecting, documenting, evaluating, and responding to patient safety data, CMS core measures data, patient satisfaction data, and more have been added onto the daily practice reality for nurses today. It is no mystery why there might be resistance to implementing patient-centered care practices, given the potential for them to be viewed as "yet one more thing to do."

There is an ironic aspect to this viewpoint, however, given the health care industry's well-deserved reputation for a seemingly insatiable appetite for "flavors-of-the-month." This well-recognized phenomenon refers to the ongoing cycle of short-lived, quick-fix programs initiated by management to address perceived deficiencies in or problems with organizational culture. Most of these programs apply discrete and simple approaches like customer service training, scripting, and recognition-and-reward systems. Although each of these has something to contribute, they are the proverbial Band-Aid on a gaping wound.

Health care is an industry in crisis on many levels, not the least of which is the level of meaning and purpose. As explored in Chapter One, the quality of human relationships that support the very fabric of a healing environment need deep and fundamental attention and repair. Using a holistic model like Planetree to critically examine every aspect of the patient and staff experience and then address culture change in a broad, comprehensive manner is hard work. It takes a longer-term vision and commitment to seeing that vision through. The case study in Chapter Twelve, describing Aurora Health Care's integration of Planetree into its ten-year strategic plan, is a case in point, but frankly a rarity in health care. Our flavor-of-the-month mentality continues to present significant obstacles to wider-spread adoption of practices that cannot effectively be mandated by policy but must be allowed to develop organically from within the organization itself over time, with a balance of staff and management involvement. Unless changes in practice have true buy-in from staff, can we really be confident that it is happening on third shift when no one is watching? The need for broad staff involvement and buy-in is both the most challenging and the most rewarding aspect of effective and maintainable culture change.

Changing to a more patient-centered system of care is also mistakenly seen as being more costly in time and resources. In fact, organizations that have implemented a patient-centered culture have found that it not only is the right thing to do but that it is cost-effective too. Patient-centered care involves providers partnering with patients and their family members to identify and satisfy the full range of patient needs and preferences and focusing on supporting the professional and personal aspirations of staff members, who can more effectively care for patients if they are cared for themselves. This focus on partnering with patients and reengaging staff has tangible financial benefits, as described in more detail in Chapter Ten, Building the Business Case for Patient-Centered Care.

The change in human interactions that is the core of a patient-centered approach requires a monumental shift in attitudes. This change in attitudes is undoubtedly priceless, but not costly. The cost of not changing the attitudes is much higher and is reflected not only in dissatisfied patients but also in disillusioned staff, who will routinely change jobs to work for the highest bidder. Many aspects of patient-centered care require only this change in attitude, and many of the aspects that involve new services can effectively be implemented by volunteers. Even patient-centered design can be accomplished within the traditional facility renovation budget. In designing its innovative ICU in the early

1990s, Griffin Hospital was required by the state certificate of need agency to complete the project without spending any more money than a traditional renovation and was able to accomplish that goal. Patient-centered care does not necessarily involve an infusion of financial resources. It involves engaging an organization's most powerful resources—the hearts and minds of its staff, patients, and community—more effectively.

NEW STRATEGIES TO OVERCOME THE BARRIERS

Since 1978, Planetree has been working with health care organizations to define and implement patient-centered care. It has been an amazing journey, with many twists and turns: from Angelica Thieriot's "radical" vision, to health resource centers, model hospital units, recognition of patient-centered care by the Institute of Medicine, and the rapid growth of a vibrant network of hospitals and other health care providers all working together toward a common goal. As of this writing, the Planetree community consists of more than 140 Planetree members in thirty-two U.S. states, the Netherlands, and Canada. The growth of the Planetree network is extraordinary considering that Planetree does not advertise its services. Instead, members have found Planetree.

Working within this Planetree community to define patient-centered care and to continually develop new ways to meet the needs of patients and staff has helped break down the barriers to patient-centered care in Planetree member sites, but as national interest in patient-centered care has grown, new strategies have been introduced to help more broadly break down the barriers to patient-centered care. These include the Patient-Centered Hospital Designation Program and the Patient-Centered Care Awareness Month.

Patient-Centered Hospital Designation Program

The Patient-Centered Hospital Designation Program is a voluntary program that was created by Planetree to recognize the achievements of individual hospitals in implementing and sustaining a culture of comprehensive patient-centered care. The program is based on the core patient-centered care elements discussed in this book, as well as additional elements related to organizational structures and measurement. For each core element, there are specific criteria that hospitals must meet in order to demonstrate that they have implemented that aspect of patient-centered care. The criteria were developed with extensive input from Planetree-affiliated hospitals, under the oversight of a designation advisory committee composed of leadership from affiliated hospitals, Planetree staff, and outside experts. The criteria are designed to provide a level of consistency in what it means to be a patient-centered hospital while continuing to promote individuality and innovation.

In order to achieve designation, a hospital must undergo a rigorous, yet collaborative, process to verify that it has successfully implemented programs that meet the designation criteria. An applicant hospital initially conducts a self-assessment and then submits documentation to Planetree. If the hospital appears to meet the criteria after the documentation has been reviewed, a site visit is scheduled to verify the hospital's implementation. During the site visit, Planetree tours the facility, meets with hospital leadership, and conducts detailed focus groups with patients and staff. Following the site visit, the hospital receives a status report and recommendations related to opportunities to further enhance patient-centered care. A designation committee of national health care experts makes the final determination on designation. Designated sites are recognized by The Joint Commission, who includes designation status as one of the few national awards eligible to be included in the profiles of hospitals on The Joint Commission's Quality Check Web site, along with such prestigious achievements as the Malcolm Baldrige Award and Magnet status.

A commonly cited barrier to the implementation of patient-centered care is the lack of understanding of how to go about implementing it. The designation program helps address this uncertainty by providing a concrete framework for implementation. Whether or not they intend to apply for designation, hospitals can use the designation criteria as a self-assessment tool to identify where opportunities exist to build and reinforce a culture of patient-centered care. The designation criteria provide a tangible goal for organizations to achieve—effectively transforming patient-centered care from a nebulous "soft" aim to a definable goal that can be set, measured, and achieved. As Laura Gilpin, a nurse on the first Planetree unit and a passionate Planetree staff member, observed, "What patients want is not rocket science, which is really unfortunate because if it were rocket science, we would be doing it. We are great at rocket science. We love rocket science. What we're not good at are the things that are so simple and basic that we overlook them" (Planetree, 2007).

For those hospitals that already have achieved high levels of performance in patient-centered care, the designation program provides an incentive to tackle some of the more challenging aspects, such as open charts and twenty-four-hour patient-directed visitation, that otherwise might not be addressed. Each of the hospitals that participated in the pilot hospital designation program identified new areas to work on, even though they had been focused on patient-centered care for several years. The rigorous criteria are not deterring organizations from applying. Since Planetree announced the first designated hospitals in 2007, several other hospitals have begun working on their applications. In addition, there has been demand from other providers to create similar programs, and Planetree is developing designation criteria for rehabilitation, behavioral health, continuing care, and outpatient settings.

In the future, this patient-centered goal setting may even be reinforced by payers. The Centers for Medicare and Medicaid Services (CMS) has explicitly identified promotion of patient-centered care as a goal of its national pay-for-performance program, and the American College of Physicians recently called for patient-centered care to be the focus of pay-for-performance (Snyder and Neubauer, 2007). Patient-centered care does not lend itself to quantitative measurement in the same way as other quality metrics—such as the percentage of acute myocardial infarction patients who receive aspirin on arrival—but the recent expansion of the CMS public reporting system to include results of the HCAHPS patient experience of care survey is an important step in capturing these aspects of care. The designation program provides an additional mechanism for evaluating whether systems are in place to reinforce a patient-centered culture and whether those systems are working. The strong performance of the designation pilot hospitals on HCAHPS described in Chapter Ten is promising. Excellence in patient-centered care can and should be rewarded, and Planetree will continue to pursue these opportunities.

Patient-Centered Care Awareness Month

In addition to seeking recognition opportunities for those organizations that have achieved excellence in patient-centered care and providing a roadmap for other aspiring organizations, Planetree has recently begun working to change consumer expectations. In October 2007 organizations celebrated the first annual Patient-Centered Care Awareness Month, an international awareness-building campaign coordinated by Planetree to commemorate the progress that has been made toward making patient-centered care a reality and to build momentum for further progress through education and collaboration. Planetree encouraged hospitals and health care organizations in the United States and internationally to celebrate by empowering patients, strengthening their patient-centered practices, and publicly proclaiming to their patients and communities their commitment to patient-centered care. Health care organizations around the world displayed the Proclamation for Patient-Centered Care (see Figure 15.1) to educate their patients and communities about what they should expect from their providers, and several hundred "I Am an Expert About Me" patient stickers (see Figure 15.2) and "I Am Listening to You" staff stickers (see Figure 15.3) were distributed to reinforce partnerships between providers and patients.

The celebration of Patient-Centered Care Awareness Month is not limited to Planetree members, nor do the commemorative activities have to be limited to the month of October. Several hospitals that are not affiliated with Planetree have requested copies of the proclamation, and many organizations have chosen to post the proclamation year-round, finding it to be an effective tool for communicating the organization's commitment to patient-centered care. In 2007, governors from twelve U.S. states also commemorated Patient-Centered Care Awareness Month by issuing proclamations formally recognizing the event in their states, and more are expected to join in future years. As the public and policymakers become more aware of what is possible, hospitals will face increasing demands from informed consumers, who will accept nothing less than a comprehensive patient-centered approach.

YOUR ROLE IN OVERCOMING THE BARRIERS

Planetree has created tools to help organizations determine how to begin to implement patient-centered care, but another key barrier that must be overcome is the feeling of powerlessness on the part of many individuals who would like to see a change but feel that they do not have the authority to make that happen. You may be reading this book, thinking that it sounds ideal, but it could never happen in your hospital or your community. You may feel that there is nothing you can do to make this a reality—that it is someone else's responsibility and that the barriers are insurmountable. The fact that you have come this far in the book proves that you are wrong. You already have dedicated several hours to thinking about patient-centered care; at a minimum, you took the time to get this book and read it.

As children, we believe that we can do anything, but as we grow, we lose faith in our ability to change things. We may grumble about it,

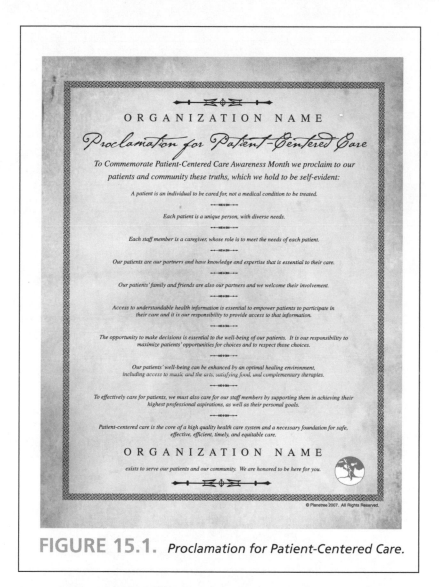

FIGURE 15.1. *Proclamation for Patient-Centered Care.*

Source: © Planetree 2007. All Rights Reserved.

but we tend to accept "that's just the way it is." We also point fingers at those we perceive are responsible without taking a look at our own behavior. Patients blame the hospital, hospital staff blame administrators, administrators blame payers and other market forces. Everyone

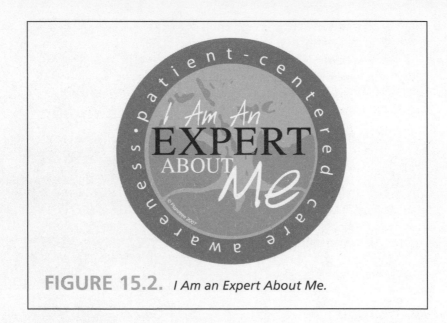

FIGURE 15.2. *I Am an Expert About Me.*

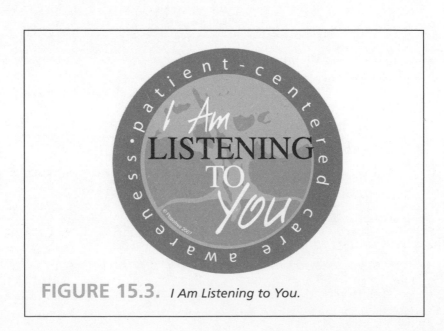

FIGURE 15.3. *I Am Listening to You.*

acknowledges the system is not working, but in the end no one takes on the challenge of fixing it.

You have more power than you think. Angelica Thieriot was one patient with a vision. Thirty years later, her vision is guiding the work of health care organizations around the world. What is your vision? Spend some time thinking about what you would do if you had a magic wand and could change things in an instant. At this stage, do not reject any idea as too crazy or unrealistic—after all, things like open medical records and twenty-four-hour visitation were once dismissed as impossible. Do not temper your expectations with reality. Dream big. What would be the ideal health care experience for you as a staff member, a patient, a family member? Write down your ideas.

There is no doubt that you *can* change the world. Leaders of all kinds have been teaching the same message for generations:

"You must be the change you wish to see in the world."

—Mohandas Gandhi

"Go confidently in the direction of your dreams.
Live the life you imagined."

—Henry David Thoreau

"If you think you can do a thing, or think you can't do a
thing, you're right."

—Henry Ford

"Not everyone is called to be a physician, a lawyer, a
philosopher, to live in the public eye, nor has everyone
outstanding gifts of natural capacity, but all of us are
created for the life of social duty, all are responsible for the
personal influence that goes forth from us."

—Vittorino da Feltre

"Never doubt that a small group of thoughtful, committed
citizens can change the world. Indeed, it is the only thing
that ever has."

—Margaret Mead

Now take your vision and break it down into smaller parts. What can you do today that would help move toward that vision? Make a commitment to yourself and write that down. "To help make health care more patient-centered, I will . . ." The key is to believe that you can make it happen. Some ideas are included here, but they are just a starting point. Just as a patient-centered culture must grow from within a health care organization, your personal commitment must be uniquely yours. Make it as specific as you can and include a time frame. For example, instead of saying, "I will remember to *care* for my patients instead of only treating their medical conditions," you might identify specific behaviors. For instance, "Starting tomorrow, I will tell each patient at the beginning of my shift that they should let me know if they are hungry or thirsty, cold or hot, and so forth." Also, avoid using the word *try*. By putting *try* in your statement, as in, "I am going to try to . . ." you already are acknowledging that you might not succeed—*before* you have even gotten started.

FOR EXAMPLE

Personal Commitment Ideas for Hospital Leadership

- Make an explicit organizational commitment to patient-centered care and put systems in place to reinforce that commitment. Display or distribute the Proclamation for Patient-Centered Care. Consider using the proclamation as part of the employee selection process or new employee orientation to reinforce that patient-centered care is an essential part of the organization. (To request a complimentary copy of the proclamation, please contact Planetree.)
- Distribute "I Am an Expert About Me" stickers to patients and "I Am Listening to You" stickers to staff to reinforce that patients are respected partners.
- Host a celebratory meeting or meal to honor the staff members who make patient-centered care a reality.
- Create a patient and family advisory council if you do not already have one.
- Invite patients or family members to join the board or hospital committees.
- Share information with staff and the community about patient perspectives on their experiences, as well as patient suggestions that have been implemented.
- Host an open house for patients and families.

- Write a letter to the editor of your local paper describing your organization's commitment to patient-centered care and identifying the opportunities for patients and families to get involved.
- Determine how you can make it easier for your staff to be the kind of caregivers they wanted to be.

Personal Commitment Ideas for Hospital Staff

- Share the Proclamation for Patient-Centered Care with your colleagues and discuss how these principles could be exemplified in your unit or by your team. (To request a complimentary copy of the proclamation, please contact Planetree.)
- Encourage patients and families to ask for what they need. Whenever you can, say yes to patient and family requests. If you can't say yes, explain why and see if you can come up with an alternative way to meet the need.
- Share the positive. Hospitals have extensive systems for capturing and responding to complaints, but often the positive comments do not get shared. Remember to thank your colleagues, nonclinical and clinical, for the work that they do. If a patient or family member makes a positive comment, share it with the people involved.
- Think about why you chose health care as a field. Be the kind of professional that you wanted to be.
- Recognize that your attitude is contagious and that what you do has an impact not only when you do it, but forever. Think about how your words and actions will be perceived by patients, families, and colleagues. Be present, smile, and connect with others as people, not "to do" list items. If there are "rules" in place that limit your ability to effectively care for your patients, work with your colleagues to change the rules.
- Share your creative talents with the hospital (for example, gardening, photography, art, music).
- If there is something that you would like to try but need administrative support to do it, make the suggestion. If the answer is no, ask why, and work with your colleagues to overcome whatever barriers are identified.

FOR EXAMPLE

FOR EXAMPLE

Personal Commitment Ideas for Patients and Families

- Contact your local hospital and ask how you can get involved. Offer to participate on a patient/family advisory committee, other committees, or in focus groups for patients to provide feedback.
- Wear "I Am an Expert About Me" stickers when you interact with your health care providers to remind them and you that you are an essential partner in your care. (Please contact Planetree for stickers.)
- Proactively take charge of your health so you are in a position to make informed decisions about your care. Many hospitals offer community education classes about particular medical conditions. Consider taking one of the classes if you or a loved one has that condition. Create a list of your medications and keep it updated. Keep a medical history file with key information, including physician names, medical conditions, prior surgeries, hospitalizations, and so forth.
- If you have a choice of hospitals, review the list of questions to ask your hospital, contact the hospitals to ask about the items that are important to you, and let the hospitals know that their answers will affect your decision.
- When you are hospitalized, do not assume things are not possible. Speak up and ask for what you need. For example, if you are hungry, do not wait for the next scheduled mealtime. Ask for something to eat.
- Share your talents with hospital patients. If you are a musician, offer to play your instrument. If you are an artist, offer to do small art projects with patients. If you like to read, offer to read aloud to patients. If you are a gardener, offer to plant or maintain a healing garden at the hospital. Share the things that bring you joy with hospitalized patients.

FOR EXAMPLE

Questions to Ask Your Hospital

Patient Preferences and Comfort

- What do the patient rooms look like? Will I be able to see outside? Will I be able to adjust the lighting and the temperature myself? If I am not in a private room, is there a place that I can go to have a private conversation?
- Are there any activities other than television available, such as music or reading material?
- Are there lounges available for me, my family, and friends to use? Are there patios, gardens, or other outdoor spaces for patients and families?

- Is it possible for you to adjust mealtimes and routine checks around my schedule? For example, if I am a late sleeper, can I receive my breakfast and have my temperature taken later in the morning instead of being awakened?
- Is food available to me twenty-four hours a day if I am hungry? Can my family and friends cook food for me at the hospital? Will I have a variety of food choices that take my personal or ethnic preferences into consideration?
- Are complementary and integrative therapies such as massage available? What types of services? How would I arrange for those services?

Access to Information

- Do you have a consumer health library?
- What type of information will you provide to me about my condition and treatment options? If I would like more background information, how could I obtain that information?
- What process would I use to access my medical records while I am in the hospital? Will someone review the records with me and answer any questions I have? Do I have the option to add my own information and perspectives into my record for my health care team to read and review?

Involvement of Family and Friends

- Are there any limitations on when I may have family and friends with me? Can they stay overnight?
- If I want them to be involved, can my family and friends be trained to help care for me while I am in the hospital? If a family member or friend will be caring for me after discharge, what type of information and training is available to him or her before my discharge?

Responsiveness to Patient or Family Concerns

- What process should I (or my family member or friend) use to raise a concern while in the hospital?
- Do you have a process for a team to rapidly assess a patient who is deteriorating? Can a patient or family member initiate the team?

Involvement of Patients in Hospital Processes

- What processes do you use to get input from patients and family members?
- Do you have a patient and family advisory council?

- Are patients involved on other hospital committees?
- Do you conduct patient focus groups?
- What type of orientation and support do you provide for patients and family members involved in hospital processes?
- How do you use the feedback obtained from patients and families?

Patient Feedback
- How do patients rate their experience in your hospital? (Patients also may view this information directly using the federal government's Hospital Compare Web site: [www.HospitalCompare.hhs.gov])

The first edition of this book sold more than ten thousand copies, and several of those copies were read by more than one person. If Planetree had asked for a personal commitment in that edition, there would be thousands more people doing their part to make health care more patient-centered. More providers would be partnering with patients and their families, and more clinical and nonclinical staff members would be achieving their personal and professional goals. We invite you to be part of this growing community of people dedicated to transforming health care. Individuals and organizations around the world are making the dream of patient-centered care a reality. You can too.

REFERENCES

Balas, E., and Boren, S. "Managing Clinical Knowledge for Healthcare Improvements." In V. Schattauer (ed.), *Yearbook of Medical Informatics.* Stuttgart, Germany: Schattauer, 2000.

Health Resources and Services Administration. "The Registered Nurse Population: Findings from the March 2004 National Sample Survey of Registered Nurses." Washington, D.C.: U.S. Department of Health and Human Services, 2006.

Institute of Medicine. *Crossing the Quality Chasm: A New Health System for the Twenty-First Century.* Committee on Quality of Health Care in America. Washington, D.C.: National Academy Press, 2001.

Planetree. *Creating Patient-Centered Care in Healing Environments* (DVD). 2007. [www .planetree.org].

Snyder, L., and Neubauer, R. L. "Pay-for-Performance Principles That Promote Patient-Centered Care: An Ethics Manifesto." *Annals of Internal Medicine,* 2007, *147*(11), 2007.

EPILOGUE

As a former health care worker; an activist for patient, family, and clinician rights; and most important, a patient, I can tell you that the term *patient-centered care* deeply resonates with me. Yet for years, it was a completely foreign concept, which was surprising considering my personal health history. I was born with bilateral club feet and have had more than twenty surgeries. I even worked in health care over the years in various capacities. Like the founder of Planetree, I had an experience with health care that nearly took my life. This event led me on a path to a true understanding of what patient-centered care can mean for patients like me.

On November 18, 1999, I was scheduled for a right total ankle replacement. This was to be my twentieth surgery. At the age of thirty-seven and having experience working in an OR, I thought I was well positioned to make requests about my preferences and needs. I naively requested an attending—no residents (I knew that I had a choice in that)—and made it known that I wanted medicine for the nausea that always followed my surgeries. In retrospect, I can see that the attitude conveyed by many of the staff was that this patient is demanding and pushy. On this day, however, none of this mattered. The anesthetic nerve block that was supposed to numb me from my knee down inadvertently entered my blood stream. I went into cardiac arrest, and a code was called. Luckily for me, there happened to be a cardiac suite available and a primed bypass machine awaiting another patient. They were able to get me hooked up to a cardiopulmonary bypass machine within thirty minutes, which saved my life. Looking back at the hospital stay that followed, I knew it was anything but *patient-centered,* even though at the time, I hadn't even heard the term.

The emotional impact of an event like this is staggering. It affected my children, my husband, my family, and my friends. Nonetheless, throughout my entire hospital stay, not one person referred to "the event." There was no mention of contacting social work or chaplaincy, and no one tried to prepare us for the emotional fallout that would eventually come. This was a marked difference from previous experiences. After my other surgeries, I had always received a phone call from hospital staff, asking how I was doing and if I needed anything. In this instance, I almost died, and yet I received absolutely no follow-up. I couldn't stop thinking about how very wrong this was. But I had to focus on my physical recovery and my family's well-being.

Six months later, I was lucky enough to have a candid and ultimately healing conversation with the doctor involved with my event. At the time, I didn't understand the rarity of conversations like this, due to the culture of secrecy that unfortunately persists around medical errors. There were many peaks and valleys of emotions that needed to be experienced for me to get to the other side, and this open dialogue with my physician was a crucial starting point. What's more, it began my understanding of what a patient-centered approach to health care feels like, and it served to raise my awareness of how little consideration my expertise about my own body and needs was given throughout my experiences with the health care system.

In November 2003, four years to the day of my event, I needed surgery on my right ankle to get it in position for a replacement. I met with the anesthesiologist to discuss the type of anesthesia that would be used. I told him I wanted general—I knew that spinals were not always successful on me—and I certainly didn't want a block. He was quite obviously not happy with my choice and told me about blocks and how easy they were. I firmly reiterated my choice. He persisted, trying to convince me that blocks were safe and easy. When I refused for the third time, he asked why I was so against the block. When I told him about my previous experience, his jawed dropped, and he blurted, "*You're* that patient, my God, we learned all about that case." We then agreed on a general anesthetic. Why, though, were my wishes not accepted the first time? Also, looking back, I realized that had he done his job and looked at my surgical history, he surely would have understood my choice.

Following this same surgery in post-op, I was experiencing bladder pain. I shared this with the nurse and told her that I had had this problem several times following other surgeries. I was told this was normal and not to worry. After I had gone back to the floor, I mentioned this several times to the nurses over the course of the next five hours. Each time, my concerns were ignored, to the point that I began to second-guess my own judgment. Finally, after I had been sitting on a bed pan for more than one hour, feeling extremely vulnerable and crying in excruciating pain, a new nurse listened to me and took the appropriate action. She kept saying, "Mrs. Kenney, I am so sorry." I was so relieved that I wasn't crazy and that the pain wasn't in my head that I couldn't be angry. Here, I was trying to advocate for myself, but my "complaints" were dismissed.

What continually amazes me is that even though I am forty-five years old and even though I have had at least twenty-three surgeries, the health care community still does *not* view me as a reliable source for information about myself and my body. What does it take for me to be seen as a partner in my own care?

In June of 2007, I finally got my ankle. Prior to this surgery, I warned my care providers about the problem I have with my bladder following surgery. When I got to my room after the procedure, not surprisingly, it started again. This time, when I mentioned it to the nurse, he immediately did an ultrasound and explained how much urine was in my bladder and told me that I had a couple of choices. He told me that if he put in a catheter then, he would have to remove it immediately. Alternatively, if I could wait an hour, he could leave it in overnight and give my bladder a rest. I was amazed. Choices? Who knew? I thought this nurse walked on water! It was a few days later, at home, that I came to the realization that a nurse doing his or her job and engaging me in my care was viewed by me as "amazing" and Godlike. What was wrong with this picture? I could see that my expectations of health care were extremely low. Today, I know I should expect no less than patient-centered care and neither should anyone else.

Surviving the adverse medical event that nearly took my life and being grateful to be alive weren't enough for me. I needed to do more, and I made a personal commitment to change the system that not only had failed to support me but also had neglected to support the clinical staff involved in my care. This was my new path: from a suburban housewife raising her three children to an advocate for health care change. In 2002, I founded Medically Induced Trauma Support Services (MITSS), with the help of a wonderfully caring group of friends and the physician involved in my care during that fateful surgery. The mission of MITSS is to support healing and restore hope to patients, families, and clinicians following adverse medical events.

My journey has been very similar to that of Angelica Thieriot, the founder of Planetree. I met with many incredible and knowledgeable individuals along this journey, both those who believed passionately in what MITSS is all about and others who started out apprehensive but have since become some of our biggest champions. It was through my work with MITSS and the Health Research and Educational Trust (HRET) Patient Safety Leadership Fellowship that I first learned about Planetree and about how Planetree hospitals are incorporating patient-centered care into everything they do.

Everything Planetree stands for is so close to my heart. I believe every hospital should be incorporating the core components of a patient-centered approach to care. Though I can't rewrite my own personal history, I can't help but think of how some of the experiences I've described here may have been different had I been considered a knowledgeable partner in my own care. What is extremely exciting to me is the fact that Planetree affiliates are showing the link between patient-centered care and patient safety and quality. This connection will only help to spread this important work.

In early 2007, I was approached about the possibility of joining the Planetree board of directors. I had every intention of declining because I did not want to be overextended, but after going through all the materials that I had been sent about the organization, including the first edition of this book, I knew I couldn't pass up the opportunity to be a part of the effort to advance the practice of patient-centered care. I joined the Planetree board in the spring of 2007. I feel honored and privileged to be part of an organization with human-centered values.

As a patient myself, I am not surprised that the Planetree model was first conceived by a patient. It is my hope that in my story and that of Angelica, patients and their loved ones recognize that the time has come for us to collectively raise our expectations for how health care is delivered, demanding that our expertise as the owners and operators of our bodies be acknowledged and heeded, and that our intellect and emotions be treated in concert with our physical symptoms. By definition, patient-centered care is for and about us, but as patients, we too bear responsibility to be active participants in our care. We must not shy away from raising our voice, demanding to be listened to, and speaking up when we have questions or when something does not feel "quite right." And we must acknowledge that as "the patients," oftentimes we are in a vulnerable, overwhelmed state, and we may need to turn to our family and friends to help advocate on our behalf. As such, we must insist on a health care system that accepts this important role that our loved ones may play. We must not underestimate the influence that our voice can have, for it was one patient's experience that inspired the Planetree model, and it will continue to be the voices of patients and their loved ones that define and refine a patient-centered approach to care that treats us, as patients, with respect, dignity, caring, and compassion.

Linda K. Kenney
president and founder,
Medically Induced Trauma Support Services

NAME INDEX

SUBJECT INDEX

A

A La Carte Meal Service (Kadlec Medical
    Center), 89–90
Adherence, 221
Adverse events, 261–262
Advisory Board, 206
Agency for Healthcare Research and
    Quality, 199–200, 251, 253, 276
Alameda County study, 15
Albany Stratton VA Medical Center, 259
Alberta Children's Hospital, 58
Alcoholics Anonymous, 32
Alegent Health, 17–18
Alliance Community Hospital, 158, 159
Allopathic (traditional) medicine, 115
Ambulatory Quality Alliance, 277
American Academy of Family
    Physicians, 274
American Academy of Pediatrics, 274
American College of Physicians,
    274, 291
American Hospital Association, 250
American Hospital Association Survey of
    Hospital Leaders (2007), 206
Architectural design. *See* Facility design
Aromatherapy, 124, 232
Art
    artist and designer preferences for visual
      images and, 136
    behavioral health and healing power of,
      231–232
    biophilia theory on health outcomes and,
      132–133, 136
    continuing care enhanced through,
      237–238
    emotional congruence theory on health
      outcomes and, 133–134
    general public preferences for visual im-
      ages and, 134–135
    guidelines for selecting health care,
      141–143
    patient preferences for visual images and,
      135–136

Planetree art programs, 143–145
as positive distractions, 144
stress-reducing effects of viewing,
    137–139
See also Visual images
Ask Me 3 Web site, 251
Aurora BayCare Medical Center
    integrated health care journey by,
      242–246, 288
    lessons learned and future challenges
      facing, 246–247
Aurora Medical Center Oshkosh
    café of, 162–163
    healing garden of, 160
    integrated health care approach used by,
      242–247
    rooftop garden of, 158
Aurora Sinai Medical Center (ASMC),
    252–253, 254–255

B

Baby boomer generation, 197, 206
Baked goods, 163
Balanced Budget Amendment
    (BBA), 197
Banner Health System, 108
Bayhealth Medical Center, 58
Beck Depression scale, 124
Bedside report, 34, 36
Behavioral health
    access to information related to, 231
    allowing family, friends, and social
      supports for, 230–231
    human interactions focus of, 230
    Moral Treatment approach to, 228–229
    New York—Presbyterian Medical Center
      adoption of patient-centered care for,
      229–232
    patient safety, food, and healing arts for,
      231–232
    spirituality, human touch, complementary
      therapies, and health communities
      for, 232

311